AGEISM
Problems and Prospects

AGEISM

Problems and Prospects

Edited by

Ramesh Sharma

C. Joshua Thomas

AKANSHA PUBLISHING HOUSE

NEW DELHI-110002 (INDIA)

AKANSHA PUBLISHING HOUSE
4649-B/21, Ansari Road
Darya Ganj, New Delhi - 110 002
Ph.: 23263193 / 9811582579 / 09435116718
Fax: 011-23263193
Email: ektabooks@yahoo.com
www.akanshapublishinghouse.com

Ageism: Problems and Prospects

First Published 2010
ISBN 978-81-8370-203-4

PRINTED IN INDIA

Published by Akansha Publishing House, New Delhi and Printed at Mehra Offset, Delhi.

Contents

Foreword

It gives me immense pleasure to write a foreword to this book entitled *Ageism: Problems and Prospects.* Aging is a multi-dimensional phenomenon involving changes in physical, mental and social aspects of a person's life. It is also a natural and universal phenomenon which is experienced by all the individuals' world over but its magnitude and manifestations are not the same everywhere. Thus, governments all over the word are taking special care to alleviate problems of the aged in their respective states.

The present publication – *Ageism: Problems and Prospects* is based on the proceedings of a National Seminar on Aging in India with Special Reference to North East India organized by the ICSSR North Eastern Regional Centre with financial assistance from National Institute of Social Defense (NIDS) of the Ministry of Social Justice and Empowerment, Government of India, New Delhi, North Eastern Council (NEC), Shillong and the Indian Council of Social Science Research (ICSSR), New Delhi.

I understand that India is the home of second largest number of elderly population in the world with about 77 million elderly and more than 80% of its elderly population resides in the rural areas. However, very scant information is available about the health status particularly of rural elderly in our country, which is very important for planning health services to them.

This publication is a unique one in the sense that it contains contributions from all aspects of ageism such as bio-medical, socio-psychological and socio-economical dealing with the problems and prospects of aging phenomena under these categories. It is highly appreciative of the fact that this book will have a great impact onto its readers to collate the information on various aspects of ageism from one such publication.

I wish that this book will be used to improve planning and implementation of programmes and services for the welfare of the aged and make a difference to the millions of older people in India and more particularly in North-East India.

Prof. Pramod Tandon
Vice-Chancellor, NEHU
and
Chairman, ICSSR-NERC

Preface

Old age is a natural process. It is part and parcel of every human being. It is a natural phenomenon which affects each society. Today the elderly population is growing at a fast pace all over the world. This phenomenon is not restricted to the developed world, where this demographic transition started earlier, but is fast spreading to the developing countries. Advances in medical science, better nourishment, and improved standards of public health have all contributed to prolonging human life. What is common is the fact that extended longevity, due to decline in death rate and improvement in medical care, is the universal cause of rise of the elderly population. The problem of aging (becoming old) is a global problem in the sense that it is experienced by all the societies, but its magnitude and its manifestations are not the same everywhere. According to the United Nations (1988), the most dominant trend from the mid-eighties to the middle of the 21st century is likely to be the aging of the population in the developed as well the developing world. The United Nations Principles for Older Persons were evolved in recognition of the fact that *in all countries, individuals are reaching an advanced age in greater numbers and in better health than ever before*. Recognizing the importance of this particular age group, in 1990, the UN General Assembly designated October 1 as the *International Day of Older Persons* for celebrating and acknowledging the contribution of elderly people to society. The United Nations then declared the year 1999 as the International Year for Older Persons. The number of elderly persons in India has increased at a faster rate as compared to the growth of the total population. According to the Research, Reference and Training Division, Ministry of Information and Broadcasting, Government of India, the population of elderly persons 60+ in India ranks fourth highest in the world and by the end of the present century it will be second only to China. In India, the age of 60 years had been adopted by the National Policy for Older Persons (1999), for the purpose of classifying a person as old. Today India is home to one out of every ten senior citizens of the world. At present, the world's elderly population is nearly 600 million and by the year 2025, it is expected to be 1,100 million (United Nations, 1999). According to the Indian census figures, the proportion of elderly persons in India has risen from 5.63 per cent in 1961 to 6.58 per cent in 1991, to around 7.08 percent in 2001 and will be somewhere 9.87 percent in 2021.

Thus the population of 60+ is assuming an enormous size and the tremendous growth of the population of the elderly and its growing proportion in the total population are creating new problems for the society and for themselves. Old age is generally accompanied by a number of problems that the elderly have to face and adjust with in varying degrees. Loss of economic independence and physical vigour and the emergence of various types of degenerative diseases change an elderly from an independent self-supporting individual to one who needs help from his children, members of the family and the society in general. Since the time the United Nations dedicated the year 1999 to the aged/elderly as the International Year for Older Persons, a large number of literatures have flooded the global print market focusing on a wide range of issues and concerns related to the elderly population of the world. India for its part has not been lacking behind in its approach to its elderly. This is reflected in the amount of literature appearing regularly. But as far as India's Northeast is concerned, there is very little information on issues regarding the elderly. Understanding the lacunae in this aspect, the ICSSR North-Eastern Regional Centre had organised a series of seminars on each of the Northeastern states and thus brought out the proceedings in a book form on each seminar. Apart from these publications, not much has been written on Aging in North-East India. In this regard, the Centre with the support from the National Institute for Social Defence (NISD) of the Ministry of Social Justice and Empowerment, Government of India and the North-Eastern Council (NEC), Government of India organized a two-day national seminar on Aging in India with Special Reference to North-East India during October 1 – 2, 2008 at Shillong and addressed some of the following issues:

- the growth in population of the elderly persons
- the status of living arrangements, family life and inter-generational adjustment of the elderly
- the social and economic status of the elderly
- the health condition and access to health care services
- to review the existing services, policies and facilities by the Government for the welfare of the elderly.
- to make suggestions for implementation

The seminar was formally inaugurated by Smt. Subbulakshmi Jagadeesan, former Minister for Social Justice and Empowerment, Government of India, New Delhi and her speech is included in this volume. This book contains the various research articles presented in the two-day seminar. It has three sections under the following titles: Bio-Medical Aspects of Agism, Socio-Psychological Aspects of Agism and Socioeconomic Aspects of Agism. Altogether there are 22 papers in this volume and we sincerely desire that this volume finds wider readership and make a difference to the millions of older people of the country and more particularly in the North-Eastern region of India.

We are grateful to NIDS, New Delhi, NEC, Shillong and ICSSR, New Delhi for extending the financial assistance towards this programme. There are many people directly and indirectly involved in the preparation of the national seminar on Aging and also in the publication of this volume, we owe our sincere thanks to all of them. We put on record the valuable advice and direction which we received from Professor Pramod Tandon, Vice-Chancellor, North-Eastern Hill University (NEHU) and Chairman, ICSSR-NERC, during the seminar and also writing the foreword for this volume. We appreciate much the contribution of each of the paper writers in this book and all the staff of the ICSSR-NERC deserves special appreciation for their helps not only in the seminar but also during the preparation of this volume. Mr. M.P. Misra, Akansha Publications, New Delhi, deserves our appreciation for bringing out this publication on time.

- Editors

Our Contributors

1.	A.B. Dey	: Professor, Department of Medicine and Chief of Geriatric Services, All India Institute of Medical Sciences, New Delhi
2.	Ashish Goel	: Department of Medicine and Chief of Geriatric Services, All India Institute of Medical Sciences, New Delhi
3.	Arun P. Bali	: Consultant, Indian Council of Social Science Research, New Delhi.
4.	A. Lanunungsang Ao	: Professor, Department of Sociology, Nagaland University, Nagaland
5.	Chandana Sarmah	: Assistant Professor Department of Anthropology Gauhati University Guwahati, Assam
6.	C. Joshua Thomas	: Director, Indian Council of Social Science Research, North Eastern Regional Centre Shillong

7. Ch. Priyoranjan Singh : Associate Professor
Department of Economics
Manipur University
Canchipur, Imphal

8. Debendra Kumar Nayak : Professor, Department of Geography, North-Eastern Hill University, Shillong

9. Elizabeth Sangliana : Assistant Professor, State Institute of Public Administration and Rural Development (SIPARD), Tripura

10. F. T. Diengdoh : Programme Officer, Indian Council of Social Science Research, North Eastern Regional Centre, Shillong

11. G.S. Saun : Director, Indian Council of Social Science Research, New Delhi

12. G.K. Medhi : Scientist C, Regional Medical Research Centre, N.E. Region (ICMR), Dibrugarh, Assam

13. H.S. Ranhotra : Department of Biochemistry, St Edmund's College, Shillong

14. Indira Jai Prakash : Consultant Gerontologist, Bangalore

15. Indrani Chakravarty : Director, Calcutta Metropolitan Institute of Gerontology (CMIG), Kolkata.

16. J. Mahanta : Director, Regional Medical Research Centre, N.E. Region (ICMR), Dibrugarh, Assam

17. Jayanata Choudhury	:	Senior Lecturer and Coordinator, Centre for Rural Studies, Tripura University, Tripura.
18. K.K.Lakshmanan	:	Retired Professor, Department of Botany, Bharathiar University, Coimbatore, Tamil Nadu
19. K.L.Sharma	:	President, Indian Gerontological Association, Jaipur
20. Kalluri Subba Rao	:	Professor, Centre for Biotechnology, Institute of Science and Technology (IST), Jawaharlal Nehru Technological University, Kukatpally, Hyderabad
21. Linus Neli	:	Visiting Professor, Oriens Theological College, Shillong and Institute of Oriental Canon Law, Dharmaram Vidya Kshetram, Bangalore, Vicar General of the Roman Catholic Archdiocese of Imphal
22. Lianzela	:	Professor, Dean, School of Economics, Management and Information Sciences, Mizoram University, Aizawl
23. M.K. Thakur	:	Professor, Department of Zoology, Banaras Hindu University, Varanasi
24. Manoshi Das	:	Research Officer, Association for Research on People and

Nature (ARPAN), Agartala, Tripura

25. Paramita Saha : Lecturer, Department of Applied and Analytical Economics, Tripura University, Tripura

26. Ramesh Sharma : Professor, Department of Biochemistry, North Eastern Hill University, Shillong

27. S. K. Chakravarty : Calcutta Metropolitan Institute of Gerontology (CMIG), Kolkata

28. Vanlalchhawna : Reader, Department of Economics, Mizoram University, Aizawl

29. Wilma Wilson : Department of Medicine and Chief of Geriatric Services, All India Institute of Medical Sciences, New Delhi

30. Z.C. Visielie : Research Scholar, Department of Sociology, Nagaland University, Nagaland

Inaugural Address

Aging is a natural process which involves every person and affects every society all over the world. It is a gradual process of growing old. It was observed that during the past few years, there has been a tremendous growth in the elderly population world wide. The reason behind this phenomenon is because of improved living standards due to advances in medical science, better health facilities, better nutrition etc., resulting to prolong human life expectancy and decline in mortality rates. This has become a wake up call for the Governments particularly the developed nations which initiated the process of developing an international agenda on ageing. Initially the increase in the number of this particular section of the population was felt only in the developed countries but recent studies and surveys show that there has been a serious rise in the elderly population even in the developing countries in the recent past and it is also projected that in the next few decades, most of the elderly people would be in the developing countries.

After first World Assembly on Aging in 1982, the concern for the welfare of the elderly population gathered momentum and in 1990 the UN General Assembly designated October 1 as the *International Day of Older Persons* for celebrating and acknowledging the contribution of older people to society. The United Nations in 1991 adopted the Principles for Older Persons based on independence, participation, care, self-fulfillment and dignity for the elderly society and thereby referring to adding life to the years now living. Consequently, in 1999 the UN General Assembly decided to observe this year as the International Year for Older Persons. Simultaneously the National Policy on Older Persons in India was declared the same year.

India, like many other developing countries in the world, is presently witnessing rapid aging of its population. In the year 2025 India will occupy the second rank in having the old persons in their population projected by the United Nation Population Division. According to the population projections for the next twenty year period till 2016, worked out by the expert committee headed by the Registrar General and Census Commissioner of India, the 60 plus population will grow from 56 million in 1991 to 71 million in 2001; 96 million in 2011 and 113 million in 2016. Population projections for 1996-2016 made by the Technical group on population projections (1996) indicate that the 100 million mark is expected to be reached in 2013. Projections beyond 2016 made by the United Nations has indicated that 21 per cent of the Indian population will be 60+ by 2050. The UN defines a country as 'ageing' where the proportion of people over 60 reaches seven per cent. India has already exceeded this and is likely to reach 12.6 per cent by 2025. Census reports indicate that the Indian population has approximately tripled during the last 50 years, but the number of elderly Indians has increased more than fourfold. When considering the continuation of the trend, the United Nations predicts that the Indian population will again grow by 50 percent in the next 50 years, whereas the elderly population is expected to grow another fourfold. By 2025, almost 70 percent of the world's elderly are expected to live in developing countries, most of them in China and India. While China is expected to have over 194 million persons aged 65 or over, India will house almost 119 million elderly in 2025.

The rampant increase in this particular section of the population maybe regarded as an achievement on the basis of advancement of medical technology. On the other hand, it posed as a challenge for a developing country like India with a large population in ensuring the well-being and to meet the needs of a particular segment of the society which is vulnerable to various types of diseases due to biological deterioration and familial and societal pressure leading to psychological wound in their mental being. One needs to understand that in India, ageing or growing old was not an issue as the aged were always well respected and well looked after. However with the gradual process of urbanization, modernization and technical advances, the society is witnessing a change in the traditional setup of the joint family system to nuclear families due to migration of the younger generation to different locations in search of jobs leaving their parents behind to take care of themselves even in spite of poor health. Therefore the elderly are now facing several problems whether physical, psychological or social and they are emerging as a special population group with differential needs and problems.

The rise in life expectancy will emerge as a mounting task for the Government to cater to the welfare of the older group of persons and therefore policies will be needed focusing on the entire elderly population so that they do not suffer from neglect, humiliation, abuse and poverty in the society. This becomes a challenge for the Indian government to focus only on the specific needs of the elderly. Hence a coordinated and concerted efforts from the various sections of the society involving the government, NGOs, civil society, social scientists etc. for the overall social development of this group of individuals.

The growth in the elderly population is also experienced in the North-Eastern part of the country. Few studies have been made on this particular issue in this region and these indicate an upward trend in the rise of population in this particular age group.

I am happy to learn that the Indian Council of Social Science Research, North Eastern Regional Centre, Shillong had completed a project on the Magnitude of the Problem of Elderly Persons in the State of Meghalaya for the Department of Social Welfare, Government of Meghalaya. The findings and the recommendations of this report, I understand, has helped the Government of Meghalaya in setting priority to alleviate the problems of the elderly in the State. I am also delighted to learn that the ICSSR-NERC has sponsored a series of State level seminars on Aging in various States of the North-Eastern region and has published the proceedings of these seminars in book form.

It gives me immense joy to learn that the Department of Biochemistry of the North-Eastern Hill University has produced more than ten doctoral research works on aging related issues and in this national seminar we have scholars and researchers from different disciplines like Biochemistry, Biology, Psychology, and from Social Sciences.

I have great delight in inaugurating this two-day national seminar on *Aging in India with Special Reference to North-East India* and wish all the resource persons and participants to have a fruitful discussion. I do hope that the outcome of this two-day national seminar will be beneficial to the society in general and the elderly in particular as we chalk out ways and means to make the older persons live a life of dignity and respect within the family and society.

Smt. Subbulakshmi Jagadeesan
Honorable Minister of State
Ministry of Social Justice & Empowerment
Government of India, New Delhi.

Section-I
Biomedical Aspects of Ageism

1

The Science of Aging: Its Social Impact on India

Kalluri Subba Rao

Today's population statistics tell us that earth's population has gone beyond 6.5 billion and is expected to touch 9 billion mark by 2050. India can be proud that out of this 9 billion about 2 billion are from India. That is only one aspect of the demographic story. Out of the 9 billion people in 2050, about 10% of them would be above 60 years of age, the contribution from India to this "grandparent's boom" being 150 million. What is the reason for this global "grandparents boom" in spite of the apparently decreasing rate of population surge? The answer lies in the enormous increase in the medicare, decreased infant mortality coupled with health awareness of human population—all these emanating from the advances made in medical and health sciences research.

The impact of ever increasing population of elderly people has become a subject of great debate and consequences. The 'advanced' countries of the globe are, as usual, the first to realize and respond to this transforming demography. The science of Aging and associated debilities has become a thrust area of research. To keep elderly population in reasonable health has become a social and economic priority for these nations in view of the medicare expenses for this section of society and the impending social problems.

However, India has lagged behind in implementing programs to control population and now lagging behind to take measures to covert its elderly population into a national asset. Improving the knowledge about the science of becoming old is intimately connected to keep the aging population young and convert them into a socially viable component of the society. This presentation is a small attempt to underscore the need to look into the changing demography as a composite problem involving both scientific as well as psycho-social aspects.

History has never witnessed so much information and knowledge about human body and the molecular mechanisms that dictate its miraculous function, as it is now. The two fundamental and awe inspiring natural phenomena, the birth and death had so much influence on human civilization and attracted the capabilities of the best minds to understand these phenomena. Man has gained some significant ground in the case of former. However, even though people are living longer and with the percentage of people above 60 on this planet is reaching the double digit 10, little is known about the precise mechanism behind why and how we become old and then die. According to an estimate by UN, nearly 20% of India's population will comprise people over the age of 60 years. Yes indeed, the ever-increasing population on this planet has crossed the 6.5 billion mark in the month of July 2005. Although the rate of increase of population has decreased from 2 percent in 60s to 1.2 percent to day, the nine billion mark is expected to reach around 2050. That is only one side of the story and the problem there off. Out of this 9 billion people in 2050, a large chunk of them would be from developing countries with India's share being close to 2 billion. Secondly the "grandparents boom" would become clearly visible and pose a major problem to the countries concerned and to the world at large. This means a significant percentage (according to my rough estimate-10%) of this 9 billion people would be in the age bracket of 60 and above. More than 150 million of this global aging population will be from India.

What are the reasons for this demographic change? It is but obvious that the reasons are scientific in nature. Because of the advances in medical and biological research during the last 100 years, infant mortality has grossly reduced and health care has vastly improved. People have become aware of the benefits of good nutritional habits. All these resulted in extended life span of people all over the globe. For example in India the life expectancy in 1970 was 49 years which has increased to 68.6 years today. The trend is the same in many other countries as well (Table 1) This demography is likely to bring up peculiar challenges including the national budgets for aged, health care problems, retirement policies, and utilization of the elderly and social management of the aged. It is a challenge that greets this millennium. It is a challenge whether the rapid advances in science and technology would enable maintenance of good health and the postponement or reversal of that type of old age marked by debilitating diseases and frailty. Would it be possible to preserve youthfulness for the later years in life? In other words, the problems of managing ever increasing elderly population must be based on science and technology as was the case in improved longevity of the human population. This means the science that has enabled us to live longer must also be used to see that proper health is maintained during the extended period of life span. The socio-psychological and economic problems would become easy to be tackled once the aging population is fit enough to basically manage themselves through the fruits of the scientific research. In fact a healthy elderly population could be converted into a national asset through proper utilization and management.

Advanced countries have sensed this imminent "grandparents boom" almost 50 years ago and launched measures to alleviate the pressures that this demographic change could bring in. The reasons for the expected changes were looked into. It was obvious that reduction in the infant mortality coupled with improved nutrition and health care, resulting from the fruits of medical and biological research, are the reasons. It would be unwise and even uncivilized to make any effort to reverse these achievements. On the other hand emphasis was turned to see why we become "old" and what is the molecular mechanism(s) of this fascinating yet undesirable process. Would it be possible to modulate/control this process? The Science of getting "old" was born with a bang. Separate Institutes and centers were created both from philanthropic and Governmental initiatives to understand the science of aging and age associated debilities as well as to formulate innovative and humane management of elderly. Above all to examine how to prolong the "health span" of aging populations and convert them into a national asset. To day aging is one the thrust areas of research in almost all the developed nations and many others are following the suit.

For example, USA has created a new Institute for Aging Research, called National Institute on Aging (NIA) almost 40 years ago. Japan, European and many other countries have followed the suit. In fact, the European countries have got together and formed a European Research Area in Ageing (ERA-AGE, Gerda Geyer, *Experimental Gerontology*, 40, 759-762 2005). Apart from the State supported new Institutes, already existing centers, universities have created divisions and centers for gerontological research. These initiatives are yielding rich dividends. Tremendous progress is being made in understanding the biological, clinical and behavioral aspects of the phenomenon of getting 'old'. To day about 250 genes are identified to be associated with the aging process and therefore the life span. Attempts are also being made to examine whether the process of 'aging' can be modulated at genetic, molecular and social levels. Extensive research is also going on to examine the possibility of attenuating the deleterious effects of age dependent disorders including neurodegenerative (Alzheimer, Parkinson, Huntington, Stroke etc.). It is no exaggeration to say that there is no university in USA, which not have a center or institute for gerontology researches (see Tables 2-5).

Independent India is just 60 years old. At the time of independence, the average life expectancy in India was around 40 years. Clearly old age was not a problem to worry about. On the other hand, the average life expectancy of an Indian to day is reported to be around 68 years and this figure is fast improving. Never before have had so many people lived for so many years- thanks to the amazing progress made in medical and biological research. As such to day India has nearly 80 million people over sixty and this number is suspected to go up to 117 million in 2010 and further up in the years to come (Registrar General of India and National Commission on Population, 1996; http://populationcommission.nic.in). As already mentioned above, it is projected that there will be more than 150 million people above 60 years of age by 2050. This changed demographic profile is likely to exert immense pressure on the Government and the people themselves in many ways that are being experienced by the nation to day as a result of mere increase in the population-not to talk about the bulging portion of the aged population.

Yet India does not seem to show any urgent concern about the fast changing demography. It has lagged behind in this aspect for obvious reasons. If the increasing 'aged' population of the country is not taken care of and looked after well and maintained at reasonable health levels, then it would eventually become an extraordinary cost burden of no returns to the Government and the society at large. On the other hand, the 'ageing' population can also be converted into a national resource and asset with proper planning and imaginary inputs. Thus the older people in any country would pose a challenge as well as an opportunity. It is time that India takes an initiative to make it an opportunity because of the advantage it enjoys in mere numbers. This can be termed as Wisdom Resource (preservation and) Development (WRD) and through this the country can derive the *longevity dividend.* Thus it pays to keep the people with extended longevity in good health and spirits. It is encouraging that the Government of India has indeed started looking seriously at this problem (responsibility) in recent past and announced a policy for senior citizens as below.

The National Policy on Older Persons seeks to assure older persons that their concerns are national concerns and they will not live, unprotected, ignored and marginalized. The National Policy aims to strengthen their legitimate place in the society and to help older people to live the last phase of their life with purpose, dignity and peace. The National Policy on Older Persons inter alia visualizes support for financial security, health care and nutrition, shelter, emphasis upon education, training and information needs, provision of appropriate concessions, rebates and discounts etc. to Senior Citizens and special attention to protect and strengthen their legal rights such as to safeguard their life and property. The National Policy on Older Persons confers the status of senior citizen to a person who has attained the age of 60 years.

This above avowed policy has been capped very recently, in December 2007, by a bill passed by parliament. This bill is named "The maintenance and welfare of parents and senior citizens bill-2007". I would like to describe this bill as an historical one in that the Government of India has perhaps for the first time taken the maintenance and welfare of the senior citizens rather seriously and mooted steps to be taken for dignified living of senior citizens. This bill provides a provision for judicial authority to jail children for three months if the parents complain their negligence by children. This may sound peculiar to Indian society, what is important is that the Govt. has taken cognizance of the plight of some parents and created a deterrent in the form of a law for such social offence. The bill also envisages establishing old age homes in every district and a tribunal to look into the difficulties of senior citizens in that district.

The above bill sounds so good as to raise suspicion about its implementation. Be as it may, this is only one way of tackling the problems of senior citizens and there is yet another and perhaps more important way to empower the aged population in terms of their health and quality living and make use of their expertise in different needs of the country. Concrete steps and inputs are necessary. One such step is to establish one or more (in view of the vastness and diversity of the country) Institutes or Centers for a multidisciplinary scientific study of the phenomenon of aging and the associated diseases/problems. Such Institutes would also prepare a database for the clinical and biological profiles of the populations around particularly of the senior citizens to begin with.

It is heartening to note that finally Government of India has decided to start two National Institutes of Aging research and some regional centers. Some budgetary provisions have also been made by the finance ministry but it is to be seen when the proposals will become a reality. Meanwhile it is the responsibility of all the intelligentsia of the country to see that the public at large are engaged in realizing the fruits of aging research and then mould the life styles in a manner that is useful to them and the people around. The management of the elderly should not become a vested tool in the hands of some but it should grow on a scientific and sociological basis.

Table 1
A glimpse global life expectancy in 2008

Country	*Life Expectancy in Years*
India	68.6
USA	78.0
Australia	80.6
South Africa	42.5
China	72.9
Russia	65.9
Saudi Arabia	75.9
UK	78.8
France	80.6

Data Taken from World Life Expectancy.com

Table 2
Longevity & time taken for reproductive maturity

Spcies	*Longevity (Years)*	*Age of Puberty (Years)*
Human	100	12-14
Elephant	70	12-14
Chimpanzee	40	10
Dog	30	1
Rhesus Monkey	25	3
Cat	252	1.5
Rat	3	0.25
Mice	3	0.20

Table 3
Aging is genetically programed

- Hayflick's limit for in vitro grown cells
- Fixed Life Span of Species
- Aging Begins at discrete stage of Life
- Premature Aging Syndromes
- Gerontogenes (Genes affecting life span)
- Immortalization of cells in Laboratory

Table 4
The number of genes when mutated, known to either extend or shorten the life span in different species

Organism	*Total number of genes known to modulate life span*	*No of genes that shorten life span*	*No. of genes that extend life span*
C.elegans	116	12	104
S.cerevisiae	94	48	46
Drosophila	35	5	30
Mice	24	13	11
Humans	8	8	NIL

Information gathered largely from University of Washington, Seattle, WA. USA data base.

Table 5

A selection of Evolutionarily Conserved Longevity Determinants. A small number of genes or interventions are known to increase life span in different model organisms. Some are mentioned here

1. Antioxidant enzymes – Increased expression of antioxidant enzymes, such as superoxide dismutase and catalase increase life span in yeast, flies, and mice

   Resveratrol – Increases life span in fish, worms, and flies Resveratrol is a polyphenolic compound found in red wine and grapes that acts on several cellular proteins and acts as antioxidant.

2. Dietary restriction- (calorie/caloric restriction) – Dietary restriction increases life span in yeast, worms, flies, mice, rats, and other organisms. Increased activity of Sir2 orthologs increases life span in yeast, worms, and flies.

3. Insulin/IGF-1 – Mutations that decrease insulin/IGF-1-like signaling increase life span in worms, flies, and mice

4. Inhibition of all those pathways that promote growth and development (ribosomal proteins maturation, protein synthesis, fat synthesis etc.,) and promotion of maintenance pathways like DNA repair, reversal of oxidative damage leads to extended life span.

2

Dietary Restriction – A Way to Elixir of Youth

R. Sharma

Aging or getting old is a universal feature of most organisms and has been a global concern of every society. The maximum lifespan of an organism is a constitutional feature of speciation to polygenic controls and to environmental influences. There is a progressive functional decline of physiological functions associated with decreased fecundity and increased vulnerability to diseases. In the current times, the fountain of youth seems no longer a legendary fairy tale. There are now scientific evidences to suggest that the age-related impairments can be reversed by dietary and other interventions. Among various intervention strategies, dietary restriction (DR), a reduction in calorie intake without malnutrition, has been shown to be the most powerful modulator of the aging process in diverse groups of organisms. It is an efficacious means of increasing longevity and reducing age-related pathology. A manner in which dietary restriction help extend human lifespan and reduce age-related diseases has been of immense interest to the scientific community. These studies strongly support the role of DR in increasing longevity, enhancing functional capacity and reducing diseases of old age in wide group of experimental animals. Studies in humans and other experimental animals indicate that good nutrition and regular physical exercise not only contribute significantly to health and well-being, but also prolong mean and maximum lifespan. Indeed, these interventions are now accepted as a natural way to tackle a number of diseases of old age. One of the major goals of gerontologists is to prolong health-span part of the lifespan and have healthy old age without disability. In my opinion, if one can follow a strict regimen of 15-25 per cent of reduction in what she/he normally takes, it could provide a better health and longer lifespan. Some of the biochemical changes that happen during such intervention in experimental animals are presented herein.

Various theories have been put forward to explain the phenomenon of aging, however, none has yet accounted for all phenotypes, though many have attempted to explain at least some of the major and most frequent aging phenomena.[1,2] These theories have been grouped as molecular, cellular and systemic theories. *Molecular theories* envisage that the genes (specific DNA sequences) govern the lifespan of any species in a close knit with the environmental factors. It may result from changes in DNA template activity, which regulates the formation of the final cellular products. The molecular theories include codon restriction, somatic mutation, error theory, and gene regulation theory. They also include antagonistic pleiotropy, dysdifferentiation and soma disposal hypothesis. *Cellular theories,* on the other hand, relate to changes that occur in structural and functional elements of cells with the passage of time. These theories include wear and tear, age pigments, free radicals, cross-linking and membrane alterations. *System level theories* include the endocrine and neuroendocrine and immunological systems. These theories relate overall performance of an organism to the efficacy of a variety of control mechanisms that regulate the interaction between different organs and tissues. Adaptation to external and/or internal stress depends on the control mechanisms orchestrated by the joint interplay of the nervous and endocrine systems. Complete surveillance to foreign invaders is looked after by the concerted efforts of the immune system. The failure of which leads to a reduced adaptability of an organism to the pathogenic challenges in old age. Healthy aging and maximum longevity may thus depend on the genetic make-up of an organism under a strict control by the nature and nurture. The impact of dietary restriction has been associated with most of the mechanistic approaches of various theories proposed for causation of aging.

A manner in which dietary restriction help extend human lifespan and reduce age-related diseases has been of immense interest to the scientific community. After an early work of McCay and his collaborators,[3] many more experimental studies have been undertaken using a wide range of strategies.[4-6] These studies strongly support DR in increasing longevity, enhancing functional capacity and reducing age-associated diseases in experimental animals. Studies in humans indicate that good nutrition and regular physical exercise not only contribute significantly to health and well-being, but also prolong mean and maximum lifespan. Indeed, these interventions are now accepted as a natural ways to tackle a number of diseases of old age. One of the major goals of gerontologists is to prolong health-span part of the lifespan and have healthy old age without disability.

Biochemical Changes During DR

DR influences animal's reproduction to endocrine and neuroendocrine responses, immunological systems, metabolic responses, gene expression profiles, and also pathophysiological conditions. It has been postulated that DR by reducing the secretion of pituitary hormones, such as growth hormone (GH), lowers the oxidative damage of tissues, thereby reduce the age-related pathologies and extend lifespan.[7] Moderate caloric restriction in rodents delays puberty without loss of fertility and enhances longevity[8]. This has been correlated with retarded maturation of the hypothalamo-pituitary-gonadal (HPG) axis. The anti-aging property of DR seems to have evolutionary significance and might have evolved in nature in response to food scarcity[9]. During such periods, inbuilt resources would be diverted from reproduction to maintenance of the adult body and thereby increase survival until the next period of food availability. Another neuroendocrine axis that appears to be influenced by DR is the hypothalamus-pituitary-adrenal (HPA) axis. During periods of restriction, the axis is stimulated possibly due to a feeling of stress by underfeeding leading to an increased level of circulating glucocorticoids. Although transient increase in glucocorticoids improves performance at spatial memory tasks and helps synaptic efficacy, long-term elevations of glucocorticoids are associated with decreased cognitive performance, attenuated synaptic efficacy and neuronal atrophy. Elevation of glucocorticoids during aging is also associated with mild cognitive impairment and hippocampal atrophy. DR paradoxically increases plasma glucocorticoids and also prolongs lifespan. It has been suggested that the beneficial effects of DR outweigh the deleterious effects of glucocorticoids. It is proposed that the lifespan extension in rodents by DR could be an example of hormesis (having a beneficial effect in response to a low-intensity stressor) and that sustained moderate hyperadrenocorticism helps life prolongation. Hormesis thus refers to a phenomenon of beneficial biological action from a factor that is generally viewed as detrimental in nature. The anti-aging action of DR could be viewed as a nutritional stress, which might stimulate metabolic responses for better survivability. During mild stress, the organism regulates its metabolism to allocate more energy for its maintenance and survival and could be in a better condition after the stress, if it is not too harsh. Recently, this laboratory has reported an increased level of hepatic glucocorticoid receptors during three months of alternate days feeding in mice.[10] The increase in the level of hepatic glucocorticoid receptors could be a contributory factor in controlling the glucocorticoid-mediated metabolic responses during long-term DR in mice. Such rodents are found to be more resistant to a variety of other stresses such as trauma, heat shock and drug toxicity. Recently, it has been reported that an age-dependent decrease in liver and kidney glucocorticoid receptor function is reversed by DR in older mice.[11,12]

Several molecular, cellular, structural and functional changes occur in the brain during old age. Nerve cells might adapt to these changes or succumb to neurodegenerative events that result in diseases like Alzheimer's and Parkinson's. Multiple mechanisms operate to maintain the integrity of nerve circuits. These include production of neurotrophic factors and cytokines, expression of various cell survival-promoting proteins, preservation of genomic integrity and mobilization of neural stem cells to replenish damaged neural and glial cells.[13] Such neuro-protective and restorative mechanisms are compromised during aging process giving rise to neuropathological complications in elderly individuals. DR has been shown to reduce the pace of age-dependent decrease in genome integrity.[14] The adaptive responses in brain aging could be determined by the combined action of genetic and environmental factors. Neuroprotective functions thus are achieved by dietary calorie restriction, and by behavioral (physical and intellectual activity) modifications.

Numerous reports exist on the effects of DR in reducing mitochondrial damage, free radical accumulation, and lipid peroxidation. Such reduction could be possible partly by a decrease in the energy expenditure due to lower metabolic load in restricted animals and/or by an increased activity of those enzymes that are responsible for scavenging the reactive oxygen species. In fact, oxidative damage has been linked to many major degenerative diseases, including atherosclerosis, diabetes, Parkinson's disease, Alzheimer's disease, and cancer[15,16]. It is corroborated with the genetic studies on *C. elegans*, wherein reactive oxygen species (ROS) are closely attributed in lifespan determination.[17] Accumulation of oxidatively damaged proteins is evident during aging in many organisms. DR has been shown to reduce the age-related increase in the half-life of proteins, suggesting that the dwelling time of the proteins is reduced in DR animals. Thus, DR can increase turnover of proteins and thereby attenuate potentially harmful consequences of altered proteins.[18]

Reduced immunological surveillance is a major predicament for increased morbidity and mortality in old age. Hence, the restoration of immunologic function may provide a beneficial effect in reducing pathology and maintaining healthy status in old age. Among various interventions, DR has been shown to be a powerful modulator of aging process. Several mechanisms have been proposed to explain its robust beneficial effects on various physiological processes, including the immune system. Overall immunological status of rodents fed with a caloric restricted diet is superior to the status of *ad libitum* (AL) fed animals.[19] The incidence of autoimmune diseases, which increase during aging of normal fed animals, is significantly decreased in response to DR. The molecular mechanism(s) of such protective action remain(s) to be elucidated.

Orchestrated expressions of many genes provide a powerful molecular description of the normal aging process. Nearly 23% of the genome in fruit flies shows altered transcription with age. DR leads to a slower progression of normal age-related changes in transcript levels, particularly of genes involved in cell growth, metabolism, and reproduction.[20] A detailed analysis of expression patterns of genes in skeletal muscle of mice during aging revealed a greater expression of genes involved in oxidative stress, DNA-damage, neural atrophy and a decrease expression of genes leading to slower rate of glycolysis and mitochondrial dysfunction in aged animals. Most of these deficits in the expression of genes were either fully or partly reversed by DR in age-matched mice. Worth mentioning are the genes involved in protein metabolism (synthesis and turnover), carbohydrate metabolism (gluconeogenesis and pentose phosphate pathways) and fatty acid synthesis whose compromised expressions otherwise during aging were increased by DR in mice. Taken together, these observations suggest that DR may retard aging process by causing a metabolic shift toward enhanced protein turnover and lowered macromolecular damages caused by various toxic agents.[21] The health- and lifespan-extending properties of DR reveal that aging is accompanied by the altered gene expression associated with increased inflammation, cellular stress, and fibrosis and reduced capacity for apoptosis (programmed cell death), xenobiotic metabolism, normal cell cycling, and DNA replication.[22] It has been observed that both the long- and short- term DR reverses many of these changes. Hence, it seems plausible to obtain the benefits of DR in aging animals that have such functional impairments.

Human Studies Using DR

Quite some studies have been done on human subjects involving one or other regimen of DR. Islamic individuals who fast during the daylight and consume meal after sunset, their plasma high-density lipoprotein (HDL), also called good cholesterol, levels increase[23] by 30%. HDL removes cholesterol from the blood and carries it to the liver. It is inversely related to the atherosclerosis and other cardiovascular diseases. A similar increase in HDL level was also observed in DR monkeys. After 12 weeks of DR to non-diabetic healthy male individuals, the level of HDL-cholesterol is increased with concomitant decrease in hepatic lipase activity. The decrease in hepatic lipase could be a genuine link for increased HDL-cholesterol level in DR individuals.[20] A study of naturally occurring South Indian population of three age groups (young, 8-14 years; adult, 20-35 years; old, above 55 years), who were having normal and undernourished diets on the basis of body mass index (BMI) and history of their dietary intake, reveal that the DNA repair capacity was found to be higher in the lymphocytes of age-matched undernourished individuals.[24] A slower reduction in DNA repair capacity was also observed as a function of age in undernourished individuals as compared to normal fed ones. These studies provide a crucial link between DNA repair mechanisms and nutritional status in humans. It has been seen that 16 weeks of energy restriction (by 33%) results in significant reduction in body mass, lean body mass and fat mass in sedentary overweight men.[25] It is known that the people of Okinawa, one of the prefectures of Japan, have highest longevity in the world. Okinawa has the highest prevalence of centenarians in the world at 33.6 per 100,000 populations, in contrast to an average of 10 per 100,000 in most developed countries. They have high number of those who live longer than 105 years, called supercentenarians. Major contributory factors to such a higher longevity are mild climate, unique eating habits, and an active lifestyle. Among these, eating habits could be a most crucial factor influencing Okinawan longevity. Japanese living on the island of Okinawa, eat 20% less food than those in Tokyo.[26,27] Majority of Okinawans believe that proper eating is the most efficacious medicine for better health. It is being perceived that the longevity can be attributed one-third to our genes and two-third to lifestyle, of which nutrition is an important component.[27] Healthful aging may thus depend on the genetic makeup within strict control of nature and nurture. The average life expectancy of Okinawans living in Brazil is 17 years shorter than Okinawans who live in Okinawa.[27] Thus, it is quite reasonable to practice the dietary interventions to achieve better health and lifespan in humans as well.

There is a serious possibility that only few people would reduce their food intake enough to lengthen their lives, gerontologists are now looking for alternatives that could mimic the beneficial effects of DR in people who may not like to go for actual restrictions. These alternative interventions are termed as DR mimetics. DR mimetics targets improvement of mitochondrial function, use of antioxidants, administration of compounds (2-deoxyglucose) known to lower blood glucose levels and increase insulin sensitivity, regular physical exercise and maintenance of body weight over the lifespan.[28,29] In search of a DR mimetic, Howitz *et al.*[30] have found resveratrol, a plant polyphenol present in red wine, extending the lifespan of budding yeast *S. cerevisiae*, which is analogous to lifespan extension by caloric restriction in the same organism. Once, the effects of such DR mimetic agents are fully established in higher organisms, including humans, they may serve a better substitute for those having lesser compliance of DR on a long-term basis. The DR mimetic drugs, preferably from plant sources, could be a suitable alternative to achieve beneficial effects of actual DR[22] (eating food without having it). Many uses of such herbal products have been listed in Ayurveda, an ancient Indian system of medicine since 600 BC. A gum resin, called gugglu in Sanskrit, from Commiphora mukul used for the treatment of obesity and lipid disorders has its mention in the Sushruta Samitha written around 2500 years ago. The extract of resin, known guggulipid, has been successfully shown to exhibit lipid-lowering activity in normal and hyperlipidimic animals.[31] It is known to elevate HDL (good cholesterol) levels with concomitant lowering of low density lipoproteins (LDL) in rabbits on high fatty-diet and also shown to have lipid-lowering effects in humans.[32,33] Out of many such plant products being investigated, extract of aloe vera, a tropical plant, is now a familiar ingredient in variety of health formulations and cosmetics. A life-long dietary use of aloe vera extract has been found to suppress free radical induced oxidative damage and hepatic cholesterol rise in aging rats.[34] Uses of such natural herbal products may alternatively exert many of the similar beneficial effects of DR, without cutting the food intake.

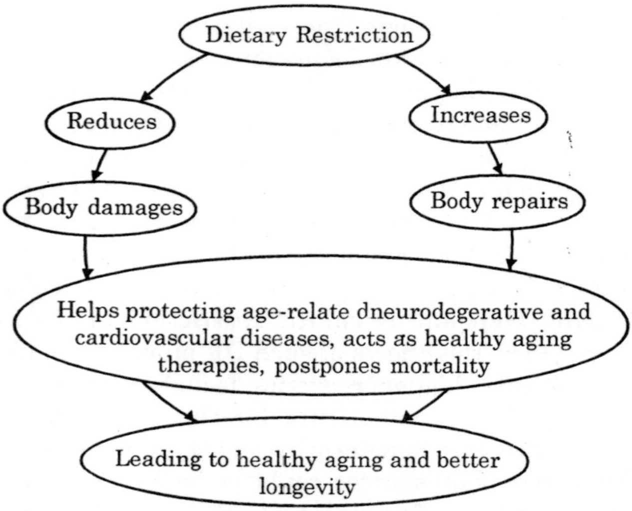

Multiple effects of dietary restriction leading to healthy aging and better longevity - a way to elixir of youth

Concluding Remarks

Though a battery of data available on the merits of DR, there are some points which are yet to be considered before it could be floated as a health care resort for humans. Among these, the most vital ones are the duration and periods of onset of such restrictions and/or the uses of mimetic pharmaceutical and nutraceutical agents. DR and its mimetics, once fully evaluated, could provide an attractive way to elixir of youth and to achieve healthy longevity in various organisms, including humans.[35]

Acknowledgements

Financial support from the Department of Science and Technology, New Delhi (SP/SO/D-33/99) and the Council of Scientific and Industrial Research, New Delhi (37/1031/99/ EMR-II) to carry out research on dietary restriction studies is gratefully acknowledged. Part support from UGC- UPE to NEHU is also appreciated.

REFERENCES

1. Sharma, R. (1994) Theories of aging, in (ed) P S Timiras, *Physiological basis of Aging and Geriatrics*, 2nd edition, CRC Press, Florida.
2. Carey, J. R. (2003) Theories of aging, in *Physiological Basis of Aging and geriatrics* (ed. P. S. Timiras), 3rd edition, CRC Press, Florida.
3. McCay, C. M., Crowell, M. F. and Maynard, L. A. (1935) *J. Nutr.* 10, 63-79.
4. Weindruch, R. and Walford, R. L. (1988) *The retardation of aging and disease by dietary restriction,* Charles C. Thomas, Springfield, IL.
5. Sprott, R. L. and Austad, S. N. (1996) Animal models for aging research, in Schneider, E. L. and Rowe, J. W. (eds.), *Handbook of the Biology of Aging,* Academic Press, London.
6. Finch, C. E. and Ruvkun, G. (2001) *Ann. Rev. Genom. Hum. Genet.* 2, 435-462.
7. Everitt, A. V. (2003) *Biogerontology* 4, 47-50.
8. Holehan, A. M. and Merry, B. J. (1985) *Mech. Ageing Dev.* 32, 179-186.
9. Holliday, R. (1989) *Bioessays* 10, 125-127.
10. Dutta, D. and Sharma, R. (2003) *Horm. Metab. Res.* 35, 415-420.
11. Dutta, D. and Sharma, R. (2004) *Biogerontology* 5, 177-184.
12. Dutta, D. and Sharma, R. (2006) *Ann. N. Y. Acad. Sci.* 1067, 129-141.
13. Masoro, E. J. (2003) *Sci. Aging Knowledge Environ.* 8, RE2.
14. Bartke, A., Chandrashekar, V., Dominici, F., Turyn, D., Kinney, B., Steger, R. and Kopchick, J. J. (2003) *Biogerontology* 4, 1-8.
15. Ramsey, J. J., Harper, M. E. and Weindruch, R. (2000), *Free Radic. Biol. Med.* 29, 946-968.
16. Betarbet, R., Shere, T. B. and Greenamyre, J. T. (2002) *Bioessays* 24, 308-318.

17. Hekimi, S. and Guarente, L. (2003) *Science* 299, 1351-1354.
18. Goto, S. (2002) *Ann N Y Acad Sci.* 959, 50-56.
19. Pahlavani, M. A. (2000) *Front. Biosci.* 5, 580-587.
20. Pletcher, S. D., MacDonald, S. J., Marguerie, R., Certa, U., Stearns, S. C., Goldstein, D. B. and Partridge, L. (2002) *Curr. Biol.* 12, 712-723.
21. Cao, S. X., Dhabbi, J. M., Mote, P. L. and Spindler, S. R. (2001) *Proc. Natl. Acad. Sci. USA* 98, 10630-10635.
22. Finkel, T. (2003) Nature 425, 132-133.
23. Maislos, M., Abou-Rabiah, Y., Zuili, I., Iordash, S. and Shany, S. (1998) *Eur. J. Clin. Nutr.* 52, 127-130.
24. Rao, K. S., Ayyagari, S., Raji, N. S. and Murthy, K. J. R. (1996) *Curr. Sci.* 71, 464-469.
25. Cox, K. L., Burke, V., Morton, A. R., Beilin, I. J. and Puddey, I. B. (2003) *Metabolism* 52, 107-115.
26. Sharma, R. (2001) *J. Okinawa Chubu Hospital* S27, 13.
27. Willcox, D. C., Willcox, B. J., Todoriki, H., Curb, J. D. and Suzuki, M. (2006) *Biogerontology* 7, 173-177.
28. Lee, I. M., Blair, S. N., Allison, D. B., Folsom, A. R., Harris, T. B., Manson, J. E. and Wing, R. R. (2001) *J. Gerontol.* 56A, 7-19.
29. Johnson, M. D., Bebb, R. A. and Sirrs, S. M. (2002) *Ageing Res. Rev.* 1, 29-41.
30. Howitz, K. T., Bitterman, K. J., Cohen, H. Y., Lamming, D. W., Lavu, S., Wood, J. G., Zipkin, R. E., Chung, P., Kisielewski, A., Zhang, L., Scherer, B. and Sinclair, D. A. (2003) Nature 425, 191-196.
31. Dev, S. (1997) *Curr. Sci.* 73, 909-928.
32. Nityanand, S., Srivastava, J. S. and Asthana, O. P. (1989) *J. Assoc. Physicians India* 37, 323-328.
33. Dev, S. (1999) *Environ. Health Perspect.* 107, 783-789.
34. Lim, B. O., Seong, N. S., Choue, R. W., Kim, J. D., Lee, H. Y., Yu, B. P., Jeon, T. I. and Park, D. K. (2003) *J. Nutr. Sci. Vitaminol* (Tokyo) 49, 292-296.
35. Sharma, R. (2008) *Oki. Well. Longev. J. 2(1)*, 15-23.

3

Alzheimer's Disease Type Dementia – Present Status and Future Perspective

M.K. Thakur

In India, the life expectancy at birth has increased by 30 years since Independence. According to the World Health Organization (WHO), India's population of those aged over 65, which was 40 million in 1997, is expected to increase to 108 million by 2025 and to 240 million by 2050. This means enormous increase in age-related problems such as dementia - a condition characterized by progressively declining memory and intellectual functions, impairment in the ability to carry out activities of daily living, and a number of neuropsychiatric symptoms. Current data from developing countries suggest that the prevalence of age-adjusted dementia in 65 year olds is high ($\geq$5%) in certain Asian and Latin American countries, but consistently low (1-3%) in India and sub-Saharan Africa. Dementia costs in developing countries are estimated to be US$73 billion yearly (Kalaria *et al.* 2008). Thus dementia is a serious health problem and social challenge.

The most common and well-known type of dementia is Alzheimer's disease (AD), which is a fatal neurodegenerative disorder that directly affects millions of people and indirectly affects the lives of tens of millions of others who must deal with many years of cognitive decline of their loved ones. It affects the ability to think, speak, reason, remember and move. It is a progressive brain dysfunction, which results in a restriction of daily activities and in most cases leads to the need for long term care. It affects not only patients, but also those related to them and on whom the patients depend for care. There is no definite diagnosis of the disease, except for brain biopsy. Insufficient evidence exists for the use of biomarkers in clinical practice for diagnosis or *disease* management, but promising discoveries are made. Optimal treatment requires both nonpharmacological and pharmacological interventions, yet none have been shown to cure the disease. Therefore, it is becoming an ever-increasing social burden for the health care system and national economy in addition to the emotional burden for the immediate family members.

Although enormous advances have been made in AD research, many questions remain unanswered and more research is needed to address the gaps in our understanding of the *disease*. For instance, although advanced age, female gender, apolipoprotein E (APOE) e4 allele, smoking, family history of AD or other dementia, fewer years of formal education, lower income and lower occupational status have been associated with an increased risk of developing the condition, the pathogenesis of AD is still largely unknown. Although progress is being made in developing new therapies for AD, no therapeutic interventions to cure or substantially modify disease progression currently exist. Here we discuss the present status and future perspective of this disease regarding descriptive epidemiology, clinical course, characteristic neuropathological changes and promising new avenues for the treatment of dementia of the Alzheimer type.

Types of Dementia

There are three most common forms of dementia - Alzheimer's disease (AD), vascular dementia and Lewy body dementia. Sometimes, a person can have more than one of these problems simultaneously. Some of these disorders progress to worse with time and cannot be cured, whereas other types can be treated and reversed.

In vascular dementia, arteries feeding the brain become narrowed or blocked. The onset of symptoms is usually abrupt, frequently occurring after a stroke. Vascular dementia often causes problems with thinking, language, walking, bladder control and vision. The progression of vascular dementia may be halted after preventing additional strokes by treating the underlying diseases such as high blood pressure. In Lewy body dementia, abnormal round structures called Lewy bodies develop within cells of the midbrain, beneath the cerebral hemispheres. It shares characteristics with both AD and Parkinson's disease. Like AD, it causes confusion and impaired memory and judgment. It often produces two distinctive physical signs typical of Parkinson's disease - a shuffling gait and flexed posture. This suggests that the three ailments are related, or that Lewy body dementia and Alzheimer's or Parkinson's disease sometimes co-exist in the same person. Some people with Lewy body dementia have experienced dramatic improvements in symptoms when treated with medications for Alzheimer's or Parkinson's disease.

There are many conditions that can cause dementia. For example, neurological disorders like Parkinson's disease, cerebrovascular disease and strokes, brain tumors, blood clots and multiple sclerosis can sometimes be associated with dementia although many patients with these conditions are cognitively normal. Some brain infections such as *chronic syphilis, chronic HIV*, or chronic fungal *meningitis* can cause dementia. Many medicines may have side effects causing cognitive impairment, especially in elderly patients. Perhaps the most frequent offenders are drugs used to control *bladder urgency* and *incontinence*. “Psychiatric medications” such as anti-depressants and anti-anxiety medications and “neurological medications” such as anti-seizure medications can also be associated with cognitive impairment. In older persons, some forms of *depression* can cause problems with memory and concentration that initially may be indistinguishable from the early symptoms of AD.

Alzheimer’s Disease Type Dementia

Alzheimer’s disease was first described in 1907 by the German physician Alois Alzheimer. AD is more severe than the mild memory loss that many people experience as they grow old. It is a progressive degenerative disease that affects areas of the brain involved in memory, intelligence, judgment, language and behavior. It causes memory loss, disorientation, depression and decay of bodily functions. It is characterized by a deterioration of both cognitive and physical abilities. It first affects memory and the ability to carry out complex, coordinated tasks. It also causes depression, inattention and outbursts of anger. It affects personality, the ability to think clearly, and the ability to carry out daily activities. In a more progressive stage, the disease can cause difficulties in the ability to perform even simple tasks such as speaking and comprehending, eating and sleeping. The affected person can even forget his name and identity (Thakur 2000, 2002).

AD predominantly occurs in the second half of lifespan, often after the age of 65 years. The probability of suffering from AD increases with advancing age from about 5% for the 65-69-year olds, to 10% for the 70-75-year olds and to more than 20% for the 85-89 year olds and about 30% of those over 90. Every third person over 90 years of age suffers from moderate or severe dementia. About half of those affected by dementia suffer from AD. Since the average life span has increased over the years, AD is becoming a more common problem. The probability is higher for women and for people having a lower standard of education. More than 18 million people are affected with AD worldwide, in India alone the figure is over 3 million. This number is projected to nearly double by 2025 to 34 million. Much of this increase will be in the developing countries, and will be due to the aging population. Currently, more than 50% of people with AD live in developing countries and by 2025, this will be over 70%. However, studies conducted in South India, Mumbai and the northern state of Haryana have reported very low rate of occurrence of AD at 65 years of age or older, ranging from about 1% in rural north-India to 2.7% in urban Chennai (the lowest reported from anywhere in the world) (Chandra et al. 1998). Such lower prevalence of AD in Indians might be due to decreased occurrence of a risk factor for AD, apolipoprotein E4, in Indian population than elsewhere. Also the study involving genetically altered mice suggests that curcumin, the yellow pigment in Indian curry spice, inhibits the accumulation of destructive beta amyloids in the brains of Alzheimer's patients and breaks up existing plaques (Lim et al. 2001). The low molecular weight and polar structure of curcumin allow it to penetrate the blood-brain barrier effectively and bind to beta amyloid.

Symptoms of AD

The onset of AD is usually gradual and progresses slowly. It attacks brain cells (where memory is stored), brain nerves and transmitters (which carry instructions around the brain). Production of a chemical messenger acetylcholine is disrupted, nerve ends are attacked and cells die. The brain shrinks as gaps develop in the temporal lobe and hippocampus, which are important for receiving and storing new information. The ability to remember, speak, think and make decisions is disrupted. Later in the course of the disorder, affected individuals may become confused or disoriented about what month or year it is, be unable to describe accurately where they live, or be unable to name a place being visited. Eventually, patients may wander, be unable to engage in conversation, erratic in mood, uncooperative, and lose bladder and bowel control. In late stages of the disease, persons may become totally incapable of caring for themselves. Death can then follow, perhaps from pneumonia or some other secondary problems that occur in severely deteriorated states of health. Those who develop the disorder later in life more often die from other illnesses (such as heart disease) rather than as a consequence of AD. After death, tangles and plaques made from protein fragments, dying cells and nerve ends are detected in the brain. This confirms the diagnosis.

Diagnosis

Dementia remains under-diagnosed largely because memory loss, the main symptom, is common in old age. There is thus a general perception that dementia is simply because of old age. But this is not true as it is a disease of the brain which can be treated. The most important issue in dementia is its diagnosis. There are no blood tests for AD, though there are for other causes of dementia such as abnormal thyroid and vitamin deficiency. Imaging helps, but only with vascular diseases such as stroke. A new brain-imaging method allows physicians to diagnose Alzheimer's before its onset. When a radioactive dye is injected in the blood, it travels to the brain and attaches to amyloid plaque deposits which look yellow in a Positron Emission Tomography (PET) scan. Researchers have developed an optical test that can determine the presence of amyloid beta proteins in the lens of the eye and help in the early detection of AD. The eye is treated with special fluorescence drops that bind to the amyloid beta proteins, which glow under an infrared light, indicating AD. Then a device called an interior laser ophthalmoscope can detect the presence of the amyloid protein.

Some biomarkers have also been suggested. It is likely that nanotechnology tools help early detection of AD because of their potential to detect ultra-low concentrations and multiple biomarkers of AD in cerebral spinal fluid (CSF) (Nazem and Mansoori 2008). Taken together, dementia can be diagnosed after a careful medical history and physical examination, evaluation of the person's mental and functional status, and selected laboratory tests and imaging tests, such as CT and MRI scans, to rule out other possible causes of the symptoms. The most important task is a good understanding of family history. Simply talking to the patient and his family members gives most of the information to confirm the diagnosis.

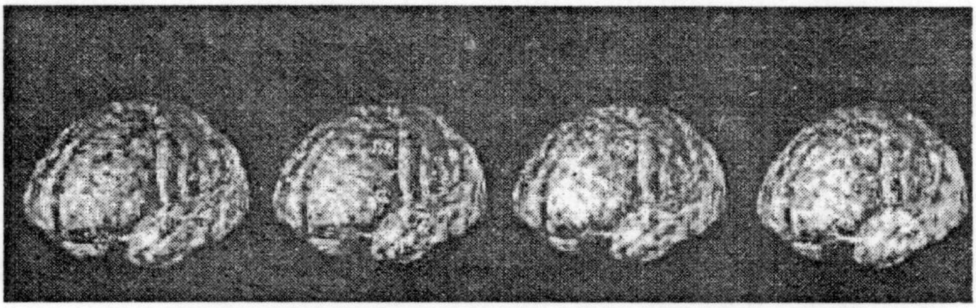

Fig 1. MRI of brain showing the dynamic wave of gray matter loss that occurs as patients progress from mild to severe AD. The blue colour indicates brain regions with no detectable tissue loss, red colour denotes regions with up to 10% tissue loss, and white up to 20% loss. Beginning in the temporal brain areas underlying memory function, the deficits spread into frontal and limbic brain regions, leaving sensory and visual cortices spared until very late in the disease. (Thompson et al. 2003).

Mechanism of AD

In AD, as in other types of dementia, increasing numbers of nerve cells deteriorate and die. A healthy adult brain has 100 billion nerve cells, or neurons, with long branching extensions connected at 100 trillion points. At these connections, called synapses, information flows in tiny chemical pulses released by one neuron and taken up by the receiving cell. Different strengths and patterns of signals move constantly through the brain's circuits, creating the cellular basis of memories, thoughts and skills. In AD, information transfer at the synapses begins to fail, the number of synapses declines and eventually cells die. In a brain with advanced Alzheimer's, there is dramatic shrinkage from cell loss and widespread debris from dead and dying neurons.

Scientists do not yet fully understand the processes resulting in the catastrophic brain damage associated with AD. According to a leading theory, called the "amyloid hypothesis," the prime suspect is a tiny protein fragment called beta-amyloid. Trouble begins when yet-to-be-identified factors trigger overproduction of beta-amyloid or reduce the brain's ability to dispose of it. The excess jams signaling at the synapses, blocking information flow and leading to a cascade of damaging events ending in cell death. Beta-amyloid fragments gradually accumulate into the microscopic "plaques" considered to be one pathological hallmark of Alzheimer's. The other hallmark is "tangles," formed when a different protein called tau twists into strands inside dead and dying neurons. Although these two pathological hallmarks were recognized more than a hundred years ago, only within the past decade have real advances been made in determining the molecular and biochemical basis of AD (Neet and Thinakaran 2008). Other abnormalities seen in Alzheimer brain tissue include inflammation and oxidative damage due to highly reactive oxygen-containing products of cellular metabolism.

Presently, it is not clear when the process of AD starts and how long the pathobiochemical processes take to develop. To explain the etiology of AD, Lahiri et al. (2008) have proposed a "Latent Early-life Associated Regulation" (LEARn) model, which postulates a latent expression of specific genes triggered at the developmental stage. This model integrates both the neuropathological features (e.g., amyloid-loaded plaques and tau-laden tangles) and environmental factors (e.g., diet, metal exposure and hormones) associated with the disease. Environmental agents perturb gene regulation in a long-term fashion, beginning at early developmental stages, but these perturbations do not have pathological results until significantly later in life. The LEARn model operates through the regulatory region (promoter) of the gene and by affecting the methylation status within the promoter of specific genes.

While many clues about the mechanism of AD have been uncovered, the exact molecular mechanism associated with the cause of this disease is not completely understood. Animal models of AD, though not perfect, offer a means to gain knowledge of the basic biochemistry associated with this disorder. The field of proteomics which focuses on identifying the dynamic nature of the protein content expressed within a particular cell, tissue, or organism, has provided many insights into AD. Proteomic studies have revealed many pathways that are associated with disease pathogenesis and that may lead to the development of potential therapeutic targets (Sowell *et al.* 2008).

Risk factors for AD

AD is a complex disease which is caused through interactions among genetic, environmental and lifestyle factors. It develops over many years, and it appears to be affected by a number of factors that may increase or decrease a person's risk of developing the disease. The biggest risk for Alzheimer's is simply age. Alzheimer's cases double with every five years of age between 65 and 85. Although most people who develop AD do not have a family history of the condition, one is at increased risk for the condition if a member of the family is afflicted with this disease. In a small percentage of cases, the disease is caused by genetic changes (mutations) in the family. Early-onset AD is a very rare form of the disease that can occur in people between the age of 30 and 60. It is caused by mutations in amyloid precursor protein (APP), presenilin (PS)1 and PS2 genes located on three different chromosomes. A person has a 50-50 chance of developing early-onset AD if one parent has any of these genetic mutations. Late-onset AD, the more common form, develops after age 65. It is influenced by apolipoprotein E (apoE) gene which may be present in three forms. For example, apoE2, a rarely occurring form, may provide some protection; apoE3, the most common form, appears to play a neutral role; and apoE4, which is found in about 40% of people with AD, appears to increase the risk.

Over the last few years, association of Alzheimer's with lifestyle has emerged. Scientists have found that what is good for the heart may also be good for the brain. The risk factors for heart disease - high blood pressure, diabetes, excess weight, high cholesterol and lack of exercise - may also play a role in AD. High cholesterol may also affect brain arteries and promote clumping of the beta-amyloid peptide, which causes neurodegeneration in Alzheimer's. A recent population study has shown that people who take statins, the most commonly prescribed cholesterol lowering drugs, have reduced risk of developing dementia.

Treatment of AD

As with numerous other diseases, there is no cure for AD but medication can improve disease symptoms. Typically antidementia or psychotropic drugs are prescribed. The medicines administered today to Alzheimer's patients focus on preventing the breakdown of acetylcholine, a chemical produced by brain cells which transmits information within the brain and is vitally involved in cognitive processes that include memory, attention and thought. Because acetylcholine-producing cells are among the first to die in

Alzheimer's patients, drug-induced elevation of acetylcholine levels partially attenuates the cognitive deterioration. The more recent antidementia agents belong to the so-called acetylcholinesterase inhibitors reminyl (galantamine), exelon (rivastigmine) and aricept (donepezil). Tumor necrosis factor-alpha (TNF-alpha), which regulates synaptic function in neural networks, increases in AD and disrupts the synaptic memory mechanisms. When an antagonist of TNF-alpha (etanercept) is administered perispinally in a patient with late-onset AD, it shows rapid cognitive improvement, beginning within minutes (Tobinick and Gross 2008). No drugs slow the rate of progression of AD, but they can only delay the deterioration of symptoms. A variety of *clinical research trials* are underway with agents that try either to decrease the amount of amyloid beta peptide produced or increase the amount of amyloid beta peptide removed. Okura and Matsumoto (2008) developed nonviral DNA vaccines and used them to obtain a substantial amyloid beta reduction in AD model mice without any side effects. It is hoped that such therapies may slow down the rate of progression of AD.

Modulation of immune/inflammatory responses by diverse strategies including amyloid-β immunization, nonsteroidal anti-inflammatory drugs and manipulation of microglial activation states has been shown to reduce AD-like pathology and cognitive deficits in AD transgenic mouse models. Human umbilical cord blood cells (HUCBCs) have also unique immunomodulatory potential. Nikolic et al. (2008) report a marked reduction in Aβ levels/β-amyloid plaques and associated astrocytosis following multiple low-dose infusions of HUCBCs into the PSAPP mouse model of AD. Moreover, microglia isolated from HUCBC-infused PSAPP mice demonstrated increased phagocytosis of Aβ.

The apparent increased frequency of AD in women has led to considerable research about the role of female sex steroid hormone estrogen in AD. Estrogen influences the expression of genes involved in AD (Thakur and Mani 2004, 2005; Mani and Thakur 2006; Ghosh and Thakur 2008a, b). As estrogen therapy shows side effects, recent studies suggest that estrogen should not be prescribed to post-menopausal women for the purpose of decreasing the risk of AD. However, these studies have some lacunae and the role of estrogen in AD still remains an interesting area of research focus.

There is overwhelming clinical evidence that antioxidants, which fight against free radicals, are effective in preventing the symptoms of both dementia and AD. In recent years, there has been a lot of interest in using antibodies against the abnormal deposits of beta amyloid in the brain. A nasal spray vaccine has also been tested in AD patients. Similarly, intensive investigation is conducted for gene and stem cell therapy to treat the people suffering from AD. As of 2008, the safety and efficacy of more than 400 pharmaceutical treatments are being investigated in *clinical trials* worldwide, and approximately one-fourth of these compounds are in *Phase III* trials, which is the last step prior to review by regulatory agencies. Unlike preventive vaccination, the putative therapy would be used to treat people already diagnosed. It is based upon the concept of training the immune system to recognise, attack and reverse deposition of amyloid, thereby altering the course of the disease. Many population-based studies suggest that lifestyle interventions may also help to slow the onset and progression of AD.

Concluding Remarks

Our knowledge is growing rapidly as researchers expand their understanding of the many factors involved in the pathogenesis of AD. People can take some actions that might reduce the effect of possible AD risk factors. These actions include: lowering cholesterol and high blood pressure levels, controlling diabetes, exercising regularly, and engaging in intellectually stimulating activities. It is advised to adopt a brain-healthy diet, stay physically and mentally active, and remain socially involved. All these strategies are useful because they lower risk for other diseases and help maintain and improve overall health and well-being. Even though there are no treatments, drugs, or pills for curing AD, early identification and intervention are the best ways to delay/ prevent and manage the disease. More in-depth research and awareness about the disease is necessary. A goal of molecular and cellular neuroscience is to bridge basic mechanisms with translational studies to help develop novel agents for pharmacotherapeutic interventions. As a result of extensive investigations, it is expected that the novel therapies targeting AD pathogenesis will appear in near future and the next few years may be exciting for AD researchers.

Acknowledgements

The author's work cited in this article has been supported by financial assistance from the Indian Council of Medical Research, Department of Science and Technology, and Department of Biotechnology, Government of India.

REFERENCES

Alzheimer A (1907) Über eine eigenartige Erkrankung der Hirnrinde. *Allgemeine Z Psychiatrie Psychisch-Gerichtliche Med.* 64, 146–148.

Chandra V, Ganguli M, Pandav R, Johnston J, Belle S and DeKosky ST (1998) Prevalence of Alzheimer's disease and other dementias in rural India: The Indo-US study. *Neurology* 51:1000-1008.

Ghosh S and Thakur MK (2008a) PS1 expression is downregulated by gonadal steroids in adult mouse brain. *Neurochem Res* 33:365-369.

Ghosh S and Thakur MK (2008b) PS2 Protein expression is upregulated by sex steroids in the cerebral cortex of aging mice. *Neurochem Int* 52:363-367.

Kalaria RN, Maestre GE, Arizaga R, Friedland RP, Galasko D, Hall K, Luchsinger JA, Ogunniyi A, Perry EK, Potocnik F, Prince M, Stewart R, Wimo A, Zhang ZX and Antuono P (2008) Alzheimer's disease and vascular dementia in developing countries: prevalence, management, and risk factors. *Lancet Neurol*. 7:812-26.

Lahiri DK, Zawia NH, Greig NH, Sambamurti K and Maloney B (2008) Early-life events may trigger biochemical pathways for Alzheimer's disease: the "LEARn" model. *Biogerontology* (in press).

Lim GP, Chu T, Yang F, Beech W, Frautschy SA and Cole GM (2001) The curry spice curcumin reduces oxidative damage and amyloid pathology in an Alzheimer transgenic mouse. *J Neuroscience* 21:8370–8377.

Mani S and Thakur MK (2006) In the cerebral cortex of female and male mice, amyloid precursor protein (APP) promoter methylation is higher in females and differentially regulated by sex steroids. *Brain Res* 1067:43-47.

Nazem A and Mansoori GA (2008) Nanotechnology solutions for Alzheimer's disease: advances in research tools, diagnostic methods and therapeutic agents. *J Alzheimer's Disease* 13:199-223.

Neet KE and Thinakaran G (2008) Thematic minireview series on the molecular basis of Alzheimer's disease. *J Biol Chem* (in press).

Nikolic WV, Hou H, Town T, Zhu Y, Giunta B, Sanberg CD, Zeng J, Luo D, Ehrhart J, Mori T, Sanberg PR and Tan J (2008) Peripherally administered human umbilical cord blood cells reduce parenchymal and vascular â-amyloid deposits in Alzheimer mice. *Stem Cells and Development* 17:423-440.

Okura Y and Matsumoto Y (2008) Novel vaccine therapy for Alzheimer's disease - recent progress and our approach. *Brain Nerve* 60:931-940.

Sowell RA, Owen JB and Allan BD (2008) Proteomics in animal models of Alzheimer's and Parkinson's diseases. *Ageing Res Rev* (in press).

Thakur MK (2000) Alzheimer's Disease: a challenge in the new millennium. *Curr Sci* 79: 101-108.

Thakur MK (2002) Molecular studies in aging with special focus on Alzheimer's disease. In K. Bagchi (es), *Alzheimer's Disease in India,* pp 83-103, Society of Gerontological Research, New Delhi.

Thakur MK and Mani ST (2005) Estradiol regulates APP mRNA alternative splicing in the mice brain cortex. *Neurosci Lett* 381:154-157.

Thakur MK and Mani ST (2004) Role of sex steroid hormones in Alzheimer's disease. In: *Proc Int Conf Biotech Neurosci,* Cochin, pp. 195-202.

Thompson PM, Hayashi KM, Zubicaray G, Janke AL, Rose SE, Semple J, Herman D, Hong MS, Dittmer SS, Doddrell DM and Toga AW (2003) Dynamics of Gray Matter Loss in Alzheimer's Disease. *J Neuroscience* 23:994- 1005.

Tobinick EL and Gross H (2008) Rapid cognitive improvement in Alzheimer's disease following perispinal etanercept administration. *J Neuroinflammation* 5:2

4

Aging in India: Health and Health Care Issues

A B Dey, Wilma Wilson & Ashish Goel

[The increasing proportion of older persons in the Indian society is well perceived from census data. The population above the age of sixty years has nearly tripled in last 50 years and this relentless increase continues in projected population figures by demographic experts. According to 2001 census, there were 75.93 million Indians above the age of sixty years of them 38.22 millions were males and 37.71 millions were females. The projections for next five census are 96.30 millions (2011), 133.32 millions (2021), 178.59 (2031), 236.01 millions (2041) and 300.96 millions (2051). Health systems are expected to care for large number of older patients with multiple diseases involving multiple organs; and multiple disabilities. The expectations of patients from health systems have also increased tremendously keeping in tune with the advances in technology. Evidence exists to suggest the effectiveness of multidisciplinary interventions in old age health care by health care professionals from different streams. Geriatric services need to have several special features usually not required for the adult population. These include multidisciplinary interventions that focus on rehabilitation by way of physiotherapy, occupational therapy, cognitive behavioral therapy; and rapid access to specialized/surgical interventions].

Introduction

Enhanced human life span as witnessed in the preceding decades has not been accompanied by good quality of life for majority of older Indians. Of the three crucial factors that determine quality of life: financial security, emotional security and health and wellbeing, the last one is supreme, as all other factors become irrelevant in poor health. Research studies in social gerontology and geriatrics in past decades have provided insight into various aspects pertaining to the status of older people in India.[1] Large volume of authentic data on demographic trends, impact of changes in the family structure and migration, physical and behavioral status, organization and dynamics of health systems exist in Indian literature. However, very little effort has been made to develop a model of health and social care in tune with the changing need and time. Absence of such a model for older people in India and other countries with similar socioeconomic situation, presents a challenge as well as an opportunity for innovation in health system development.

Magnitude of the Challenge

While population ageing is a success story of socio-economic development and good public health practice, it also denotes economic crisis, social crisis due to increased demand and inequitable supply; and progressive deterioration of health and functional status for individual leading to increase demand for services from various institutions of the civil society.

Data from focused academic research as well as three nation wide sample surveys of 1986-1987, 1995-1996 and

2004 conducted by National Sample Survey Organization have provided information on the magnitude and nature of diseases and disabilities in old age.[2] It empirically considered that health problems in old age are a constellation of problems such as; increased susceptibility to infection, inability to cope with physical and psychological stress, degenerative arthritis, atherosclerotic and vascular diseases heart and brain, cancer of various organs and cognitive impairment due to declining brain size or more importantly various types of dementing disorders.

The ICMR funded study conducted between 1984-1986 by Late Professor A. Venkoba Rao, in rural Tamil Nadu identified conditions; namely visual impairment and loco-motor disability as the leading health issues in rural elderly.[3] It may be noted here that at that point of time, the National Blindness Control Program targeting cataract related blindness was in its early phase. Nearly 90 percent of this rural older population had cataract related blindness. Forty percent of this group had loco-motor disability indicating the need for assistance in activities of daily living. Depression was detected in a tenth of the subjects. This study also detected acceptance of primary health care (PHC) services among older subjects. Over the years, however the level of satisfaction among older people regarding the PHC services have declined, which has necessitated affirmative action in strengthening the primary health care services by means of policy initiatives on the part of the Government.

While the ICMR study was based on a primary care approach, the sample surveys of 1986-87 (NSSO Survey 42nd round) and 1995-96 (NSSO Survey 52nd round) were community surveys that estimated the prevalence of chronic disease and disability. Over a decade between the two surveys, the burden of chronic diseases increased from 45% in 1986-87 to 52-55% in 1995-96. The prevalence of disabilities was assessed in the later surveys and was reported to be about

40%; visual impairment and hearing deficit being the most frequent, 25-27% and 12-14%, respectively. The prevalence of amnesia (possibly a surrogate question for cognitive impairment) was estimated at an alarming figure of 7-10.5% (urban and rural figures respectively).

The latest round of the survey (60th) reported that about 8% of older Indians were confined to their home or bed; the proportion of such immobile or home bound people rose with age to 27% after the age of 80 years and women were more frequently affected than males in both villages and cities. The 60th round of sample survey estimated the state of self perceived health status of older people. A good or fair condition of health was reported by 55-63% of people with a sickness and 77-78% of people without sickness. In contrast about 13-17% of survey population without any sickness reported ill health. It is possible that many older people take ill health in their stride as a part of "usual/normal ageing". This observation has a lot of significance as self perceived health status is an important indicator of health service utilization and compliance to treatment interventions.

In a systematic review of all relevant research projects funded by ICMR, prevalence figures of three important diseases namely: hypertension, diabetes and ischemic heart disease, were estimated and published in a land mark paper Indian Journal of Medical Research 1997.[4] The prevalence of hypertension, ischemic heart disease and diabetes were 110, 118 and 53 per thousand for the rural elderly respectively while for the urban elderly the figures were 209, 234 and 165 per thousand respectively, indicating an urban bias. The prevalence of two common disabilities studied; namely visual and hearing impairment were 172 and 141 per thousand and 597 and 613 per thousand for rural and urban areas respectively. It was projected that out of a possible 63 million older people in India in the year 1996; there were 11 million older people with visual impairment;

38 million with hearing impairment, 9 million each with hypertension and ischemic heart disease and 5 million with diabetes. These data only provided some glimpses of the burden of ill health and disability older people carry and by no means provide the total picture. It is worth noting here that there are many other health and functionality issues which have not yet been addressed scientifically.

In a publication from North-East India, the disease and disability data from a Geriatric Clinic was published.[5] The report indicated that older people have limited number of common diseases to account for most of their illnesses. The ten most common diagnoses in this clinic were hypertension (39.5%), cataract (35.3%), osteoarthritis (33.7%), COPD (20%), IHD/CAD (19%), prostate enlargement in men (16%), diabetes (15.2%), dyspepsia (11%), constipation (irritable bowel syndrome) (9.2%) and depression (8.5%) which accounted for 81% of all diagnoses while 95% of all diagnoses were accounted for by 20 common problem in a dedicated facility in a tertiary care center. Most people had multiple diagnoses; two diseases were diagnosed in 29%, three in 25% and four in 15% of older patients in this facility. In addition 87% of patients had one acute health problem or the other in the preceding one month. The report also noted physical dependence, stroke, osteoporosis, fragility fractures, heart failure and dementia as common health problems among the very old people. In addition to the diseases mentioned above, several disabilities were also detected in the clinic population. These included impaired vision (48.5%), impaired hearing (32%), inability to pursue activities of daily living (7%), impaired arm function (6.5%) impaired leg function (5%), cognitive impairment (5%), depressed mood (20%) urinary incontinence (20% mostly in women). Conclusively, multiple diseases (from common conditions), multiple disabilities and frequent acute health problems were found to be the hallmark of old age health.

The mortality data of older people in India is vague and may not provide a clear picture of the actual causes leading to death.[6] In rural India pneumonia and bronchitis account for 27% of all deaths in old age while IHD (12.5%), stroke (9.8%), tuberculosis (7%) and cancer (5.8%) are the other common causes of death. Whereas in urban India cardiovascular disease (IHD and stroke included) account for 39% of deaths in old age, while infection (13%), lung diseases (possibly chronic bronchitis and cancer- 10%), cancer (7%) ill defined conditions account for 27% of all deaths. However, as indicated earlier accurate collection of data with clear definition of each diagnosis as a cause of death is required for a better understanding of the issue. The above paragraphs are adequate to provide a clear picture of the challenges in hand. While confronting the needs of such a large group people with a multitude of disease and disability, clarity in planning and strategy is mandatory.

Principles and Processes of Old age Care

Health in old age is affected by social and economic issues apart from the inherent disadvantage of biological decline. The aim of health care system for older people is to provide qualitative service closest to their home, to keep them functional and to help them return to their normal lives as soon as possible after illness. Hence the health system catering to the needs of older people must have full knowledge of its users, their financial status, social and cultural resources and living arrangements, apart from other disadvantages they might be facing. The care provided should be tailored to meet every individual's need. A comprehensive care package that includes promotive, preventive, curative and rehabilitative service is essential for this group of population. Easy accessibility, continuity and good quality of care can only earn respect and satisfaction among the older generation. A high degree of coordination is essential in such a model so that different services do not function at cross-purpose but are complementary to each other. Most importantly, the services should be complete in terms of physician consultation, paramedical services, drugs and restorative interventions.

Illness in old age calls for rapid access to high quality medical care. Older people have multiple related and unrelated diseases, non-specific and often confusing presentations, high incidence of complications and rapid deterioration if untreated or inadequately treated. The value of early interventions in terms of saving life and limiting disability is well-established in older people. However, unlike other age groups, older patients need active and early rehabilitation. Adverse environmental factors, absence of family and community support and lack of economic resources can make care difficult and more challenging.[7]

The process of assessment of older people is a complex task. In addition to usual assessment for health and illness, an evaluation of their functional ability (physical, mental and social) and resources (economic, social, educational and community) is essential as case management is greatly influenced by such factors. It is important that a goal for care is set which would strike a balance between what the patient aspires to have and what the health system can provide by way of therapeutics and prosthetics. This process of assessment is continuous, as with the biological decline newer illnesses and disabilities would appear from time to time. Consequently, a constant review of the management plan is a very important part of the care process.[8]

The health system for older people requires several levels of interventions, e.g. primary care at community level, specialized care by an internist or a geriatrician, and specific interventions by a specialist physician or a surgeon (cardiologist, neurologist, urologist, cardiovascular surgeon, ophthalmologist, etc.) at tertiary level. The process of care is a dynamic where an older individual may be moving between the community and the hospital in early stages of ill-health or disability. However, patients with severe disabilities and incurable diseases may require long-term care and institutionalization. The concept of day care and day center is an innovation in the care of older people where healthy as well as disabled persons spend time in a quasi-health-care setting with recreation and rehabilitation facilities.

From the above discussion, it is clear that in large health-care settings, several medical and paramedical professionals would have to be involved to provide a variety of services. In developing societies, focused interventions for common physical illnesses and disabilities are essential as development of specialized services may not be economically feasible and logistically manageable. The design of services for older people has been an object of debate in most developed countries. Till now, no consensus has been reached on whether these services should be age-based or need-based. What would be ideal: to have all people above the age of 60 to be cared by these services or only those people with multiple disabilities to be included in the system? For a society like ours, probably a balanced mix of both these models should be more pertinent and of great value.

Community Health Services

The majority of older Indians live in the community they grew up and prefer to continue living there till the end. Various data on met and unmet health needs among community living older people has been collated in surveys and studies.[8] The health needs of community living older individuals are related to: vision, hearing, ambulation, cognition, behavioral, activities of daily living, continence and common non-communicable disease like hypertension, ischemic heart disease, diabetes, cancer, cerebrovascular disease, chronic obstructive pulmonary disease etc. As most of these needs are chronic and non-communicable in nature, they are unlikely to change drastically over short periods of time. Prioritization of the felt needs of the older people is useful for planning of services, training of medical and paramedical workers, caregivers, family members of the older people and the aged themselves in providing knowledge and skills for better care provision.

To provide first contact geriatric services, screening of the patient and curative and rehabilitative services can be provided at primary health care levels. Screening of the older patients can be done for general medical problems like diabetes, hypertensions, ischemic heart disease, high cholesterol, anemia etc. Curative services in primary health care must address to day to day health needs of older people. Acute health problems both communicable and non-communicable and follow-up services for chronic health problem are part of curative services. Quality of curative services determines the acceptability of the community of all other heath promotion and preventive services. The health care professionals must have sensitivity towards the problems of older people to make the curative services effective. Rehabilitative services are an essential part of care among older people. Unfortunately physicians often underestimate the role of physiotherapist and occupational therapist in the care in older patients and consequently there is a great deficiency of qualitative therapists in both these fields. Ideally a physical therapy unit must exist least at the Community Health Care (CHC). Community rehabilitation needs to be strengthened effectively for quality care of the older people. Camp approach of services for cataract surgery and specialist care for common health problems in old age by a team of ophthalmologist, dentist, physician, urologist is an alternative for older people living in community with no access to good quality of secondary or tertiary care.

The in service training of medical professionals and paramedical personnel working in the community is necessary to provide better health care for the elderly. There should be a program on skill up-gradation of multipurpose workers; they can be given training in providing curative, preventive and promotive aspects of the health care needs of the elderly. The skills of these community workers need to be enhanced. Special training focusing on identification and treatment of common problems in the elderly needs to be imparted to multipurpose workers who can carry out these tasks easily along with their routine work.

Currently the state of primary health care in India is in a dismal state. A qualitative assessment by the author revealed several reasons for non-utilization of PHC services namely; inaccessibility, inability to travel, lack of faith in the doctor or the system, fatalistic attitude, lack of motivation, inability to afford cost of treatment, lack of carer support and unavailability of better alternatives. The most frequent suggestions for improvement were free drugs, ensuring availability of doctors, continuity of care, supervision of field workers and improvement of sanitation which implies an overall improvement of services. An alternative model of PHC is mobile health units reaching out to the user in the community. The author assessed the role of such units run by an NGO. The services were appreciated but on the long run people desired the need for a permanent structure providing them health care.

To fulfill the need of providing quality health care to the elderly, a review of the existing community based models is required. The model of specialization and service delivery that is to be developed must be appropriate in the local context it will operate. The recently launched National Rural Health Mission can play a big role in improving the quality of care available to older Indians in the community level if implemented as envisaged.

Hospital Services

Despite all measures of health promotion and protection

older people will require domiciliary as well as hospital care from generalists as well as specialists. The main objective of providing hospital services to the elderly is to render specialized health care not available in PHC. The other objective is to reduce mortality and minimize morbidity and complications. The value of multidisciplinary approach in improving the quality of life of older people has been re-emphasized by an ICMR study conducted by the author#. The multidisciplinary team of geriatricians should be ably supported by: physiotherapist, occupational therapist, nursing assistants, social workers, nutritionist, pharmacists etc. along with specialists such as cardiologist, psychiatrist, ophthalmologist, orthopedic surgeon, urologist, surgeon and ear-nose-throat specialist etc. A regular follow-up of all the patients should be maintained.

It has been always debated whether the enhanced longevity as witnessed in past decades has been matched by quality of life in the extra years. To alleviate these concerns for health and well being in later years there is an urgent need for health professionals trained in care of the older people at all levels of health service. Thus certain issues require urgent attention in developing the academic discipline of geriatric medicine, which produces such health professionals. These issues include:

a) Multiple disciplines of medicine need to be involved in health care of the elderly.

b) Specialized training to physicians for geriatric care of older people from training centers in the country.

c) Geriatric units must be created and made functional in all teaching hospitals and selected non-teaching hospitals in different parts of the country.

d) Specialized OPD services and extra dedicated beds in in-patients facilities are a necessity.

e) The concept of day care centers and long stay centers is alien to our health care system. There is need for creation of such facilities in selected areas and centers to begin with which can be extended further later on.

f) As a resources are scarce there is a need to utilize existing community based services, social service agencies, voluntary workers in the care of older people who can be a part of a support system for emotional and social well being of older people.

g) Research in the discipline of geriatrics and gerontology in non existent. There is need for stimulating research in this area by organizing fellowships in established centers.

h) In view of the resource crunch it may be a good idea to start geriatric services within the existing health services

i. To create a large base of carers it would be a good idea to include nurses, paramedical workers and community health workers for care of the older people.

Old age care in undergraduate curriculum of health professionals is scant and needs immediate augmentation. Linked with this is the development of post graduate courses to produce teachers and practitioners for geriatric medicine. Development of hospital services and academic geriatric medicine are linked to each other. Urgent action in this direction is the need of the hour.

Long Term Care

Long term care is a system of activities undertaken by informal caregivers (family, friends and/or neighbours) and/or professionals (health, social and others) to ensure that a person who is not fully capable of self-care can maintain the highest possible quality of life, according to his/her individual preferences, with the greatest possible degree of independence, autonomy, participation, personal fulfilment and human dignity. Long term care for older person in India has always been a matter of great concern in the family of an individual. However, with increasing longevity, advances in medical technology and people living into very old age, severe physical and mental disability, long term care by family has emerged as a challenge in India. Currently there is no system of long term care in Indian society apart from the institutions of family. In gross terms long term care denotes long stay institutions for mentally and physically disabled older people. None of the old age homes or senior citizen accommodation provides services for older people with mental and physical disability requiring assistance in activities of daily living and intense nursing care. Irrespective of economic status the care givers of such individuals undergo great stress in managing the care for such disabled relatives and their own personal lives. Older people living alone without any surviving carer also need long term care at some point of time or the other. Though there are a few high profile cases highlighted in the media; the plight of large majority of the individuals remains unnoticed. Out-of-box thinking is essential to create a provision for long term care funding in India. This includes creation of a trust to receive funds from diverse sources and utilize them for people in need of long term care.

Agenda for Research and Development

Research is the cornerstone of policy formulation and implementation. It also influences allocation of resources for developmental activities. In addition, research provides evidence for scientific practice of medicine. Currently, the research base for the care of older people in India is not adequate for evidence-based practice. The importance of evaluation and maintenance of a database on various aspects of care of older people has been emphasized time and again. The components of such a database would include demographic profile and projections; and activity profiles of the population. The double burden of communicable and non-communicable diseases is an essential determinant for resource allocation in health services. In addition, operational research on health needs, service utilization and user satisfaction needs to be promoted in the research agenda. To gather a large volume of data in a short period of time, a multi-centric approach would be useful. Finally, for the continuous promotion of research in geriatrics and gerontology publications in journals would be a major requirement.

REFERENCES

1. Ramamurti PV. 2003. Perspectives of research on aging in India. *J Aging Soc Policy.* 15:31-43.
2. National Sample Survey Organization. Government of India: 42nd, 52nd and 60th Round.
3. Rao AV. 1990. *Health Care of the Rural Aged.* Indian Council of Medical Research, New Delhi.
4. Shah B, Prabhakar AK. 1997. Chronic morbidity profile among elderly. *Indian J Med Res.* 106:265-72.
5. Dey AB, Soneja S, Nagarkar KM, Jhingan HP. 2001. Evaluation of the health and functional status of older Indians as a prelude to the development of a health programme. *Natl Med J India.* May-Jun;14(3):135-8.
6. Ageing population in India . An analysis of the 1991 census data. A study report in the Analytical Study Report Series based on the 1991 Census Data. Registrar General, India. 1999.
7. Dey AB. 2007. *Handbook of Geriatrics.* Paras Publications, Hyderabad.
8. Kumar V. 1997. Ageing in India—an overview. *Indian J Med Res.* 106:257-64.

5

Modulation of Serum Biochemistry in Aged *Khasis* of High Altitude Location

H. S. Ranhotra & R. Sharma

[The indigenous *Khasis* inhabit different geographical and climatic locations of Meghalaya and have a unique dietary habit, lifestyle and perhaps gene pool. This study was intended to find out whether habitation in moderately high altitude place has any effect on the levels of few serum biochemical parameters in aged *Khasis*. The levels of few serum biochemical parameters of aged male *Khasi* residents of low (Byrnihat town) and moderately high (Shillong city) altitude were analyzed and compared. Blood collected from overnight-fasted old male *Khasi* volunteers (65-70 years) were analyzed for lipid profile and liver function tests. Results obtained showed a decreased total serum cholesterol (29%) and triglyceride (27%) level in old *Khasi* resident of Shillong compared to Byrnihat. Furthermore, the alkaline phosphatase (AP) activity was significantly raised (~2-fold) in old *Khasis* from Shillong as against Byrnihat. The decreased level of total cholesterol and triglyceride in old *Khasis* from Shillong could be due to living and acclimatization in high altitude place with low annual temperature in contrast to the low altitude and warm climate of Byrnihat. Lipid metabolism has been shown to be altered with exposure to high altitude. Hence, high altitude residence could have acted as a stressor thereby reducing the level of serum cholesterol and triglyceride, which also may put them at lower risk of cardiovascular diseases (CVDs). On the other hand, residents of Byrnihat with high cholesterol and triglyceride levels may increase their risk of suffering from coronary complications. The raised AP activity amongst the old *Khasis* of Shillong could be due to increased bone and/or intestinal turnover as a result of living in high altitude, which, however, may elevate the risk of osteoporosis. Thus, it may be concluded that low cholesterol and triglyceride levels, accompanied with high AP activity amongst the old *Khasis* of Shillong could be due to the influence of high altitude with mild climatic condition that prevails, and which may reflect a biochemical adaptation for survival.

Keywords: Altitude - serum biochemistry - aged - *Khasis*]

Introduction

It is now widely believed that aging operates at the cellular and molecular levels.[1] The ability to adapt to internal as well as external variations declines during this phase, leading to fall in homeostatic balance.[2] Although numerous research have and is being carried out to find out the causes of aging, however, till date, little is known at the molecular level as to what triggers aging.[3] Aging is a complex and gradual process, and its ongoing operation is present to some degree in all individuals. It is a journey to the maturity, as well as to the degeneration of the body.

Aging has become an important area of study due to the rapid increase in number of old age people that has enormous social implications. By 2020, there will be 1 billion aged people, with over 700 million living in the developing world.[4]

Improvements in sanitation, housing, nutrition, medical innovations etc have contributed to the steep increase in the number of people reaching older age. Human aging and the biochemical, molecular and physiological variations associated with it has received increased focus particularly in the western countries, including Japan. In Japan, for instance, detailed clinical studies have been undertaken amongst the aged inhabitants of the island of Okinawa, which has the world's highest longevity.[5-7] However, fewer scientific investigations have been directed especially towards the indigenous tribes of the world, who are considered to harbor a rich gene pool. Hence, biochemical and molecular data from the aged populations of such indigenous people are extremely insufficient.

Modern clinical research on the elderly population in India is still in its infancy. Hence, insufficient data is being generated, which is hampering the understanding of clinical changes in the older population, thereby putting them in a disadvantage. This is applicable to the growing number of older people in India. Additionally, the Indian subcontinent in particular, boasts of a diverse community of ethnic tribes, inhabiting different geographical locations with contrasting climate. Again, it's an irony that negligible clinical studies have been undertaken amongst these indigenous populations.

One of such tribes of India, the *Khasis* represents an indigenous inhabitant of the North-Eastern part of India.[8] They possess unique lifestyle, social customs, dietary habit and perhaps gene pool.[9] In the state of Meghalaya, the *Khasis* inhabit different geographical regions including the Shillong plateau and Ri Bhoi (Byrnihat) bordering the state of Assam.[10] The Shillong plateau has a cool and a mild climate as it is located at a moderately high altitude with low annual temperature. Byrnihat has a low elevation with high annual temperature compared to the Shillong plateau. Almost negligible biological or clinical studies have been undertaken on this ethnic group within the same or different inhabiting locations. Also, no age-related clinical, biochemical and molecular variations study has been reported from this tribe. Therefore, perhaps there is no relevant clinical data originating from this particular tribe. Furthermore, no data are presently available which compares the levels of different blood biochemical constituents within the tribe's old population. In our study, we assumed that there could be variations in the levels of some of the key blood constituents amongst the old *Khasis* residing in two different geographical and climatic locations. Hence, this study is perhaps the first that has attempted to evaluate the levels of few clinically important blood constituents from the old *Khasis* residents of two contrasting climatic conditions. There are few reports available which shows that people inhabiting moderately and high altitude regions from around the world have significantly different levels of many serum biochemical elements compared to low altitude inhabitants. Therefore, the aim of the present study was also to reveal whether variable physical and environmental factors such as altitude and temperature can be contributory factors that modulate the levels of some of the key blood elements in aged *Khasis* from the two regions.

Materials & Methods

Blood sampling from donors: This study was approved by the Institutional Ethics Committee (IEC) of North-Eastern Hill University, Shillong, to which the college is affiliated. Blood collection from subjects was carried out according to the applicable guidelines of the IEC and Indian Council of Medical Research (ICMR). Brief questionnaires were prepared during survey from multiple individuals that included the age, profession, residency, martial status, dietary habit etc. Subjects were randomly selected, non-related individuals, who have been resident of respective locations for at least 15 years. Finally, blood was obtained from the chosen twenty (n = 20) old (65-70 years) *Khasi* males who were residents of Shillong and Byrnihat town (Ri Bhoi). Blood sample were also collected from ten (n = 10) young male subjects (15-20 years) of respective locations in order to have age-related correlations. Only informed consent individuals became the subjects and were volunteers. Participant inclusion criteria included subjects in stable clinical conditions, similar dietary habit and other lifestyles in order to minimize experimental variations. Participant exclusion criteria were subjects with no known liver/kidney diseases and no intake of lipid-modifying drugs. Five milliliter of blood was collected from overnight-fasted subjects using sterile, single-use disposable syringe (Dispovan) by a trained nurse. All biochemical tests were carried out in duplicate with a single blood sample drawn from each subject.

Serum biochemical tests: Sera from the blood drawn from each subject was isolated by centrifuging glass tubes containing 5 ml blood in a laboratory centrifuge at a moderate speed for 5 min. Serum isolated was then be analyzed for Liver Function Tests (LFT) that included total serum protein, albumin, globulin, total bilirubin, serum alkaline phosphatase, aspartate aminotransferase (AST) and alanine aminotransferase activities (ALT). Lipid profile (total cholesterol, triglyceride, LDL- and HDL-cholesterol levels) of each subject's serum were also determined. All the above biochemical analyses was performed with a routinely used, well-calibrated Erba-Chem7 Autoanalyzer (Transasia Bio-Medicals Ltd, Mumbai, India) by trained technicians in the Pathology Department of Woodland Hospital, Shillong. The test methods employed were:

Lipid Profile

i) Total Cholesterol: By Cholesterol-DES kit method (Erba Manheim, India).

ii) Triglyceride: By enzymatic colorimetric method using Autopak kit (Bayer Diagnostics, India).

iii) HDL-Cholesterol: By two-point kinetic method (Synergy Bio, India).

iv) LDL-Cholesterol = Total cholesterol Triglyceride - (HDL- Cholesterol)/5

Liver function tests:

i) Total protein: By Biuret method.

ii) Albumin: By BCG method.

iii) Globulin = Total protein - Albumin.

iv) S.G.O.T (AST): By UV kinetic (IFCC) method.

v) S.G.P.T (ALT): By UV kinetic (IFCC) method.

vi) Alkaline Phosphatase: *p*NPP-AMP (IFCC) kinetic assay using Autospan kit (Cogent, India).

vii) Total Bilirubin: Jendrassik and GROF method.

All the tests under LFT were performed using Autopak kit (Bayer Diagnostics India), unless otherwise indicated. IFCC (International Federation of Clinical Chemistry) denotes IFCC recommended tests.

Data analyses: Level of each of the blood constituents was compared and analyzed statistically using Student's *t*-test. A *P* value of less than 0.05 is considered as statistically significant.

Results

The present study attempted to evaluate and compare the levels of some of the clinically significant blood constituents between the old male *Khasi* subjects of two contrasting climatic region of Meghalaya, the Shillong plateau and

Byrnihat. The geographical and climatic feature of the two regions show significant differences and are being shown in Table I. There is a huge difference in the altitude (above sea level) between the two regions, with the Shillong plateau exhibiting six times higher elevation compared to Byrnihat. Hence, Shillong has a cooler climate through out the year compared to Byrnihat as shown in the comparison of maximum and minimum annual temperature in Table 1. Hence, the *Khasi* inhabitants of the Shillong plateau are exposed to a mild, cooler climate as opposed to Byrnihat, where the climate is warm and tropical.

Table 1
Altitude and temperature profile of Shillong and Byrnihat

Features	*Shillong*	*Byrnihat*
Altitude* (m)	**1495**	**250**
Average Temperature (°C)		
Maximum	**20**	**30**
Minimum	**14**	**22**

*above sea level

The old *Khasi* males chosen for the present study from the two different places were between the age group of 65-70 years. In order to have age-related correlations, various serum biochemical parameters were also investigated in young *Khasi* males (15-20 years) of the respective locations. The mean and median age of young and old *Khasis* of Shillong and Byrnihat are shown in Table 2.

Table 2
Mean and median age of young and old *Khasis* from Shillong and Byrnihat

Age (years)	*Shillong*			*Byrnihat*
	Young	*Old*	*Young*	*Old*
Mean ± S.D	17.8 ± 5.90	68.1 ± 15.62	18 ± 6.0	68.25 ± 15.65
Median	18	69	18	69

The various serum biochemical tests performed under the lipid profile and liver function tests on the blood samples collected from young and old *Khasis* of the two regions are summarized and compared in Table III. We found that the lipid profile data obtained from the old *Khasis* of Shillong and Byrnihat shows significant difference in the levels of total cholesterol and triglyceride. There is a remarkably higher level ($P<0.05$) of serum cholesterol (29%) and triglyceride (27%) amongst the old *Khasis* of Byrnihat (O_B) as compared to the old *Khasis* of Shillong (O_S). In other words, the O_B subjects appear to be hyperlipidemic. In addition, quite interestingly, a decreased (~ 2-fold) ($P<0.05$) serum alkaline phosphatase activity was detected from old *Khasis* of Byrnihat (O_B) compared to Shillong (O_S). However, no statistically significant differences were observed in other serum biochemical parameters analyzed between O_B and O_S.

Comparison of the biochemical data between the young age group from Shillong (Y_S) and Byrnihat (Y_B) show a 39 % decreased triglyceride level in Y_S compared to Y_B (Table III). Also, a significantly higher (29%) LDL-cholesterol level and a 23% increased alkaline phosphatase activity were detected in Y_S compared to Y_B. Age-correlation data between the young and old *Khasis* of respective region shows definite correlation. A 28% higher ($P<0.05$) triglyceride level was detected from O_S compared to Y_S. Additionally, the LDL-cholesterol level was significantly decreased (28%) in O_S as opposed to Y_S. However, the level of various biochemical parameters measured between Y_B and O_B show no differences.

Table 3

Levels (mean ± S.D) of serum biochemical parameters obtained from young (n = 10) and old (n = 20) *Khasis* of Shillong and Byrnihat

Biochemical parameters	*Shillong*		*Byrnihat*		*Normal*
	Young (Y_S)	*Old (O_S)*	*Young (Y_B)*	*Old (O_B)*	*reference values*
Lipid Profile					
Total Cholesterol (mg/dl)	150 ± 50	142 ± 32	168 ± 56	200 ± 46[a]	120 - 220 mg/dl
Triglyceride (mg/dl)	97 ± 32[d]	134 ± 30[g]	158 ± 52	184 ± 42[b]	< 200 mg/dl
LDL-Cholesterol (mg/dl)	74 ± 24[e]	53 ± 12[h]	57.3 ± 19	51 ± 12	<130 mg/dl
HDL-Cholesterol (mg/dl)	40 ± 13	44 ± 10	45.5 ± 15	40 ± 9.2	30 - 70 mg/dl
Liver Function Tests					
Total Protein (g/dl)	6.3 ± 2.1	6.7 ± 1.54	6.2 ± 2.0	6.1 ± 1.4	6.7 - 8.7 g/dl
Albumin (g/dl)	3.8 ± 1.2	3.9 ± 0.9	3.9 ± 1.32	4.0 ± 0.96	3.5 - 5.5 g/dl
Globulin (g/dl)	2.5 ± 0.8	2.8 ± 0.6	2.3 ± 0.76	2.1 ± 0.48	2.3 - 3.6 g/dl
AST (IU/l)	29.5 ± 9.8	31.6 ± 7.2	30 ± 10	29.1 ± 6.7	0 - 42 IU/l
ALT (IU/l)	30 ± 10	25.5 ± 5.8	26.5 ± 8.8	25.6 ± 5.9	0 - 42 IU/l
Alkaline Phosphatase (IU/l)	91 ± 30[f]	114 ± 26.1	70 ± 23	60 ± 14[c]	15 - 120 IU/l
Total Bilirubin (mg/dl)	0.70 ± 0.23	0.61 ± 0.13	0.52 ± 0.17	0.43 ± 0.10	0 - 1.0 mg/dl

Y_S-Young subject of Shillong; **O_S**-Old subject of Shillong; **Y_B**-Young subject of Byrnihat; **O_B**-Old subject of Byrnihat.

***a*:** 29 % more total cholesterol in O_B compared to O_S ($P < 0.05$), ***b*:** 27 % more serum triglyceride in O_B compared to O_S ($P < 0.05$), ***c*:** ~2-fold less alkaline phosphatase activity in O_B compared to O_S ($P < 0.05$), ***d*:** 39 % less triglyceride level in Y_S compared to Y_B ($P < 0.05$), ***e*:** 29 % more LDL-cholesterol in Y_S compared to Y_B ($P < 0.05$), ***f*:** 23 % higher alkaline phosphatase activity in Y_S compared to Y_B ($P < 0.05$), ***g*:** 28 % more triglyceride in O_S compared to Y_S ($P < 0.05$), ***h*:** 28 % less LDL-cholesterol in O_S compared to Y_S ($P < 0.05$).

AST-Aspartate aminotransferase; **ALT**-Alanine aminotransferase; **IU**-International Unit.

Discussion

The evaluation and comparison of the levels of some of the clinically significant blood constituents amongst the young and old male *Khasi* subjects from the two different climatic region of Meghalaya was challenging, as no such clinical study was previously undertaken or reported from this ethnic group. Data obtained from the various clinical tests performed amongst the old *Khasi* participants from the two locations shows a few significant differences. It is now widely believed that interplay between environmental exposures and human biology limits longevity and quality of life[11]. More precisely, it is now acknowledged that healthful aging in human may depend on polygenic regulation as well as environmental influences[12,13]. It has been observed that human adaptation to moderate and high altitude places induces physiological changes.

The higher level of total serum cholesterol and triglyceride that was reported from O_B as compared to O_S population might suggest a modulatory role of environmental factors prevailing in the respective region. The *Khasis* from these two location shares similar gene pool, however, they are under the influence of opposing climatic conditions. Amongst the environmental influences, it is now widely acknowledged that high or low temperature does modulate the metabolic rate of an individual. Increased level of serum total cholesterol and triglyceride as observed in case of O_B may be perhaps due to higher environmental temperature prevalent in Byrnihat, which increases the metabolic processes and ultimately the metabolic rate. A possible explanation for this increase in metabolic rate may be as a result of increased mobilization of cholesterol and triglyceride through the blood plasma to various tissues. Hence, perhaps a higher cholesterol and triglyceride level is detected in O_B, which may reflect a biochemical adaptation. Additionally, lipid metabolism has been shown to be altered with exposure to high altitude. It is reported that exposure to high altitude led to increased circulating triglyceride levels and reduced or unchanged plasma cholesterol concentrations,[14] which corroborate with our finding, whereby the O_S population have reduced cholesterol level but not triglyceride. The effects of exposure to high altitude on lipid metabolism appear to be complex, interrelated processes involving multiple responses by the body. The report of elevation of serum total cholesterol in people from high altitude areas by few investigators[15,16] is however not supported by our findings, where a decrease in cholesterol level in O_S subjects was observed. Our finding is also in contrast to a report[17] which showed that there is a significantly higher serum triglyceride level in subjects who are inhabitants of moderately high altitude.

Lipid profiles, among other factors, are associated with risk of cardiovascular disease (CVD). Ironically, a higher cholesterol and triglyceride level in the blood of O_B populations may elevate the risk of CVD such as coronary heart disease and stroke as compared to the O_S population. A lower level of total serum cholesterol and triglyceride in case of O_S may be perhaps due to the mild climate prevalent in Shillong. In other words, the O_S populations may be a little better protected against CVDs. The other explanation could it be that at high altitude, people has to work hard, even for daily routine work, hence, less triglyceride and cholesterol levels for Os as compared to O_B. Residence in hilly area seems to have a "protective effect" from coronary mortality. Increased physical activity from walking on rugged terrains under conditions of mild hypoxia among the hill residents of Shillong could explain these findings, which is supported by the observation of Baibas *et al.*[18] Another report[19] from study on inhabitants of high altitude populations of Peru showed no differences in total cholesterol level, whereas, the triglyceride level was markedly elevated in comparison to low altitude, which is also corroborated by other findings.[20] Furthermore, the ~2-

fold higher activity of serum alkaline phosphatase (AP) in O_S with respect to O_B may be due to high bone and/or intestinal turnover in high altitude O_S population leading to increased AP release into the blood plasma. The report of higher AP activity in subjects of moderately high altitude was reported earlier[17,21] which corroborate with our findings. Higher AP activity, however, may also correlate with increased risk of osteoporosis in O_S population.

The age-correlation data between young and old *Khasis* of respective region show a definite pattern. The higher triglyceride level along with decreased LDL-cholesterol level was observed in O_S as opposed to Y_S, which could be due to multitude of influences. It is now well-known that changes in energy regulation occur during human aging. There are also changes in patterns of dietary intake and a reduction in the variety of foods consumed in old age. These alterations in the level of triglyceride and LDL-cholesterol in O_S and Y_S could be due to differences in the mean age of young an old population. The Os having more triglyceride compared to Ys could be correlated with greater risk of diseases associated with high triglyceride level in elderly population compared to young. In contrast, the lower LDL-cholesterol level in Os could be correlated with lesser risk of atherosclerosis in elderly population compared to young.

Analysis of biochemical parameters between the young age groups of the respective locations showed some interesting variations. The decreased triglyceride and increased LDL-cholesterol level along with higher alkaline phosphatase activity observed in Y_S compared to Y_B may have a definite environmental influence. This modulation in the levels of lipids and AP activity amongst the young *Khasis* could be due to the effect of high altitude and low annual temperature of Shillong as opposed to Byrnihat. Additionally, modifiable factors such as quality and quantity of nutrition intake could also be attributed for these differences. Furthermore, the demand for these serum constituents may be different in the young *Khasis* from Shillong and Byrnihat as they are exposed to opposing climatic conditions.

The work reported in this paper is preliminary, nevertheless; it is a first report on any clinical study undertaken amongst the old *Khasis*. Taken together, results from this study shows that there are indeed significant differences in the level of three blood biochemical constituents between the old resident *Khasis* of Shillong and Byrnihat, which may be reflect a biochemical adaptability for survival in the respective region.

Acknowledgement

The authors acknowledge the financial support (No.F-5-01/2006-07/MRP/NERO) from the University Grants Commission, India.

REFERENCES

1. Luckinbill LS, Foley P. (2000). Experimental and empirical approaches in the study of aging. *Biogerontology, 1*: 3-13.
2. Roth GS. (1998). Mechanisms of altered hormone and neurotransmitter action during aging: the role of impaired calcium mobilization. *Ann N Y Acad Sci; 521*: 170–176.
3. Kanungo MS. (1994). Genes and Aging. Cambridge: Cambridge University Press.
4. World Health Organization (1999), *Ageing and Health*. Geneva (Switzerland).
5. Sharma R. (2004). Dietary restriction and its multifaceted effects. *Curr Sci; 87*: 1203- 1210.
6. Akisaka M, Asato L, Chan YC, Suzuki M, Uezato T, Yamamoto S. (1996). Energy and nutrient intakes of Okinawan centenarians. *J Nutr Sci Vitaminol; 42*: 241-248.
7. Willcox BJ, Willcox DC, Todoriki H, Fujiyoshi A, Yano K, He Q, Curb JD, Suzuki M. (2007), Caloric restriction, the

traditional Okinawan diet, and healthy aging: the diet of the world's longest-lived people and its potential impact on morbidity and life span. *Ann N Y Acad Sci; 1114*: 434-55.

8. Roy S, Rizvi SHM. Khasi tribe of Meghalaya. Calcutta: B.R. Publishing Corp; 2006.

9. DIPR; Government of Meghalaya (2002). *Meghalaya - Land and People*. Shillong (India).

10. DIPR; Government of Meghalaya (2003). *The Dwellers of the High Hills - The Khasis of Meghalaya*. Shillong (India).

11. Schwartz D, Collins F. (2007). Medicine. Environmental biology and human disease. *Science; 316*: 695-696.

12. Manolio TA. (2007). Study designs to enhance identification of genetic factors in healthy aging. *Nutr Rev; 65*: S228-33.

13. Libert S, Pletcher SD (2007). Modulation of longevity by environmental sensing. *Cell; 13*:1231-4.

14. Young PM, Rose MS, Sutton JR, Green HJ, Cymerman A, Houston CS (1989). Operation Everest II: plasma lipid and hormonal responses during a simulated ascent of Mt. Everest. *J Appl Physiol; 66*: 1430-5.

15. Temte JL (1996). Elevation of serum cholesterol at high altitude and its relationship to hematocrit. *Wilderness Environ Med; 7*: 216-224.

16. Savourey G, Garcia N, Caravel JP, Gharib C, Pouzeratte N, Martin S, Bittel J. (1998). Pre-adaptation, adaptation and de-adaptation to high altitude in humans: hormonal and biochemical changes at sea level. *Eur J Appl Physiol Occup Physiol; 77*: 37-43.

17. Ramirez G, Bittle PA, Colice GL, Foulis PR, Agosti SJ. (1991). Biochemical adaptations to moderately high altitude living. *J Wilderness Med; 2*: 287-297.

18. Baibas N, Trichopoulou A, Voridis E, Trichopoulos. (2005) *Residence in mountainous compared with lowland areas in relation to total and coronary mortality*. A study in rural Greece. *J Epidemiol Commu Health; 59*: 274-278.

19. Mohanna S, Baracco R, Seclen S. (2006). Lipid profile, waist circumference, and body mass index in a high altitude population. *High Alt Biol Med*; *7*: 245-255.

20. Brito J, Siqués P, León-Velarde F, De La Cruz JJ, López V, Herruzo R. (2007). Chronic intermittent hypoxia at high altitude exposure for over 12 years: assessment of hematological, cardiovascular, and renal effects. *High Alt Med Biol 8*: 236-244.

21. Rawal SB, Singh MV, Tyagi AK, Roy J, Dimri GP, (1999). Selvamurthy W. Effect of time exposure to high altitude on zinc and copper concentrations in human plasma. *Aviat Space Environ Med*; *70*: 1161-5.

6

In the Domain of Health: Issues and Elderly Concerns

Arun P. Bali

Population aging will constitute a serious challenge for societies, as it has very important socio-economic and health consequences. Among other things, the importance of health of older persons in society is highlighted. It implies growing health care needs and associated costs of health provisions. These constitute especially a burden for countries like India, with already limited resources.

There has been a growing awareness of the neglect of elderly persons' health. We find that health is the most common domain cited in terms of disadvantages of the ageing process. Health concerns are, however relevant across the life-course, not just in later life. The process of ageing will be accompanied by increased vulnerability to illness, disability and death. All these features of ageing will imply that the problems of the elderly will need a special focus and approach. In the present century, the most pressing issue may well be the health of the elderly.

This paper seeks to address some of the key issues relating to health and elderly in India. It examines the nature and extent of health needs of the elderly; issues relating to health care including facilities of health care, and their utilization. The paper looks at the health care system in the country, and the challenges it faces, as ageing of population takes place. An agenda for action for elderly people therefore needs to address these issues.

All societies face important dilemmas, but none is as critical and consequential as the health conditions of their people. Ageing brings inevitable decline in capacity, and greater vulnerability. All these assume great importance in view of the fact that India, like other developing countries, is experiencing a rapid increase in the number of its elderly persons. The importance of understanding the specific health needs of older persons is beginning to be felt.

The world over, there has been a rapid increase in the number of elderly people, and this trend continues to accelerate. Countries have experienced and are experiencing quite different rates of ageing, and therefore the challenges it presents are varied. In India, the "aged" population (60 years and above) is the second largest in the world. It is estimated that the proportion of elderly people will increase from 7.7 per cent (76 million), in 2001 to about 11 per cent (142 million) in 2020 and 177 million in 2025. In 2002, 8 per cent of the older population was over 80 years of age and by 2050 this proportion is expected to go up to 15 per cent. Life expectancy at 60 for men and women is 16 and 18 years respectively. The extent to which these added years would be free of disability is subject to debate.

Population projections for India for the next twenty years show that ageing process will gradually gather momentum. India will experience rapid population aging. This phenomenon will demand that a higher proportion of financial resources be allocated for health care services in the coming decades. It is likely to demand a great deal of human resources to cope with the rapid increase in the number of elderly who need intensive human care. With age, the medical and health care expenditure increases and their own resources shrink thereby increasing their dependence on their adult children. 10 per cent of the elderly in India, i.e., about 8 million people are in need of psycho-geriatric services.[1]

As more people will be reaching old age and living longer, the dominant and most critical need for them will be in the health care domain. A life-course perspective on aging is indispensable to an understanding of the process of aging in all its dimensions: physical, social, psychological, and spiritual. A population of elderly persons embedded within a general population will include a wide array of states of health, of mental and physical capacity appearing in a fluctuating way to affect them, of social support, and of need. This would involve: (i) increased understanding of older people's experience of everyday environments; and (ii) a more comprehensive analysis of the role and coping styles and health care beliefs in determining psychological adjustment. "Nutrition, access to health care, immunization, immediate attention to health problems, healthy lifestyle, physical exercise and genetically endowed constitution determine health status at any stage of life" (Indira Jai Prakash 2004:7).

The World Health Organization (WHO) defines health as "a state of complete physical, mental and social well being and not merely absence of disease or infirmity". Health is a key contributing factor to the quality of life and thus liveability. It is a "generalized condition of the bodily and mental well-being, a multi-factor response to spatially viewed physical, biological and socio-economic environment" (Fellman, 1988). Health and well-being is of prime importance to both the individual through the life-course, and the society. For the individual, it determines his or her ability to perform those tasks, which facilitate his or her participation in social and economic life. While the society, on its part, depends on the good health of its members to enable them to perform their roles adequately, be they in the economy, community, or family. Equally, the society is concerned about the health care provisions it has to provide.

Health in elderly persons is a product of life experiences and environmental factors. Many interwoven aspects of their life and physical environment, ranging from lifestyles and family structure through social and economic support systems and the organization and provision of health care affect the health and well-being of the elderly. Elderly persons have different exposures to life situations that affect health and access to health care and have differential power to influence decisions regarding the provision of health. Majority of the elderly need a wide range of supportive and restorative health services and social services. Much of their health in later life depends on the availability, accessibility.

Health in old age is greatly determined by the patterns of living, exposure to health risks (such as consumption of tobacco, intake of high fat diet, leading an unhealthy lifestyle) recognized or unrecognized and opportunities for health protection over the life-course (Natarajan and Selvaraj: 2003:67). Cumulative effects of such risk behaviours often result in coronary heart disease, stroke, various types of cancers, chronic obstructive lung diseases, all of which are common in old age.

The growth in the elderly population means an inevitable increase in age-related diseases such as dementias. In addition, changes in social patterns will alter the role of the elderly and the ways they are valued. These conditions can lead to poor mental health outcomes, such as depression, anxiety, suicide, and can cause serious constraints on the quality of life of elderly individuals.

Health Status of the Elderly

The health status of elderly persons is a matter of concern, particularly in the context of the ageing population due to increase in average lifespan. Further, with increases in the proportion of elderly, developing countries like ours will have to learn how to deal with a new set of health challenges. The health care system will become increasingly strained as this elderly segment increases in numbers and demands more time and services. It would, in future, be hard pressed to maintain quality of care well into old age.

Health is a productive asset that influences economic growth significantly. In India, evidence is impressive on both health status as the well as access to health care. It indicates the nexus that exists between poverty and ill-health. The main problem with the elderly in India is poverty. This impacts their quality of life in that they experience difficulties in meeting their basic needs. Because the elderly have little money, they suffer from malnutrition, leading to depression and mental morbidity. Not only does poverty affect a substantial proportion of elderly people, but also when it does, it is likely to be an enduring experience. The high incidence of poverty and low-income levels among older people is reflected in other measures of deprivation. The majority of older people still live in or on the margins of poverty.

The elderly are prone to chronic and non-communicable diseases and disabilities. The ten most common diseases are: hypertension, cataract, osteoarthritis, chronic obstructive pulmonary disease, ischaemic heart disease, diabetes, benign prostatic hypertrophy, dyspepsia, constipation and depression. The five most frequent causes of death in the elderly are: bronchitis and pneumonia, ischaemic heart disease, stroke, cancer and tuberculosis.

According to the 52nd Round of National Sample Survey Organisation (NSSO) data about 55 per cent elderly in urban areas were afflicted with chronic diseases, 34 per cent reported joint problems, 22.6 per cent reported blood pressure problems,

7.5 per cent suffered diabetes and 6.1 per cent suffer from heart disease.[2] Chronic illness was reported by 45 per cent males and 44.8 per cent females, being nearly identical for both urban and rural areas. Urban population reported hypertension, heart diseases and diabetes more than rural population.

A.Venkoba Rao (1990) in his study found that the top five most commonly reported illnesses were visual handicap, pain in joints, sleeplessness, vague bodily pain and backache. Urinary problems ranked 8th while cough was ranked 9th. Kothari and Sinha (2002) in their study on general health status of persons residing at a rural area of Jaipur, in the state of Rajasthan, India, all persons reported to be chronically sick and 11.5 per cent were acutely ill. The most common illness reported was bronchitis. Anaemia, vitamin deficiencies, cataract and hypertension were other disorders that were observed among the population. In addition to physical limitations, a significant proportion of elderly have mental health problems.

Health care provisions and elderly services are highly age sensitive. On average, their ability to perform daily tasks slowly erodes until, at some stage, they become dependent on others for home help, or possibly residential care or long-term care in a hospital. Estimates of future health-and disability-related expenditure depend crucially on whether the longevity revolution is adding healthy life years or years of illness and dependency to human life span.

First, our average life span continues to grow, and the rate of population growth in the oldest age groups remains high. In total, over the period 1960-91, women reaching the age of 80 saw their future average lifespan increase by almost two years, and men reaching 80 now had an expected further one-year.

Secondly, observed trends in health status indicate that our capacity to live longer is not consistently matched by our ability to prevent or delay disabling conditions. In the longer term, this trend may be influenced by healthier lifestyles, new medical discoveries or better rehabilitation services. Medical advances, however, cut both ways, by overcoming common causes of disability, or by helping to keep alive people with serious illnesses.

Normally the health status of the rural elderly varies greatly due to the following factors (Vijaya Kumar 2003: 106):

1. The nature and conditions of work, i.e., hard work combined with poor nutrition leading to a state of disability and most older persons suffering from "deficiency illness";
2. Environmental conditions such as poor sanitation, lack of basic amenities like protected drinking water, housing, and lack of proper drainage system making the environment a health hazard;
3. Inadequate and unbalanced malnourished diet and
4. Availability of and accessibility to quality health services at an affordable cost."

Owing to illiteracy, ignorance and poverty, a large majority is not even aware of the seriousness of the illness and diagnoses are often done very late. On all these accounts, the benefits of available medical science are not fully utilized.

Disability may be congenital or a result of illness, injury, or physical deterioration, especially in old age, when many find it difficult to manage without the support of others. The prevalence of disabling conditions increases sharply after the age of 75, and the consequent loss of independence in daily activities leads to a corresponding growth in the need for care, at an increasing rate in the older age groups. There is a growing concern about the future provision of care for elderly people who are frail or disabled. Frailty is multifaceted, and is the combined result of the physical, mental and social well-being. For the elderly transitions of advancing years are frequently compounded by health concerns, depression, anxiety, cognitive changes and family mobility.

Becoming vulnerable to illnesses and disabilities and/or losing economic self-sufficiency, the elderly have often reduced the freedom of those on whom they rely. The health status of older persons, for example, is intimately related to access to transportation, livelihood strategies that affect ability to pay medical fees.

There are significant variations within India, as regards existing patterns and levels of care provision. These variations affect the policy agenda. Not only existing levels of provision determine the challenges facing India but also the nature of their health and social welfare systems. Health personnel, particularly those involved in primary health care and in community health, need to be oriented to the health needs of the elderly. It is also important to ensure that the elderly have access to adequate health services.

Health is a function, not only of medical care but also of the overall integrated development of society-cultural, economic, education, social and political. Each of these aspects has a deep influence on health, which in turn influences all these aspects. Hence, it is not possible to raise the health status and quality of life of people unless such efforts are integrated with the wider effort to bring about the overall transformation of a society. This is possible only when supportive services such as nutrition, environment and education reach a higher level. The common beliefs, customers and practices connected with health and disease are intimately related to the treatment of disease. It is necessary to make a holistic view of all the cultural dimensions of the health of a community. In most of the tribal communities in India, there is a wealth of folklore related to health. Documentation of this folklore available in different socio-cultural systems may be very useful and could provide a framework for appropriate health and sanitary practices in a given eco-system. Health and treatment are closely interrelated with the environment, particularly the forest ecology.

Health Care Institutions

Elderly persons constitute a distinct population that requires interventions very different from those of younger persons. Medical care for managing diseases is the intervention most often used. The existing health services are geared toward acute rather than chronic care. Ray and Singh (2003) observe, "The health system in India faces the challenge of caring for its older population from a position of disadvantage as it has to bear the burden of communicable infectious diseases while trying to provide quality care for the disabling noncommunicable diseases".

There is a range of health service providers in India. This includes government services, private practitioners and voluntary organizations. While there has been considerable investment in government health infrastructure, this has been heavily biased in favour urban curative services. At the same time, when urban — rural differentials in hospital coverage have widened (21 per cent of hospitals were in rural areas in 1986 compared to 39 per cent in 1956) and intended coverage of primary health centres (PHCs) and subcentres has not been achieved. In 1987, there was one PHC per 40,215 population on average, compared to a target of one per 30,000. In 1985, only 15 per cent of PHCs fulfilled the prescribed norms in terms of population coverage and supplies.

The mainstay of rural health care delivery system established by the Government of India is a network of subcentres supplemented by secondary care and tertiary care medical/health institutions. An impressive network of 1,37,000 subcentres, 23,000 primary health care centres (PHCs) and 3,000 community health centres (CHCs) spread over semi-urban and rural areas, have been set up. These are manned by 1,33,570 health workers female, 62,656 health workers male, 15,917 health assistants, 5,638 block extension educators and five lakh doctors, 16,000 hospitals and 8,70,000 beds. In a recent survey it was noticed that only 38 per cent of all PHCs have all the essential manpower and only 31 per cent have all essential supplies, with only 3 per cent of PHCs having 80 per cent of all critical inputs.[3] Tertiary medical care is provided at multi- and super-specialty hospitals and medical colleges.

PHCs operate in a pluralistic system peppered by multiple systems of medicine and diversity of practitioners. Concerted efforts should be made to ensure effectiveness of such a pluralistic system. The practitioners are addressed to as *ojhas, vaidraj*, quacks, homeopaths, *hakims* depending on the system of medicine (folk medicine, ayurvedic, homeopathic, *unani,* allopathic) they owe allegiance to, as well as its dispensation. They also coexist, provide health care and cater to a cross-section of the population. Generally, people first resort to these forms of health care before approaching the PHCs for medical aid and referral services.

Poor and worsening coverage and quality of care in government health services has led to a mushrooming of the private health sector. In 1974, 16% of hospital beds were in the private sector; by 1988 this figure had risen to 30%. Recent data suggest that 84% of expenditure on health is privately rather than state financed.

Voluntary agencies have also played a significant role in health provision and particularly in promoting alternative models of community health care. Government is increasingly encouraging non-government health agencies to take on implementation of its programmes.[4]

While welcoming the participation of the private sector in all sectors of health activities, the National Health Policy 2002, encourages the setting up of private insurance instruments for increasing the scope and coverage of the secondary and tertiary sectors under private health insurance packages.

The post-90s saw a paradigm shift in health care, from accessibility, affordability and equity, to efficiency in investment. This came about following the pressure exerted by the IMF and the World Bank.

The National Rural Health Mission launched on 12 April 2005 seeks to address a few issues relating to the design of a health care delivery that 'fragments resources and dissipates energies'. The NRHM attempts, at least at the strategy level, a major shift in the patterns of governance of public health by empowering the Panchayati Raj Institutions (PRIs) to take decisions in all matters related to health at the district and sub-district levels. The Mission aims at establishing synergistic district health plans integrating nutrition, sanitation and safe drinking water.

Health care is one of the principal areas of intervention and action identified by the National Policy on Older Persons(NPOP)[5]: Affordable health services, very heavily subsidized for the poor and a graded system of user-charges for others; facilitating a judicious mix of health service providers comprising the State, NGOs and private medical care; assisting trusts, charitable societies and voluntary agencies to provide health insurance schemes with provision of state subsidy for packages which cater to lower income groups; strengthening the public health structure at all levels; expanding geriatric facilities; facilitating access to and utilization of health services by older people; training and orientation of medical personnel in geriatric care facilities; developing educational materials on health care and nutritional needs in old age and disseminating them.

Health Service Utilization by the Elderly

As in most developing countries, the health care system in India is characterized by "four toos" – "too far from home, too few trained attendants, too poorly equipped to identify or handle complications, and too deficient in quality of care" (J.Jackson, 1993). These often prevent people from seeking care. To compound these problems is the widespread prevalence of poverty, which often inhibits people from seeking health care. Even where facilities are available, they may not be made use of, due to factors such as lack of emotional support, and privacy, linguistic and cultural barriers between health professionals and health care-seekers, or even poor relationships between them.

The high prevalence of chronic conditions among the elderly, and the functional limitations that result, generate a high demand on the health services. The elderly are considered to be intensive users of health care services. Recent research has emphasized that the distribution of health utilization among the elderly themselves is very skewed, with a relatively small proportion accounting for a major share of total use of health resources. In India, there exist no specially organized health services meant for older segments of the population. There is no separate health scheme specially designed to cater to their needs. Retired government employees do enjoy the facility of health care services under the Central Government Health Scheme (CGHS), by making a nominal payment. Similar facilities do exist for some categories of retirees in the organized sector also. There is a definite suggestion that the health needs of the elderly are not being met adequately. Recent years witnessed the setting up of a few geriatric clinics in a few government-run hospitals.

Shortages in the availability of health services–health personnel, medicines, life-saving drugs, and lack of infrastructural facilities and time-consuming practices in seeking medical attention – all affect the degree to which the needs of elderly are met.

A high percentage of the poor elderly do not seek care when ill; for example the evidence from NSSO 52nd round indicates that about 24 per cent of the poorest quintile do not seek care compared to 9 per cent of the richest quintile (World Bank 2001). It is also clear that there is a higher prevalence of acute illness among households (22.6 per cent) as compared to chronic illness (17.6 per cent). Acute illnesses are more prevalent in rural households whereas chronic illnesses are more prevalent in the urban population (NSSO 52nd round).

An overwhelming majority still prefers to use private facilities for hospitalization in India, in both rural and urban areas. The percentage of individuals visiting a private facility in the urban areas is about 65 per cent, whereas this number is about 55 per cent in the rural areas.

Generally the assessment health conditions of population, it is often restrict to a few measurable aspects, such as mortality, morbidity, and nutritional status. The health status of individuals affects their capabilities both in gaining access to socio-economic opportunities and therein community at large. Other things being equal, a better health status enhances the capabilities and productive skills of individuals. Differentials in the health status of individuals in a population, in tandem with differentials in other basic endowments, will have a bearing on their pattern of access and utilization to health care services. Surveys of utilization of health services revealed sordid stories of absent personnel, irregular and erratic hours of work, leaking roofs, missing drugs, negligible consumables, obsolete equipment and the like.

Health inequities in India

The most recent review of health inequities in India is by Peters *et al* (World Bank 2002), and also a report on India prepared for the Commission on Macroeconomics and Health (Misra *et al.* 2003) which puts together findings from a number of studies on India's health system.

Evidence from several studies indicates that a high percentage of the poor do not seek care when ill. The evidence from NSSO 52nd round indicates that about 24 percent of the poorest quintile do not seek care, compared to 9 percent of the richest quintile (World Bank 2001). Further, a much lower percentage of the poor seek institutional care.

Determinants of Ill Health

Wealth clearly is a passport to health. Several studies (Ramamurti, 1996; Jamuna, 1999; Reddy and Ramamurti, 1996) have revealed that the maintenance of health in old age is linked with knowledge, attitude and practice of good health behaviour among individuals. Ensuring satisfactory health of the elderly in India would need providing better medical facilities to them and ensuring that they receive adequate nutrition and follow a regular regimen of exercise and hygienic practices.

Location of residence is also a determinant of health and health care. In most developing regions of the world, older populations tend to live in rural areas and are projected to continue to do so. The effects of living arrangements on the physical and psychological well-being of the elderly have also been examined by researchers. According to them, changes in living arrangements have an adverse effect on the elderly.

Housing policies need to recognize that demographic patterns by 2010 will differ from what they were in the 1990s. Housing policies need to be adjusted to address housing shortages in cities, improve architectural designs to reduce accidents and falls within homes, and encourage multigenerational family living arrangements. In India, ensuring a secure roof is as important for health and survival of the elderly as having potable water.

Gender Bias in Access to Health Care

Older persons are foremost women. Gender issues do not diminish with age. Gender roles and expectations affect older women as much as younger women in terms of access to health care. Over the active years, women have less access to resources, which results in high levels of female poverty and poor health status of older persons, especially of women. There is no doubt a need for research and more statistical data.

Elderly women face specific health problems: they are prone to arthritis, osteoporosis, and hypertension, cervical and breast cancer, anaemia, dementia and most of all depression. In a study, it was found that 93 per cent were suffering from depression, about 83 per cent from multiple geriatric problems (Vijaya Kumar 2000). Challenge of health security is doubled by the fact that women generally tend to underplay their health problems.

It is well documented that women of all ages have not only poor access to the health care system but are also less likely to use it. Studies from several parts of India indicate that there is a gender bias in assessing and using health care. Gender discrimination continues in later life as well, where women may downplay their morbidities, attempt home remedies and seek traditional medical treatment before reaching the modern health care system. Health care systems will have to struggle hard to provide for their needs, as some of the social systems that traditionally have provided for care of the elderly are beginning to weaken and the numbers of needy aged are rapidly increasing.

Gendered access to health care is by women's constrained mobility and literacy. Direct and opportunity costs also limit elderly women's a*bility* to access health care. Another factor, which often limits elderly women accessing health care facilities, is the incompatibility between their daily schedules and the timings of health care institutions. Often their physical ill-health as well as the environmental conditions and unending queues at government hospitals deter them from availing these facilities. Instead they are compelled to rely on private health care. In rural areas, *availability* of health care is constrained both in coverage and quality. Geographical factors and differences in lifestyles and educational levels influence acceptance and adoption of health care. Other issues inhibiting access of health care facilities by elderly women are the culture and attitudes prevailing in the health sector institutions, and attitude of medical personnel (Duraisamy: 2001). In India, older people manifest considerable morbidity while health care system is relatively deficient.

Geriatric medicine is yet to develop as a strong and widely available service. Primary care is neglected, preventive geriatrics is not a priority area, and only tertiary care is available (Indira Jai Prakash, 2003:35). The only cost-effective strategy would be in the realm of preventive geriatrics (Vinod Kumar, 2000).

The availability and accessibility to health care facilities is an important determinant of the present and future health. Elderly people are generally home-bound and are unable to travel unassisted, especially when ill. Their access to health care facilities will depend on the assistance available to reach a medical centre, their financial position to meet hospitalization or health care needs and availability of home-based care for after- care and follow-up.

Access to health care is affected by income level. "Health care system at various levels in our country is designed for the general population and no special provision preferences are so far provided in the system to take care of the elderly in our society. At present, the old have to compete with other segments of the population in getting the public health care facilities. The poor strata utilize public health centres mainly because of free treatment facilities and their nearness to their residences.

Majority of the middle-income group elderly utilize mostly the private health care facilities. The advantages cited by those utilizing private sources of medical care include: good treatment, quick relief, less waiting time to see a doctor, convenient time and nearness of its location (Siva Raju, 1997).

India's health system, though it rests on a well-conceived infrastructure to make health available to its people, the paradox, however, is that in spite of the availability of facilities, their utilization is very meagre – hardly 10 to 20 per cent (Griffith, 1963). "The problem is more acute in the remote areas, where, whatever meager facilities have been made available; the people optimally utilize them. Instead, people go to practitioners of indigenous methods who are not qualified, such as faith healers and other private practitioners who live and work among them" (Siva Raju, 1986). Majority of studies conducted so far, on the utilization of existing health care services in India have revealed the very poor image the government health centres have among the people. Among the small proportion of villagers who use the facilities, a majority is dissatisfied with the services, mainly because of the non-availability of medicines and the impersonal behaviour of the health functionaries.

The health care of the elderly is not yet appreciated in India as major responsibility of the national health cares system. In fact, the health needs of the elderly are considered to be similar to those of any other adults. Health workers at the peripheral levels rarely appreciate the special needs and vulnerability of the elderly. The existing state of health services for older persons is appalling, with no dedicated facilities for them in any of the public hospitals in the country. Bajaj (1993) observes, "Health care of the elderly is now an area which requires intensive interlocking of the services offered by national health care system and the efforts of the voluntary organizations in providing social and behavioral support to the elderly."

Though health care facilities are overwhelmingly concentrated in urban areas, yet costs of health care, and social factors such as the lack of culturally appropriate services, language/ethnic barriers, and prejudices on the part of the providers, act as deterrents for the urban poor accessing these facilities. In addition, lack of health education results in an inability to identify symptoms and seek appropriate care. The current increase in the privatization of health care in parallel with the demographic and health transition in a country like India does not augur well for the future of elderly persons. The social consequences of ageing with inadequate infrastructural support are serious.

The health status of any segment of population is inferred from stratified mortality and morbidity data, derived from various sources such as Census reports, Central and State government health statistics reports, survey reports of National Sample Survey Organization(NSSO). In the absence of reliable monitoring, reporting and poor coverage of modern health services in India, most of the vital health statistics are generalizations from limited samples, are subject to various fallacies and therefore should treated with caution.

Health Promotion

Promoting health and well-being throughout the lifespan is part of the process of achieving greater quality of life (and longevity) for older persons. The challenge is to understand and promote the factors that keep people healthy with a focus on both personal and external resources. "The state of health in old age depends on one's genetic endowment, the surrounding environment and the kind of lifestyle that one has lived during childhood and adulthood," remarks Dey (2003: preface).Health promotion is a precursor to healthy ageing. A lot can be done as people age and individual differences in the ageing process will largely explain differences in health status once they reach old age. Health can also be promoted among elderly people. "It is thought important to consider that they are a special group in so far as they (i) tend to present multiple pathologies; (ii) are at increased risk of chronic diseases and disabilities; (iii) are particularly liable to iatrogenic problems (not necessarily professionals); (iv) can easily lose independence through the establishment of premature interventions; and (v) are often victims of negative attitudes from society (stereotypes, for instance through media), from professionals (denying to them the benefits of valuable procedures) and themselves who often attribute to old age problems that could be solved or improved through adequate management" (Kalache, 1994:9). Health promotion includes health education, health maintenance and disease prevention seen in the backdrop of socio-economic changes. Health for All must include equity and accessibility. People have to be educated in health and encouraged to adopt a variety of self-care practices. Incorporating a life-course perspective in preventive care would help reduce the problems of old age considerably. "It may become necessary to reserve services for those who are in need (and not to all older persons indiscriminately) to prevent services from being overwhelmed. Also different programmes need to be tailored for rural and urban groups and for male and female older persons (Indira Jai Prakash, 2003).

The elderly are a special group at high risk of losing independence and autonomy and suffering from multiple pathology and iatrogenic problems. Functional capacity can be improved through factors related to adaptability, fitness, social changes and disease prevention. While health promotion ensures better quality of life, medical intervention prolongs life but not necessarily better health. There is a four-tier care model consisting of self-care, informal care, community care and institutional care. "...With accelerated population ageing, there is a need for an affirmative action to ensure the basic needs for a comfortable existence in old age, i.e., shelter, financial security, health care and social support", says Dey (2003; preface).

NOTES

1. Vijay Chandra. The First Step in IPA's South Asia Initiative. www.ipa-online.org/ipaonlineV3/publications/bulletinarchive
2. The Aged in India: Socio-economic Profile, NSS 52nd Round (1988), NSSO, Department of Statistics, Ministry of Planning and Programme Implementation, Government of India.
3. Central Bureau of Health Intelligence. Directorate General of Health Services, Ministry of Health and Family Welfare. Health Information of India 2000 &2001.
4. There are an estimated 7000 voluntary health organizations in operation in India.
5. The National Policy on Older Persons(NPOP) was adopted by the Government of India in January 1999. The NPOP was conceived not only as a commitment by the State, but was also intended as a statement which would provide a broad framework for action and enable other agencies and older persons to carve out areas of intervention and the machinery for implementation.

REFERENCES

Bajaj, J.S. (1993). Message. In Bathla, P.C. (ed.), *Community Geriatrics: Care of the Elderly –Issues, Status, Solutions.* New Delhi: National Institute of Primary Health care.

Bali, Arun P. (1996). Intersectoral Aspects, Awareness and Health education for PHC Workers. Paper presented at the National

Seminar on Curriculum Development in Geriatric for PHC Workers and PHC Medical Officers organized and held at All India Institute of Medical sciences, New Delhi, January 28-31, 1996.

— (1997). Invoking Local Initiatives in Health Care Education of the Elderly in Rural Areas. *Research & Development Journal* 3(3):28-40.

— (2000). *Care of the Elderly in India; Changing Configurations.* Shimla; Indian Institute of Advanced Study.

Central Bureau of Health Intelligence. Directorate General of Health Services, Ministry of Health and Family Welfare. *Health Information of India 2000 &2001.*

Dey, A.B. (ed.) (2003). *Ageing in India: Situation Analysis and Planning for the Future.* New Delhi: All Institute of Medical Sciences/ Ministry of Health and Family Welfare,Government of India/WHO.

Fellman, Jerome D. (1988). Spatial patterns of disease and Health: One World or Two? In Norwina, G. and Gonzaloz, A.(ed.), *The Third World: States of Mind and Being.* Boston: Unwin Hyman, pp.112-23.

Government of India.(2001). *National Policy On Older Persons.* Ministry of Social Justice & Empowerment, New Delhi.

Griffith, D.H.S. (1963). *Final Report on Public Health Programmes.* SEA/PHA/30, Andhra Pradesh: WHO Project.

Jamuna, D. (1999). *Correlates of Quality of Life Among Indian Elderly Men and Women.* Project report. New Delhi: ICMR.

Kalache, Alex(1994). Promoting Health in Old Age. In Ramachandran, C.R. and Shah, Bela(ed.), *Public Health Implications of Ageing in India.* New Delhi: Indian Council of Medical Research. pp.7-10.

Kothari, Bela and Sinha, Rolly(2002).Life of the Elderly in a Rajasthan Village. *Indian Journal of Gerontology* 16(3 &4): 321-28.

Misra, Rajiv, Rachel Chatterjee and Sujatha Rao. (2003). *India Health Report.* New Delhi: Oxford University Press.

Natarajan,V.S. and Selvaraj, Kokila(2003). Changing Pattern of Morbidity in Older People. In Dey, A.B.(ed). *Ageing in India: Situation Analysis and Planning for the Future.* New Delhi: AIIMS, pp. 67-70.

Prakash, Indira Jai(2003). Ageing in a New Millennium. In Dey, A.B.(ed.), *Ageing in India: Situation Analysis and Planning for the Future.* New Delhi: All India Institute of Medical Sciences/ Ministry of Health and Family Welfare, Government of India/WHO, pp. 33-40.

— (2004). Health Concerns of Older Women in India. *Research & Development Journal (HelpAge India).* 10(3): Oct. 7-10.

Purohit, C.K. and Sharma, R. (1976). Study of the General Health Status of Persons Aged 60 years and above in Rural Health Training Centre, Area Naila. *Indian Journal of Medical Research* 64(2): 202-10.

Ramamurti, P.V. (1996). Health Behaviour among the Elderly. *Project Report.* New Delhi: ICMR.

Rao, Venkoba, A. (1990). *Health Care of the Rural Aged.* New Delhi: Indian Council of Medical Research.

Ramamurti, P.V.(1996). Health and attitude towards the health among Elderly. In Vinod Kumar(ed.), *Ageing: Indian Perspective and Global Scenario.* New Delhi: AIIMS, pp. 231-34.

Ray, Ira and Singh, S.(2003). Immunization in Older People. In Dey, A.B.(ed.), *Ageing in India: Situation Analysis and Planning for the Future.* New Delhi: All India Institute of Medical Sciences/ Ministry of Health and Family Welfare, Government of India/WHO, pp. 231-36.

Sharma, R. (1998). Emerging problems of elderly: Some steps for public action. *Indian Journal of Gerontology* 12:10-21.

Sinha, Archana (2004). Gender Ageing and Health in India: Emerging Problems. *Research & Development Journal* (HelpAge India). Oct. 10(3): 11-21.

Siva Raju, S. (1986). Evaluation of Health Care System: Some Guidelines. *Health and Population –Perspectives and Issues* 9(2): 80-89.

—(1997). *Medico-Social Study on the Assessment of Health Status of the Urban Elderly*. Bombay: Tata Institute of Social Sciences. (Mimeo).

—(2002). *Health Status of the Elderly: A Medico-Social Study*. New Delhi: B.R. Publications.

—(2002). Health of the Elderly in India: Issues and Implications. *Research & Development Journal (HelpAge India)*. 8(1): 25-30.

Vijaya Kumar, S. (2003). Rural Ageing: Ageing in Poverty. In Dey, A.B. (ed.), *Ageing in India: Situation Analysis and Planning for the Future*. New Delhi: AIIMS, pp.103-08.

—(2000). Elderly women in Rural India: Need for Health Policy Interventions. In Bathla, P.C. (ed.), *Lecture Series in Geriatrics*. New Delhi: National Institute of Primary Health Care. pp. 274-77.

Vinod Kumar(2000). Age-related disorders and disabilities. *Social Defence* 50: 39-45.

Willmott, P. (1986). *Social Networks, Informal Care and Public Policy*. London: Policy Studies Institute.

World Bank (1993). *Investing in Health. World Development Report 1993*. New York: Oxford University Press for the World Bank.

World Bank. (2001). *India - Raising the Sights: Better Health Systems for India's Poor*.

7

Living (IADL) Among Rural Elderly in Assam

G.K. Medhi & J. Mahanta

Background

India is the home of second largest numbers of elderly population in the world with about 77 million elderly and more than 80% of its elderly population resides in the rural areas. However, very scant information is available about the health status particularly of rural elderly in India, which is very important for planning health services to them. One of the sentinel events during older age, which affects quality of life, is the decline of functional status. Maintenance of basic function in basic activity of daily living (BADL) like bathing, eating, toileting, dressing, transferring in and out of bed and instrumental activity of daily living (IADL) like shopping, cooking and light household activities are important for living an independent and quality life. In the present paper, an attempt has been made to evaluate the BADL and IADL status among the elderly (60 plus age group) population living in the rural area of Assam.

Methods

Data was collected adopting a cross-sectional and

population-based study design. A total of 1214 (613 men; 601 women) community dwelling elderly individuals aged e" 60 participated in the study from 33 villages of Dibrugarh district of Assam, India during 2003-2004. Data on BADL and IADL status, self-reported health conditions, sociodemographic characteristics, health risk behaviours (e.g. smoking, alcohol use) were collected using a questionnaire. Functional status of elderly i.e. BADL and IADL status was assesses by asking them about their ability to perform activity of daily living on following items e.g. bathing, household activities. Bathing, dressing, transferring in and out of bed, toileting and/or eating were classified as basic activity of daily living (BADL); and shopping, cooking and light household activities were classified as instrumental activity of daily living (IADL). Descriptive statistical analysis was performed to present the data.

Results

The mean (± SD) age of participants was 66.40 (± 6.74). Altogether, 8.7% of elderly individuals had problem in performing one or more BADL. Proportion of individuals with only IADL limitation was 27%. Proportion individuals who had BADL and/or IADL limitation were 35.7%. Sex differential in favour of men was noted in BADL/IADL status in a statistically significant manner ($p<0.05$). A strong age gradient was also observed in the BADL/IADL status, BADL/IADL limitation being highest among 80+ age group (82%) and lowest among 60-69 years age group (27%). CONCLUSION: BADL/IADL is an important measure of care and support needs of elderly population. The findings of the study will help in understanding the BADL/IADL status and factors associated with impaired BADL/IADL among community dwelling rural elderly individuals in Assam.

Introduction

Population aging is a global phenomenon. India is also

experiencing a rapid increase of aging population due to demographic transition. The life expectancy at birth is continuously increasing in India due to gradual decline of death rate. Preventing premature mortality is considered as a great triumph of public health. The success story of public health itself is now creating a new challenge for developing nations like India for ensuring well being to an ever-increasing numbers of elderly populations. According to 2001 Indian census, elderly population of India accounted for 77 million, whereas in 1961 elderly population constituted only 24 million, then 43 million in 1981. The proportion of elderly persons in the population of India rose from 5.63 per in 1961 to 7.5 percent in 2001. It is estimated that by the middle of this century, one out of every five individuals in India will be an individual 60 years and above (Irudaya SR, 2006). Sixty plus age group will represent a most dominant demographic section in India.

Prolonging life is a laudable achievement in the last century. However, prolonging life will be appalling only if the increase life expectancy can be converted to the healthy life expectancy. With increased life expectancy, elder people also become more vulnerable to various age related chronic disorders and functional disability. One of the sentinel events during older age is the decline of functional status. Maintenance of basic function in basic activity of daily living (BADL) like bathing, eating, toileting, dressing, transferring in and out of bed and instrumental activity of daily living (IADL) like shopping, cooking and light household activities is important for living an independent and quality life. Function status in BADL and IADL is considered as important indicator of quality of life at older age. Assessment of functional status of elderly is not only important for knowing the quality of life at old age, but also for understanding health care needs for them.

In India, more than 80% of the population lives in the rural area. However, very scant information is available about the functional health of elderly population which refers to rural population in India, particularly form the northeastern region of the country. The present endeavor is an attempt to understand the functional status of elderly population in terms of activity of daily living of elderly population (60+ age group) from rural location of Assam.

A cross-sectional community based study was conducted in rural areas of Dibrugarh district of Assam, a province situated in the northeast India in 2003-. A total of 33 villages were selected by simple random method from the village list of the district. All the community dwelling individuals aged e" 60 years were eligible to participate in the study. Informed consent was obtained from the participants before data collection. Trained research staff collected the data from the eligible individuals by house-to-house visit.

A pre-designed and pre-tested questionnaire was developed to collect the data on age, sex, educational status, health habits (smoking, alcohol consumption) and health indicators (self-rated health, chronic morbidity and BADL/ IADL impairment).

Functional status of elderly was assesses by asking them about their ability to perform activity of daily living on seven items and divided into two dimensions i.e. basic activity of daily living (BADL) and instrumental activity of daily living (IADL). The BADL dimension consisted of five basic activities of daily living (BADL) e.g. bathing, dressing, transferring in and out of bed, toileting and/or eating. The IADL dimension consisted of other items i.e. shopping, cooking and light household activities.

Results & Discussion

A total of 1214 (men-613 and women-601) participated

in the study. The mean (± SD) age of participants was 66.40 (± 6.74). Some of the important characteristics of the participants are presented in the Table 1. Most of the elderly participants (70.5%) were in the age group of 60-69 years. Out of the total, 43.1% were illiterate.

Table 1
Characteristics of studied elderlies

Characteristics	*Number (%)*
Age (Years)	
60--69	856 (70.5)
70--79	280(23.1)
80 or above	78(6.4)
Sex	
Male	613 (50.5)
Female	601(49.5)
Education	
Illiterate	529(43.6)
Upto primary level	301(24.8)
High school	384(31.6)
Difficulty in ADL	
No difficulty	780 (64.3)
Difficulty in IADL only	328 (27.0)
Difficulty in BADL	106 (8.7)

Overall, 9.1% of men and 8.6% of women had problem in at least one BADL. The IADL difficulty was significantly higher ($p<0.05$) among women (33.4%) than men (20.7%). The prevalence of BADL/IADL impairment increased abruptly from lowest to highest age groups. Overall, 29.9% women and 41.8% men ($p<0.05$) had difficulty at least in one BADL and /or IADL. BADL/IADL difficulty also increased

(Fig: 1) abruptly lowest to highest age group. It is observed from the study that most of the older people in rural area of Assam maintain a fairly good functional health in 60--69 years age group.

BADL is more important indicator of health. Fortunately, proportion of individuals who had problem in BADL was only 9.1% of men and 8.6% of women. But, after the seventh 90% of male and 72% of female had problem in at least one IADL. Similar age trend with respect to IADL/BADL impairment was also noticed in the previous study done in Assam (Medhi et al. 2006).

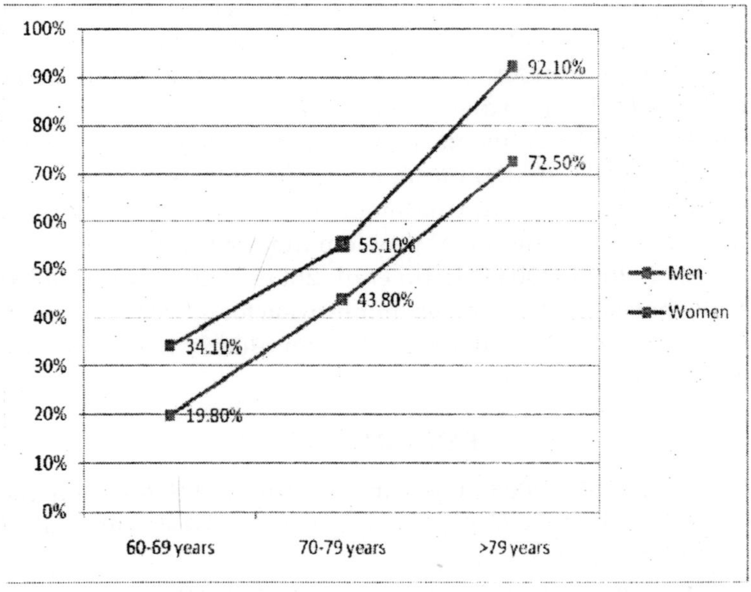

Fig. 1: Age and sex-wise prevalence of IADL Problem among Elderly

Apart from age and sex, numbers of chronic morbidities was also found to be an important indicator of BADL/IADL impairment (not shown in the table).

Conclusion

The present study has highlighted functional status of elderly population living in rural area of Assam. The main strength of the study is that it was a population based data. Maintenance of functional status is paramount important for quality of life at old age. It is revealed from the study that a high proportion of community dwelling elderly population had problem in maintaining independent life due to functional deficits in them. However, it is revealed from the study the young olds i.e. elderly in the 60-69 years age group were more or less free from functional deficit in BADL. One of the significant findings of the study is the correspondence between chronic diseases and BADL/IADL impairment. The finding implies that prevention and management of chronic disease will be important for restoring better functional health at old age. The higher prevalence of hypertension and complications related to hypertension among elderly also an important cause of BADL/IADL problem among elderly. So, creating awareness and regular treatment of hypertension is necessary for preventing functional problem among them Hazarika *et al.* 2002, 2003, 2004; Medhi *et al.* 2006). The findings of the study have important policy implication for developing health care strategy and support system for elderly living in rural area in coming years.

REFERENCES

1. Irudaya SR. (2006). Population Ageing and Health in India, 1st Ed. Mumbai: Centre for Enquiry into Health and Allied Themes, p. 1.

2. Hazarika N C, Narain K, Biswas D, Kalita H C, Mahanta J, (2004). Hypertension in the native rural population of Assam. *National Medical Journal of India.* Nov-Dec; 17(6):300--4.

3. Hazarika NC, Biswas D, Mahanta J. (2003). Hypertension in the elderly population of Assam. *Journal of Association of Physicians India.* June; 51:567-73.

4. Hazarika N C, Biswas D, Narain K, Kalita H C, Mahanta J. (2002). Hypertension and its risk factors in tea garden workers of Assam. *National Medical Journal of India.* Mar--Apr; 15(2): 63--8.

5. Medhi G K, Hazarika NC, Borah P K, Mahanta J. (2006). Health Problems and Disability of Elderly Individuals in Two Population Groups from Same Geographical Location. *JAPI*; 54: 539--544

Section-II
Sociopsychological Aspects of Ageism

8

"Agequake"- Managing the Impact of Population Aging in India

Indira Jai Prakash

Aging is no longer a personal issue for one to agitate about. Demographic changes have brought issues related to aging into sharp focus. Robert Butler, in the late 60s coined the term "*Ageism*", and the implications of ageism were much discussed in the early 70s. A more recent addition to gerontological vocabulary is the word "*Agequake*". Paul Wallace (1999), in the last decade wrote about Agequake- a demographic seismic convulsion that will impact all aspects of our lives. He noted that for the first time in human history, birth and death rates will both fall, age pyramid will turn upside down reshaping economy, shaking up business, and every aspect of social life would be affected drastically. Agequake hit developed countries first but became global very fast. Opening the World Assembly on Ageing in Madrid in 2002, UN Secretary General, Kofi Annan called upon the world community to get ready for an explosion in the numbers of old people that would strain the social systems, especially that of the poor countries.

During the 20th century, most countries witnessed high fertility and declining mortality resulting in a rapid increase in the population of older people. Later, a sharp decline in fertility ensured that the proportion of older people continued to rise while that of younger group declined (Rajan, 2003). This trend became pronounced in the Western countries with birth rates falling drastically. Figure 1, illustrates the population trends globally. As can be seen from the figure, with low birth rates and high survival rate, the population structure is rapidly becoming rectangular in shape.

Figure 1
Population Pyramids for Asia and the Pacific, 1950-2050

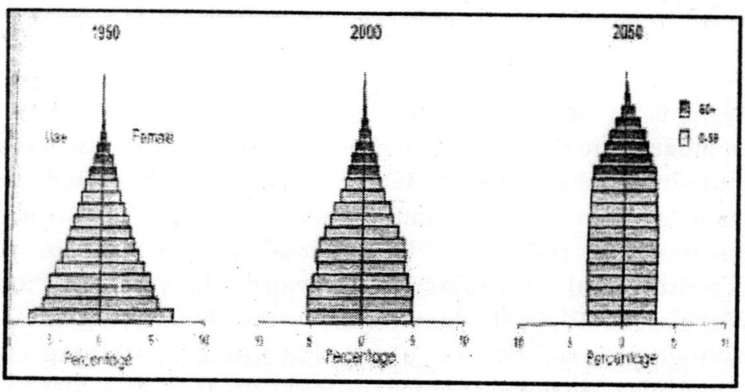

(*Source: World Population Ageing, 1950-2050,* (United Nations Publication, Sales No. E.02.XIII.3), p. 69).

In the developed world, the concerns have been focused on the burden of paying for age, health care costs, redefining retirement, dependence on immigrant workers in the absence of young people in the population, accommodating varied types of households, managing leisure time and in general, restructuring society to make it 'age-friendly'. The slogan *'Add ears to life'* changed to *'Add life to years'* and finally to *'Add quality to added life'.*

Butler (1998) points out that longevity is not a function of biological evolution, but of social and economic progress, better public health and nutrition and the application of important medical concepts. Thanks to longevity, society has experienced many positive developments. Increased productivity due to reduction of disruptive illness and premature deaths, emergence of multigenerational family, opportunity for people to generate new savings and capital and above all catalyzing basic research and investigations into aging have been some offshoots of this trend. Butler opines that like industrial-scientific revolution, longevity revolution affects everything: the family, productivity, health care system and culture. In spite of these, the initial impact has been largely negative. Lack of adequate planning for a rapidly aging population highlighted the lacunae in existing health care, social and economic welfare systems. Doomsday predictions that population aging, would lead to " 'pension bomb', 'welfare collapse', 'generation clashes', 'labour shortages'," resulted in perceiving old people as a burden to society. Even in America – the fabled land of opportunity and success - poverty, age discrimination, rationing of health care, uncertain economy and private pension crisis made one ask *"Why Survive"*? (Butler, 2002).

The process of aging of India's population is still in its early phase. In Asian countries like India and Indonesia, fertility has not come down as sharply as in China. While in developed regions of the world, the percentage of older people is around 19-20% and still rising, India registers between 7-8% (and is rapidly rising!) in the 60+ group. But in sheer numbers, (considering the billions of Indians) there were around 77 million elderly in 2001 and there is a strong possibility that it has crossed 100 million by now. There is considerable variation in the population composition given the diversity of India. The proportion of elderly is likely to be highest in South India (8.3%), and lowest (5.6%) in the North-east India. Old-age dependency ratio is, similarly high for South India (13.2) and low for the North-east (9.5). Southern region also has a favourable sex ratio (954 male for 1000 female) compared to, for example, North-east which has a ratio of 1139 male for 1000 female elderly (Rajan, 2003). Table 1 gives summary information on ageing trends for India and Meghalaya.

Table 1
Comparison between state and nation on some variables

	India	*Meghalaya*
Total Population	1029 million	2.32 million
Decadal growth	21.54	30.65
Fertility Rate	2.9	4.57
Crude birth rate	23.5	24.7
Crude Death Rate	7.5	8.0
Sex Ratio	933	975
% of Old people*	> 7%	> 4.7%*

(* 1991 census)

Longevity is the triumph of the 20th century, But why is it not greeted with more enthusiasm? Bali (2001) points out that a growing aging population will have important implications both at micro and macro-levels. At the micro-level, the concern is about the individual adaptation to transitions across life-course. At macro-level, the challenge of aging population has economic, educational, familial, health and social welfare concerns. While one is happy that Indians are living longer, the question is *"have we made the life worth living?"* The major issues with regard to elderly population in India are:

1. Nearly 80% of the older people are concentrated in rural areas where service delivery is not satisfactory. Rural aging is marked by high rates of illiteracy and poverty.

2. *Feminization of aging* implies that there are more older women in higher age groups. Widowhood (55-60%), economic dependence and higher rates of morbidity lower the quality of life of older women drastically.

3. With nearly 30% of the elderly living below the poverty line, socio-economic security cover for the masses is still a dream. Nearly 60-75% of elderly are economically dependent on others, usually their children (Prakash, 1999). There is also a *feminization of poverty* with older women being poorer. 90% of the work force is employed in the unorganized sector and the National old-age pension scheme has barely made an impact on economic insecurity of the people.

4. Increasing burden of morbidity. Increase in human life span has led to more ill-health. There is a shift from communicable diseases to non-communicable diseases in aged population and there is a considerable burden of multiple morbidity in old age. Prevalence of cognitive impairment and deterioration of physical function lowers the quality of life of people (Shah, 2003). In India, a clear policy and strategy for the development of health care for older person is not operational (Dey, 2003), preventing a holistic approach to the health care for elderly.

5. Psychiatric disorders increase *pari passu* with age. Mental disorders in old age are not just due to the ageing brain. But are due to losses associated with aging, socio-economic problems and compromised quality of life (Prakash, 2004). Figures for mental

morbidity vary from survey to survey. Community based studies report varying rates of psychiatric morbidity for the elderly ranging from 2.2% to 33.3% (Varghese, 2005). Depression ranks as the commonest disorder of old age followed by dementia.

6. Likelihood of developing dementia increases with age and the spectre of Alzheimer's diseases looms large, though exact figures are not available. Long term care of older people with dementia in the absence of known treatment will be a nightmare. Care givers of dementia patients experience severe distress due to behavioural problems of the patients (Paraswani, Sharma & Bharath, 2005).

7. Traditional family system and values are fast eroding. Nuclear and small families, dual career couple and migration of the young cause a 'crisis in caring'. (Recently a researcher added "feminization of farming"- women forced to take up agricultural work due to migration of the young and 'gero-farming' as other trends). There is a *feminization of care giving* with more women being formal as well as informal care-givers. Care giver stress could be one of the causes of increasing instances of elder abuse.

8. The existing elder care institutions house less than 1% of the elderly, community care institutions and geriatric nursing homes for chronically and terminally ill are very few (Jamuna, 2003).

9. Due to social and cultural changes, many elderly feel lonely and isolated. In a Pune -based study, 40% of the people interviewed felt totally neglected by their families. (Bambawale, 2004). The proportion of older persons, especially urban widowed women, living alone is increasing with serious consequences to their well-being (Prakash, 2003a). A summary of trends

regarding health and social situation of older people for India and the North East region is presented in Table 2.

Table 2
Health and well-being or older persons in India and North-East

Health and social well-being	India	N.E
Elderly with no disease	24.92	22.91
With one chronic disease	53.63	54.86
At least one disability	38.39	37.27
Old dependency ratio	11.9	9.5
People below poverty line	26.1	33.9*

* for Meghalaya only

These are just a few of the challenges thrown up by the rapid aging of the population in India. Most European and North American regions became affluent first and 'grey' later. For India, on the other hand, longevity came first and prosperity is yet to be achieved. At present neither the older people, nor their families, nor the society, nor the government is totally prepared to ensure a disability-free and dignified life well into ripe old age. National Policy for older people is yet to be implemented and several schemes initiated have not been sustained. Much progress has been made in the quantity and quality of health care services in the last fifty years in India. However, the development has been uneven with urban areas getting the best advantage of the advances in medicine. A Planning Commission report states that rural poverty in Meghalaya has worsened over the last decade. While Indian elders have a relatively better access to family care, they are inadequately covered by state social security programs. Growing economic problems, internal political upheavals, tensions across its borders have kept the country preoccupied with issues that appear more urgent than planning for the care of the elderly. If this trend continues, to quote D'Souza (1990), 'the simmering problem of the elderly...will burst into flames'.

Granted that we are facing an Agequake, how can we manage its impact? World Health Organization suggests that we can afford to get old if countries, regions and international organizations enact *"Active Ageing"* policies and programmes that enhance health, independence and productivity of older citizens (WHO, 2001). Active ageing is the process of optimizing opportunities for physical, social, and mental well-being throughout the life course, in order to extend healthy life expectancy, productivity and quality of life in older age. WHO adopted active ageing to express the idea of continuing involvement of elderly in social, economic, spiritual cultural and civic affairs. Maintaining independence- one's ability to control, cope with and make decisions about daily life- is a primary goal for both individuals and policy makers. An active ageing approach to policy and programme development has the potential to address the challenges of both individual and population aging. The active ageing approach is based on the recognition of the human rights of older people and the UN principles of independence, participation, dignity, care and self-fulfilment. It shifts strategic planning away from '*need-based*' approach to '*right-based*' approach. It supports both a life course perspective and intergenerational solidarity.

Determinants of active aging are—1) social factors such as education, literacy, rights, social support etc; 2) physical environment such as urban rural setting and housing; 3) economic factors such as income, work, and social protection; 4) personal factors such as biology and genetics, adaptability; 5) health and social services including health promotion, disease prevention, long term care, primary care; 6) behavioural factors such as physical activity, nutrition, appropriate medication, absence of substance abuse. Cross cutting determinants that influence all the above are: gender and culture. All these have to be addressed for prevention, intervention and rehabilitation in relation to agequake.

Is the situation totally negative or do we need a change in mindset and a different perspective to the issue? A paradigm shift from 'Population Pessimism' to 'Realistic Optimism' suggests that there are positive aspects to this trend. Longevity means longer years of work force participation by healthy elderly boosting economy. Multigenerational households may usher in new child care and family support patterns. Small families are likely to invest more in health and education of children leading to a better standard of life for the coming generations. Economists predict 'silver economy' with greater transfer of funds to young people from active and working elderly. There will be a growth in the service sectors. Older people may need less cars but require greater services which may promote local employment prospects. Longevity revolution has contributed to transformation of health care and delivery system, to development of new technology to deal with disability, frailty and also stimulated consideration of ethical and philosophical aspects of longevity, aging, dying and death. Instead of emphasizing on the negative, one may have to harness the potentials.

Preventive programs aimed at lifestyle changes help avoiding the '*explosion in health care cost*' in oldest age group. A broad range of community and public health services, strengthening of primary health care system, providing palliative and rehabilitative services have to be planned and implemented. Equity of access and cost effectiveness are key concerns of health system. Most older people still rely on their families for economic security. In the absence of this, they face the risk of homelessness and destitution. Schemes to reduce poverty, encouraging people to work as long as possible, income generating activities, retirement planning, compensation for the informal unpaid work of elderly in the family are measures to improve economic status of the elderly. Physical environment can affect aging in several ways. Rural areas need special attention, as the absence of basic amenities and poverty act as stressors on older people. In reaching the '*unreached*', Mobile medicare services and telemedicine are promising developments. Safe and adequate housing for people living alone, supportive housing, sheltered houses can be good alternatives to nursing homes or institutions. Barrier-free and age-friendly structures and services help old people maintain their independence as long as possible.

While genetic and biological factors are less modifiable, lifestyle and behavioural changes are achievable. There will be some decline in skills and functions due to age, disuse, behavioural factors like alcoholism and psychosocial factors like lack of motivation, isolation etc. These need to be addressed through awareness programs, advocacy and training. Healthy behaviour such as physical activity, nutrition, weight control and use of appropriate medication could be taught to people. Involving elders in community activities, avoiding institutionalization, providing community support networks, opportunities for life long learning, protection from violence and abuse, help overcome vulnerability due to social isolation. Special attention need to be paid to vulnerable groups such as elderly women, widows, slum dwellers, refugees and dislocated people and people living with HIV and AIDS.

Dey (2003) suggests a multi-level model of health care for older Indians. This model proposes primary care at community level, specialized care by an internist or geriatrician at the secondary level, and a specific intervention by a specialist physician or surgeon (cardiologist, urologist etc) at tertiary level. The process of care is a dynamic one with patient moving between community and hospital in the early stage of illness. Severe disability may require long term care. Day care facility helps patient spend time in quasi heath-care setting with recreation and rehabilitation. Linking the care of elderly in rural and backward areas with ICDS program is another suggestion (Prakash, 1991). Tax incentives for families caring for older persons, training for care givers, respite care, training older people as mentors and volunteers, retirement planning for workers, community based care for home-bound but independent elderly, assistive technology to compensate for disabilities, life-long learning for personal development- are other strategies.

Introducing geriatric medical facilities in all hospitals, training of geriatric nurses, volunteers, home care providers and community workers is a priority. One has to examine culturally relevant strategies to improve the well-being of the elderly. Indian culture had several elder-friendly models that may have to be reinvented. NGOs, Senior citizens clubs and pensioner's associations can play an active role in advocacy and training. Older people in India account for 12% of the vote bank. There is a need for them to get organized and lobby for their rights. American Association of Retired Persons, Grey Panthers and such organizations are powerful in the West. India too needs such senior citizen bodies to ensure rights of older people. Technology is a powerful ally that could reduce the burden of disability and add to the efficiency of health professionals. Good planning and policy making should be based on accurate information. Hence quality research on aging that is multidisciplinary in nature is recommended.

It is worth recording some of the Best practices across the different nations and learn from them. Community participation is considered a good strategy to provide services to elderly and also keep them active. In Bangladesh, the traditional *adda* (informal social gathering) combines recreational pursuits with loan collection and disbursement. In Cambodia, it is the *wat* (temple) that is the centre of social life, providing culturally accepted venue for elderly. In several Asian countries, older people's associations run community centres. Among many older Muslims, the mosque becomes the centre for social activities. In the area of social security, small credit programmes run by NGOs in Bangladesh are well known. Cambodia, India, Sri Lanka and Thailand have set up small credit programmes for groups of older people, mainly women. In some regions, community schemes are owned and managed by elder's group (Nizamuddin, 2003). National Old-Age Pension Scheme for destitute elderly, travel concessions and higher interest rates in banks for senior citizens are proactive measures.

Other examples worth mentioning are- in health care sector, there is an initiative in the Philippines to train older persons to become "community gerontologists". HelpAge India provides outreach services through mobile clinics for older and disabled persons . In the city of Karachi, Pakistan Medico International, an NGO, provides free health care services to the needy. Tsao Foundation in Singapore provides holistic health care services for low income elderly. To deal with loss of family support, home and community-based programmes for the elderly have emerged. For example, HelpAge Korea has initiated a programme of voluntary home visits by community members who help with household tasks and provide emotional and social support. In Singapore, both the Tsao Foundation and the Singapore Action Group for Elders (SAGE) offer education and training for informal caregivers. In China, day-care centres for the elderly have been set up to provide basic health and recreation (Nizamuddin,2003). In India, senior citizen's club volunteers help each other Indian Government has announced opening of day care centres and helplines for senior citizens..

It is recommended that in India, policy intervention should involve four components: basic services, social and economic security, community action, and developing supportive socio-cultural practices (Sharma, 1998). Basic services involve ensuring food, shelter, minimum income, health care and family support. Social-economic security requires instituting legislative measures for old-age pension, concessions, free health services etc. For community action, professional bodies would need to create public awareness and education about the needs, roles and rights of elderly. Supportive practices aim at changing attitudes of family and society, fighting ageism, developing skills of people, incorporating elder care in activities of *panchayats* and *nagar palikas* etc.

There are some major challenges ahead. Policy makers need to avoid viewing the elderly as a "problem", and involve them as participants in development. Mainstreaming the concerns of older persons in overall development agendas and poverty-reduction programmes is essential. Public expenditures for all older persons need to be increased. Society need to utilize the vast resources of diverse and growing population. We also need to learn from the experience of the developed countries, especially with regard to economic and social security measures. There is a need to create and maintain national geriatric programmes. The state needs to set up policy groups to anticipate, understand and plan for the growing elderly group. There is a need for capacity building and institutional development, develop data base, and use information and communication technology to promote well-being of people. This also requires close cooperation with family, community based support systems, Governmental and non-governmental agencies. Just as it is important to assess the threats posed by population aging realistically, it is equally important to explore possible solutions (Prakash, 2003b). If pessimism is a good adversary, optimism makes a good ally. There is a need to celebrate life and longevity in India. Only, we have to find ways to harness resources, use technology appropriately and find imaginative alternatives. Ultimately, individuals, families, communities should work with the Government to ensure dignity, autonomy and participation of elderly in the evening of their life. Some wise person said "Aging is mandatory, growing up is by choice". Every person should have the power to exercise this choice for which we have to create a "society for all ages".

REFERENCES

Bali, A.P (2001) *Care of the Elderly in India: Changing Configurations*. Shimla: Indian Institute of Advanced Study.

Bambawale, U (2004) Abuse of Elderly: A Myth or Reality. In P.V. Ramamurti & D. Jamuna (Eds). *Handbook of Indian Gerontology*. New Delhi. Serials Pub., pp. 243-267.

Butler, R. N (1998) *The Revolution in Longevity. Keynote at the Third International Congress on Ageing*. Paris, May 18-20.

Butler, R.N. (2002). *Why Survive? Revisited*. www//press.jhu.edu/books/butler-preface.pdf.

Dey, A.B (2003) A Model of Health Care for Older People in India. In A.B. Dey (ed) *Ageing in India. Situation Analysis and Planning for the Future*. New Delhi. Ministry of Health and Family Welfare and WHO, pp. 269-274.

D'Souza, V (1990) *The Simmering Problem of Aging in India*. BOLD (UN), 1 (1), 17-21.

Jamuna, D (2003) Issues of Elder Care and Elder Abuse in the Indian Context. In Liebig, P.S & Rajan, I. S (Eds). *An Aging India: Perspectives, Prospects and Policies*. New York: The Haworth Press Inc., pp. 125-142.

Kumar, V S (2003) *Economic security for the Elderly in India: An Overview*. In Liebig, P.S & Rajan, I. S (Eds). *An Aging India: Perspectives, Prospects and Policies*. New York: The Haworth Press Inc., pp. 45 - 65.

Nizamuddin, M (2003) Policy responses to population ageing in Asia and the Pacific. *Proceedings of the Fourth Asia-Pacific Population Conference* Bangkok, Thailand. UN ESCAP.

Paraswani, M. J, Sharma, M.P & Bharath, S (2005) Caregivers distress, Morbidity and Burden in Dementia: Rationale for Intervention. In Prakash, Indira. J (Ed) *Aging in India: Retrospect and Prospect.* Bangalore: Bangalore University, pp. 129- 132.

Prakash, Indira. J (1991) *Caring for the Disadvantaged Elderly in India: A Suggestion.* BOLD (UN) 1, (4), pp. 11-12.

Prakash, Indira. J (1999) *Ageing in India.* Geneva: World Health Organization.

Prakash, Indira. J (2003a) *Home Alone: Older People Coping with Loneliness.* In Prakash, I.J (Ed) Aging: Emerging Issues. Bangalore: Bangalore University. pp. 31-36

Prakash, Indira. J (2003b) Ageing in the New Millennium. In A.B. Dey (ed) *Ageing in India. Situation Analysis and Planning for the Future.* New Delhi. Ministry of Health and family welfare and WHO, pp. 33-42.

Prakash, Indira. J (2004) Mental Health of Older People in India. In P.V. Ramamurti & D. Jamuna (Eds). *Handbook of Indian Gerontology.* New Delhi. Serials Pub., pp. 176-207.

Rajan, I (2003). Demography of Ageing. In A.B. Dey (ed) *Ageing in India. Situation Analysis and Planning for the Future.* New Delhi. Ministry of Health and Family Welfare and WHO, pp. 3-11.

Shah, B (2003) A Perspective of Research in Geriatrics and Gerontology. In A.B. Dey (ed) *Ageing in India. Situation Analysis and Planning for the Future.* New Delhi. Ministry of Health and Family Welfare and WHO, pp. 57- 64.

Sharma, R (1998) Emerging Problems of Elderly: Some Steps for Public Action. *Indian Journal of Gerontology,* 12, 10-21.

Varghese, M (2005) Issues in Old Age Psychiatry in India. In Prakash, Indira J (Ed) *Aging in India: Retrospect and Prospect.* Bangalore: Bangalore University, pp. 15-19.

Wallace, P (1999) *Agequake: Riding the Demographic Rollercoaster,* Shaking business, Finance and Our World. London: Nicholas Brealey Pub. Ltd.

World Health Organization (2001). *Health and Ageing: A discussion paper*. Geneva. Department of Health Promotion, Non-Communicable Disease Prevention and Surveillance, WHO.

9

Aged in the North-East Region of India at the Dawn of Information Age

Indrani Chakravarty & S.K. Chakravarty

[We are going through a historic transformation in the way we live, learn, work, communicate and do business. We must not do so passively, but as makers of our own destiny. Technology has made the information age possible. Now it is up to all to build an *information society*.

Information and Communication Technology (ICT) possesses an extraordinary power. From trade to telemedicine, from education to environment protection, from new born babies to wrinkled octogenarians, ICT has the ability to improve standards of living for the *society for all*.

The task of building the information society is not about technology it is about the people with the end results of technology and their social, cultural and economic aspirations. To disseminate the blessings of ICT for a particular segment of a society, we must have a deeper focus in their lives. This paper embeds some of major aspects of the lives of elderly in North Eastern States of India (NE). NE in now getting priority in the agenda of development of government of India. As government can not bridge all the gaps in developmental works, role of NGO for providing quality like to the aged population and the concept of productive ageing along with the vision of the University of 3rd Age (U3A) is also discussed in this paper.

Key Words: Information Society, ICT; Society for all, U3A]

At the Dawn of the New Millennium

Dawn of the millennium generated hopes that we were going to embark into a new society – the information society empowered by the potentials of Information and Communication Technology (ICT). ICT is the result of the osmosis between computer and Telecommunication. Like global warming, population aging is also a prime concern of the entire human society. The problem has wide verifications and needs to be addressed from as many perspectives as possible. We need to try and to generate interest among problem solvers from whole range of disciplines in proposing new, creative and imaginative solutions. The central intention of this paper is to explore of the emerging roles ICT at this stage play for attacking the problems of aging in North-East Region (NER) of the country with district geographical and economic features. We have to bring together the heart and mind of every stake holder of the society – government, technological experts, NGOs, innovators, small entrepreneurs and other activists. The World Summits in Information Society(WSIS)-2003 in Geneva and 2005 in Tunis [1] have succeeded in bringing the concerns of all stake holders of the society to create opportunities of the end results of ICT. We will find some kind of formula to eradicate poverty and improve livelihoods. We will find ways to change environment, improve health care, reduce terrorism and bridge the digital divide.

Following points are postulated in this paper:

- Digital revolution in information and communication technologies is rapidly reducing the chasm between the knowledge and ignorance. Ignorance – the root cause of most of the miseries in the human society and aged are no exceptions.
- Paper is more inclined towards the vulnerabilities of the ageing than the aged population and therefore, it is a futuristic approach to combat the challenges of ageing in NER.
- In many action plans for social cause, there are duplicating efforts. As the task of building the information society necessitates the participation of all stakeholders of the society or in other words all hands coming together in order to reach destination have to marshal all our resources in the most efficient ways.
- This work explores more about the opportunities of ageing and efforts to attain it than detailing much about the problems.
- As the world has never witnessed such a high proportion of elderly people, we are emotionally confused in our initiatives to find solutions. Elderly are not spent force. In India there is a strength in the number of 80 millions.
- Successful aging depends upon the capacities and opportunities of individuals to fit well into the social framework of their own time.
- Adaptive technologies available within the potentials of ICT can be made as supplement to healthy ageing.

NER at the Threshold of Development

India is now in transition from poor destitute colony that the Britishers abandoned in dispair 60 years ago. The new

India is marked as different place in the world that has gained from British in August, 1947 midnight. It is now fourth largest economic state in the world. But the country is vastly populated and development and growth are not modular across the length and breadth.

The North-East Region constitutes of the states – Arunachal Pradesh, Assam, Mizoram, Manipur, Meghalaya, Nagaland, Tripura and Sikkim. The region is flanked by hills, slashed by mighty Brahmaputra river and bordering with China, Bhutan, Bangladesh and Myanmar. The North-East region is connected by Siliguri neck with the rest of the country.

The economy of North-East region has its definite identity.[2] It covers an area 2.62 lakhs sq. km. and accounts for 7.9% of total geographical area and 3.8% of the total population of country. Industrially the NER continues to be the most backward region in the country except Assam with traditional tea, oil and wood-based industries. In terms of economic indicators like GDP, Population below poverty line, Unemployed rate, per capita income, per capita domestic electricity consumption and many others the NER is behind the national standards.

Summary of Some Economic Indicators

Sectoral Share of GDP	The share of the Secondary sector in the GDP at 15% is much lower than the national average of 23.7% [1999-2000]
Population below Poverty Line	All the states in NER has much higher levels of population below poverty line [35.13%] as compared to the national average (26.1%) [2000-01]
Percentage of Urban Population	The share of urban population to total in the NER is 14.6%. The national average in this regard is 27.8% [2001 Census].

Unemployment Rate (as a % of workers)	The region represents one of the highest rates of unemployment in the country, with an unemployment rate close to 12%, against the national average of 7.7% [1999-00].
Gross Per Capita industrial output	The region has one of the lowest gross per capita industrial output at around Rs. 3313, (in Assam) which is much below the national average of Rs. 9111[2000-01]
Per Capita Domestic Electricity Consumption	The average per capita domestic electricity consumption in the NER works out to 20.4 kwh, against the national average cf 75.2 kwh. [1999-00].
Per Capita Credit Deposit ratio	This works out to 35% in the NER, against the national average of 66% [2004-05].
Per Capita Income	NER as a whole is placed amongst the poorest regions in the country. The per capita income at Rs.12409/ is less than the national average of Rs. 17978/-[2001-02].

Literature Review

For aging and the aged some matured researchers, Academicians and activists have made the beginning of gerontological studies in northeastern region. C.B. Majzumder and Paromita Saha[3] in Tripura perspective; A. Lunununsang Ao in Nagaland[4]; TARASANIKA SOCIETY in Assam[5]; R. M. Pant in Arunachal perspective[6]; Dayabati and Bagga on women NER [7]; Lianzela and Valachhawna in Mizoram[8] De, Utpal Kumar and Ghosh, Bhola Nath on Women of Khasi Society, Meghalaya[9] have thrown sufficient light on the generic issues of aging in North-Eastern region. By generic issues we conceive the common problems like declining of traditional values of respecting and caring the aged in the family, health, emotional aspects, loss of income and above all inadequate social securities. Dayabati and Bagga made some special effort to measure the miseries of the elderly women of NER whereas some mythical problems for the elderly were indicated by Lunununsang for the aged in Nagaland. Activists of TARASANIKA Society reported abandonment and elderly abuse in Assam – Abuse is really a difficult subject because it remains as a latent vice in the society like many other crimes.

Winds of Changes

Both the State and Central Government are attaching a great deal of importance to create an investment friendly climate and are offering a whole range of subsidies and incentives to set up industrial unit in the state with the Central Government earmarking 10% of Union Development Budget for North-East India. The rationale behind this initiatives are clear.

- NER is strategically placed in the global map. Since the world is flat and there is no Berlin wall now to mask the eyes of those who live at the margin of development, one has to go for changes or China will do it in Arunachal and upper Assam. NER is emerging as destination of investment for another reason as well. India is flourishing in offshore IT and BPO business. But there are few hubs in the metros in the country contributing the 85% growth in IT Sector.[10] Now due to rising inflation the main advantage of *labour arbitrage* in our metros and their developed countries are closing. This generates the urgency to go for IT business in the hinterland of the country where labour rate is low but people are equally intelligent and educated. Education is the parameter where NER is equal or more than the national standard. In Sikkim, for example, literary is above 82% compared to All India standard which is around 65%. Another advantage of

NER is the climate, the ambient temperature of places in Sikkim, Nagaland, Arunachal, Mizoram and upper Assam will cost far less in AC related load of high technology areas of Electronics and Telecoms. Thus the initiatives are on to connect NER with the resilient Optical Fibre Cable Grids, Extensive Mobile Coverage, Broadband in Wire and Wireless. Corporate Networks are realities and growing in strength and stability in the difficult terrains of NER. Can we create Information Society in the NER ?

Healthy Aging framework for the NER

NER is a focus for overall development in the government agenda; for ageing and the aged a healthy framework may be drawn once their diverse needs are well understood. It is not government alone, a broad participation in the development of healthy ageing framework is essential. At the national level we have National Institute of Social Defence(NISD) under the Ministry of Social Justice and Empowerment. *At the state level it is recommended to have one advisory council on Aging and Senior Citizens consisting of seniors and others with the interest in gerontological issues from all regions of NER in advising government on matters related to the quality of life of seniors, as well as facilitating public discussion. Healthy ageing in NER in the 21st century is intended to be the food for thought. To identify the priority issues, consultations, comments will come from all around beyond the physical presence through websites, e-mails, SMS etc. This is a major role of ICT for creating healthy ageing framework in these early years of the 21st century.*

Can we resolve the contradiction – bless or wish someone to live long and then look it in a negative way with little thought given to many positive things that life experience brings? *A snap study*[11] *amongst the middle class Nagamis in the capital city of Nagaland was made by co-author of this paper during his techno-economic survey for telecom during this year (2008). It is stricking that the middle class aged of the Nagaland suffer from the combination of ailments common to the aged anywhere in this country, but they are less prone to fatal ailments because of wisdom driven restrictions on their food habits and routine physical movements in the households or walking. Almost a similar observation can be made in Ketshukietuo Dzievichu's study on the health problems of the aged among Angami Nagas.*[12] *Another important finding of the snap study is the decline alcoholism amongst the elderly in NER.*

Gerontological studies have paid insufficient attention to the degree to which the aged are socially constituted[13] and the ways in which both aged and ageing are currently being transformed as a result of globalization.[14] Perfect health is unlikely with adding years in life but learning to live well in spite of one's limitations is undoubtedly a true mark of healthy ageing.

In this context, the concept of U3A is an important landmark.

Indian Society of U3A(ISU3A) as a networking conglomerate of voluntary bodies working for the cause of the elderly in India, was formally launched on March 29, 2008. It will act as an united forum to mobilize, organize and empower the elderly and to offer them opportunities for continued learning and working ensuring them active and graceful ageing. The main purpose of ISU3A is threefold: (1) to provide learning opportunities for the sake of knowledge; (2) To offer opportunities to grow old gracefully and (3) To promote volunteering for any Sewa to the mankind. Elders for the cause of elders are quite significant, but elders are not adequately trained in computer based Internet applications. In order to promote U3A vision in NER, some specially designed computer courses may be organized in this region. We can start some special modular training courses for the members of U3A and help them to have networking with NER forums for ageing population.

In NER a Framework of Partners should Grow for Healthy Ageing

Community organizations, including local clubs, recreational and cultural groups, may play a crucial role in the health of the senior citizens across the states of NER to provide important services, to develop friendships and collaborative relationships and pursue common interests. They will also be an outlet for self-expression. It is foreseen that as our population ages and the number of seniors grows, participation of such community organizations will flourish. As seniors tend to have more time available, compared to their middle years, community organizations will increasingly benefit.

Additional partners, including the corporate sector, governments and the health authorities, provide many of the services used by the aging population. They too need to plan and respond to the changes happening around us.

Contributions of community organizations, cultural groups, governments and corporates are nothing new for any social cause. Question is how to marshal these resources in NER perspective. October 20, 2004, in a major initiative towards redeeming the promise of giving the country an effective tool of ICT, national government rolled out the State Wide Area Network (SWAN) policy to facilitate the creation of necessary infrastructure by the state government to reach the fruits up to block level and gradually beyond the remotest part of rural India. Many states are advancing in their SWAN. Total project is around Rs. 14,000 cr. This huge ICT structure should be used by the professionals in the field of gerontology for their innovative applications. In NER, telecom infrastructure are growing now Thus important is the role of academics in training the workforce of tomorrow, including caregivers to take into account the aging population and its needs. Researchers also have an important function in ensuring a healthy aging population. We rely on their work to keep us informed of safe and healthy living practices. *Gerontology, which refers to the study of aging, must be promoted and supported in NER.*

NISD realized the importance and designated number of courses for the functionaries of NGOs, working for the elderly to achieve a proper blend of theoretical and practical knowledge. Such courses need expertises and academic resources. So far these courses are centralized in Kolkata for the East Zone of the country. But disseminating the knowledge would be faster if ICT tool like video conferencing; point to point, point to multipoint be applied for any Nodal Centre, knowledge centre of resources.

Interaction with the activists of NER transpires that the societies in the region hold many negative attitudes towards older people and the ageing process. NISD training model are driven to break the mythical barriers of attitude towards the ageing. Beneficiaries of the training course find the pause for thoughts to change their mind set.

Pause for Thought

- How can we, as a society, foster a positive image of aging?
- What will relationships between generations look like in the future?
- How do seniors contribute to your community or organization? How could they contribute differently in the future?
- Does your community or organization recognize the contributions of seniors? If so, how?

Engaging Elders of NER

Historically senior involvement in issues of the environment can probably be traced to the role of elders in any tribal society in passing along respect for the earth or mother nature [15]. As unemployment rates remains high in NER, employment of seniors in the retirement years remains a complex economic and ethical challenge and is likely to expand. NER is the richest region in the country for biodiversity, minimum pollution level and largest reserve of hydro electric power. Once action plan begins, NER would be a prime destination in tourism industry. It is expedient to promote in elderly persons of NER an environment ethic that results in expanding their knowledge, commitment and active involvement in protecting and caring for our environment for present and future generation.

Task harder than Tools

29th December, 2007, Ministry of Social Justice and Empowerment, Government of India awarded the senior citizens of the country with a tool – The Maintenance and Welfare of Parents and Senior Citizens Act, 2007. This act provides effective provisions for the maintenance and welfare of parents and senior citizens after 58th year of Republic of India. But an Act in paper and a tool under ground realities is altogether a different definition. Many states are offering best effort to draw their frameworks for this tool. NER has to accomplish by the participation of all resourceful persons in this part of the globe. A website, well planned opinion polls, forums of experts and experienced persons should be optimally marshaled. Physical distance, geographical constraints of difficult terrains of NER should not cause any problem in the information Age.

Computers and Elderly in NER

In general Economic Parameters NER is behind the

national standard but in literacy, this region is no less than national standard. Sikkim & Mizoram are ahead of the national standard, other provinces also are at per with the national parameter.[2] *There is no reason to believe that NER will be behind the nation in Internet and other Computer applications.* Telecom connectivity was a bigger issue in NER but we have discussed how & why this region is getting linked with the rest of the world by resilient optical fibre links.

Special issue of the speculations in Science and Technology – "Computers in the fight against ageing"[16] explored what roles the computer, the most versatile tool that the human brain has so far invented can play in attacking this issues of elderly. Surely computers can not be a wonder tool for all, remain restricted to a certain class who can buy it and use it. But India is altogether a different place. With teledensity of 5 in early 90's, 400 millions started talking over phones when franchisee PCOs appeared along the Indian roads. Same is the response for computer users through the Internet Kiosks.

The number of Internet users in India has gone up to 3.85 crore (38.5 millions) with 54% growth rate whereas average number of computer per 100 Indian is 1.5.[1]

In the fascinating book of recent time by ABP group, Kolkata " Sixty years after Indian Independence"[17], some master minds like Prof. Amartya Sen, the noble laureate in Economics; Prof. Tapan Ray Chaudhury, the Oxford Historian; Prof. Andre Beteille, the leading sociologist have contributed their essays.

Prof. Andre Beteille indicated the growth of middle class in India. A self assured middle class is one of the clearest markers of this new India.

Middle class ageing population should not ignore the potentials of computer particularly in the places of NER where geography is an issue, loneliness is a growing syndrome of ageing, poor eye sight is unavoidable with adding years in life.

Computer with Internet Connectivity can act as a companion for aged as:

- Pastime
- Gaming
- Magnifying the size of the text which otherwise is difficult to read by a person weaker in their sights – so common for the elderly
- A computer can create a neurobics personnel work-out station (NPWOPS) for health and vigour

Specifically, NPWOPS performs the following functions :

(1) Exercise the cardio-vascular system.

(2) Exercise the musculo-skeletal system.

(3) Exercise the immune system (by requiring the subject to act out positive emotional states and exercise the sense of humor and the erotic sense).

(4) Exercise reaction time and inspection times (time taken to absorb information).

(5) Exercise the sensory system (the definition of senses is extended to include the kinaesthetic sense and the sense of temperature).

(6) Exercise language centres, powers of imagination, mathematical faculty and long and short-term memory.

- Connectivity in Internet opens up entirely new possibilities. Qualified doctor servicing *1000 persons expels the vulnerability of the population growing in age. Diagnostics and advice that rely on experts and experts systems residing elsewhere or anywhere in the world is now available in the world of ICT.*[2]

- The computer can not only connect in to the real world but also to the virtual worlds. It offers unlimited opportunities for developing the imagination and experiencing simulated events. If a 90 year old chooses to ski down Mount Everest, say, then the computer will soon be able to provide such a think in a highly realistic way. The exploitation of virtuality has strongest possible implications for maintaining performance with age.

The Digital Genie is Yet to Come Out

Need to communicate is one of the basic needs of human beings just like life, food, shelter and clothing. Telephone is not accessible to everybody in the world and it is accessible which may not be affordable to have one to buy. Affluent society could enough margin, a revolution may take place just by sharing a telephone by millions. It happened in India at the status of less than 5 tele density could change the situation when 40 millions started making a call just by sharing the device. Voice, just application of ICT made by God. PCOs is the great success story of voice application in India followed by Gramin Telephone in Bangladesh – Mobile telephones and Telephone Ladies under Micro-credit model of professor Muhammad Yunus. This success story was repeated in many model like GRASSO in the State of West Bengal, India and other rural non-initiative in different states and this vastly populous country.

Mr. Waiverman used same model to examine the impact of fixed telephones in the development during 1970s and 1980s. The result was positive to indicate that penetration of fixed line could enhance the output significantly. Two recent study, one by London Business School and another one is supported by Qualcom, USA indicates that each 1% increase in Mobile penetration GDP per capita income comes $ 240 whereas each 1% increase in Internet penetration GDP per capita income comes up at $590. It has to be a Fishermen or Farmers at a distant village in India can check prices at different market at the district or state level before selling their product. This is just one example of many innovative ways in which a mobile phone is being used in the poorest part of the world.[1]

God's application voice has proved its strength. Now data has to prove it in multiples but the digital device capable of dealing with the data must be very simple and it can be handled even by a poor woman, or frail elderly. Professor Muhammad Yunus writes 'the ultimate design of an ICT device should be like an Aladdin;s Lamp in the hand of a poor woman. As she rubs the lamp, a digital genie comes out of it and asks; "what can I do for you, ma'am?" She commands the genie to get the information or support she needs, which would enable her to use her creativity to take care of her life.

Whatever ICT exists today, with all its glories, it is still in its infancy. But we must make absolutely sure of what it should grow up to be. If we think of it as a digital genie, it is not yet of the bottle. But soon it will be. Under whose command will this genie be? The Centre that I am proposing will work to ensure that the poor get an equal share of the command."[1]

REFERENCES

1. International Telecommunication Union (ITU), 2005. "*Digital Reach*".
2. NER Data Bank, 2006.
3. CB Mazumder and Paramita Saha (2008), *Ageing in North East India, Tripura Perspective.* Akansha Publishing House, New Delhi.
4. A Lunununsang AO, (2007) *Ageing in North-East India, Nagaland Perspective.* Akansha Publishing House, New Delhi.
5. Village of Old Age; Tarasanika Society in Assam www.tarasanikasociety.org

6. R.M. Pant (2008), *Ageing in North-East, Arunachal Perspective.* Akansha Publishing House, New Delhi.

7. Devi, S. Dayabati and Bagga, Amrita, *Ageing in Women. A Study in North-East India.*

8. Lianzela, Valalchhawna (2007), *Ageing in North East India, Magnitude of the Problem of Elderly Persons in Mizoram,* Akansha Publishing House, New Delhi.

9. De, Utpal Kumar and Ghosh, Bhola Nath; *Status of Women in the Rural Khasi Society of Meghalaya.*

10. Telecom Journal *'Data Link'*, March 2008.

11. Techno Economic Study made by Telecom professionals, (Unpublished, 2008).

12. Ketshukietuo Dziivichu, *Health Problems of the Aged among the Angami Nagas.*

13. J. Barrs (1991), *The Challenge of Critical Gerontology.*

14. Thomas L. Friedman, *The World is Flat.*

15. Modi Ishwar, *Ageing, Human Development,* pp. 244-254.

16. *Speculations in Science & Technology: An International Journal for Innovation & Creativity,* Vol.19 No.1, March, 1996, Computers in the fight against Aging.

17. *Freedom: Sixty Years after Indian Independence,* Art and Heritage Foundation, 2007.

10

A Geographical Perspective on the Patterns of Aging in North-East India with Special Reference to the Tribal Areas

Debendra Kumar Nayak

Introduction

Few areas of research in social sciences, particularly in demography, have received as much attention in recent years as aging. The subject is attracting increasing attention from Indian social scientists too. This is not surprising considering the phenomenal increase in the proportion of the aged population as noticed since the results of Census of India 1991 was made public.

While aging research is fairly well developed and well documented in Europe and other developed countries including Japan, not much interest in the past was shown by scholars and policy makers in most Asian countries including India. The reasons are not far to seek. This lack of research on aging in Asia relates to the firm belief that the robustness and continuance of the family system "is and will continue to be a full proof insurance against all problems faced during old age" (Dhar Chakraborty 2004: 26). But we are now slowly waking up to the reality that joint family, long held as our answer to the problems of aging, is neither as widespread as popularly believed, nor does it seem capable of accommodating pressures created by demands of a modern urban and industrialized lifestyle.

Initially observed in the more developed countries, the process of aging is now rapidly approaching the developing world. Although not a global phenomenon yet, various predictions indicate that population aging is going to become a major global issue in years to come. Virtually all countries will face population aging, albeit with varying intensity and at different points of time. The inter-generational balance seen today may not be observed in future. The changing balance between age groups would make the aged more of a burden on society and as resources are diverted from the young to the old, the world may experience unpleasant inter-generational conflicts and tensions. With improvements in life expectancy (and these improvements will take place at a faster rate for females than for males) there is, and will be, a progressive aging of the older population, and interestingly a majority of them will be females.

The issues that are likely to be confronted by all developing nation-states include the implications of an ageing population for socio-economic development programmes, health care, savings, investments, consumption patterns, work force participation, migration and social security. It may also include the role of the family in supporting the aged. According to Dhar Chakraborty, "...when the Western world is reshaping the world for the elderly, in order to contain costs as well as to mitigate the inter generational conflict, many Asian countries have barely begun to think about their elderly, and given the pace of population aging in Asia and the corresponding lack of adjustment mechanism, a 'time bomb' and 'agequake' may not be very far" (2004: 27).

The ongoing process of demographic transition is having—and will continue to have—profound effects on the size and age structure of its population. Slower pace of population growth has been an important factor in significant alteration in the age structure of the population. Globally, the share of the young is falling and that of the elderly rising- a process termed as aging. However all countries and regions are not experiencing these changes uniformly. Different countries and regions are at varying stages of this demographic transition. In most advanced countries, the aging process is already well under way, and it is expected that a number of developing countries in East and Southeast Asia and central and Eastern Europe will also experience significant aging from about 2020. In other developing countries, however, the demographic transition is less advanced.

Prior to 1900, the world population growth was relatively slow. The age structure of the population too was broadly constant. Fewer people lived beyond age 65. Dramatic changes in life expectancy that was witnessed during the first half of the twentieth century resulted in unprecedented population growth. This unprecedented population increment however did not significantly alter the age structure of the population at least in the initial period. But phenomenal drop in the fertility rates in the second half of the twentieth century significantly slowed down population growth resulting in a decline in the share of the young in the population with a corresponding rise in the share of the elderly. The last century thus has proved to be a watershed in terms of significant demographic transformation of the global population. The most significant of all developments is the phenomenal increment to the total size of the global population accompanied by unprecedented hike in population growth rate—a demographic event unlikely to be replicated in the coming years.

The spatial pattern of population growth was however not uniform across the developed and the less developed countries. Most developed countries had by the middle of the 20th century, witnessed major reduction in both in death rates and then in birth rates leading to not only slower population growth but also a phenomenal decline in child population. Population began to age in such countries. In sharp contrast, the less developed countries continued to experience high fertility rates in spite of large decline in mortality and significant rise in life expectancy particularly in the post World War years. This contrasting population transitions resulted in significant population redistribution across countries and continents.

By the early 21st Century a larger number of countries have joined the ranks of low fertility regime leading to a worldwide fall in growth rates to about 1.2 per cent per annum and is expected to fall further in years to come as more and more countries shall experience lower fertility. A net outcome of this vital demographic transformation is the slow but a definite change from more youthful societies in many countries to more demographically mature populations- a phenomenon variously described as the process of aging or greying. In strict demographic terms, the nations witnessing these transitions will be relieved of child dependency to a great extent while they will be faced with a greater burden of old-age dependency. This shift of dependency as reflected in the changing age-structure of such nations may be similar in quantity- decrease in child dependency compensated by increase in old age dependency- but not in quality. It may be noted that the increase in life expectancy is not only due to greater life expectancy among the younger age-group but also rising life expectancy of the older segment.

A significant fact about aging is that it increases the total number of aged persons compared to other age groups and that the pace of this change is more rapid now in developing rather than the developed countries. Though all countries in the developing world have not uniformly received the full impact of this rise in the proportion of the aged and a corresponding decline in the young age population, it is expected that nearly all countries will experience, by the beginning of the next century, a gradual demographic shift towards an older segment exceeding the proportion of the young for the first time in history (UNFPA: 1998) - a situation that has already taken roots in more developed countries.

The aging process in India is no exception but reveals remarkable regional diversity in the manifestation of the process. India presents baffling diversity in its cultural, linguistic, racial and ethnic composition. Modernization and globalization have led to a widening of the gap between the rich and the poor and has enhanced the differences in access to social and economic opportunities and resources available to different sections of the society. The resulting intensification of competition among the groups for societal resources has adversely affected older people, especially the poor, who are more vulnerable than others to social and economic hardships. Pervasive poverty and inequalities of income, coupled with a very inadequate safety net, has meant that a majority of older persons become marginalized or even destitute. The poor among the elderly people have been losing out even as economic development is taking place in the country as a whole. It is important therefore that the aging process and its impact on society be understood well, so that appropriate measures may be undertaken to minimize the negative effects and to develop appropriate policies and programmes for the welfare of older persons. As the United Nations in its International Plan of Action on Aging of 1982 states: 'Countries should recognize and take into account their demographic trends and changes in the structure of their populations in order to optimize their development' (United Nations: 1999).

The present study aims at assessing the dimension of aging among the tribal population in the Northeast India, a region which experiences a peculiar demographic situation of continuously high fertility rate coupled with an increase in life expectancy resulting in a sizeable number of old people in the total population. However this trend is not spatially or socially uniform calling for a geographical perspective on the problem. The areas which have experienced a demographic transition are already experiencing a significant alteration in the age structure that contains a sizeable proportion of aged people and declining proportion of child population. The case of Kerala, Himachal Pradesh and a few states in South India can be cited as examples of this nature of a transition. But this is not true of the Northeast India where the fertility rate continues to be high despite a significant decline in mortality. Interestingly the fertility and mortality indicators illustrate that in some of the states the socio-demographic conditions are at par or close to that of the more developed Indian states such as Kerala. Recent survey data indicate that fertility level has improved in all the states following better health facilities and longer life expectancy. The decline in mortality has been a response to improved medical facility and better spatial coverage in the provision of health care. But the fertility rate has not responded adequately to these improvements and continues to be extremely high in areas that support a sizeable tribal population. As is well known, the Northeast part of India has very high concentration of scheduled tribes in the hilly areas. The only areas where the tribes are less in number are the plains consisting of the Brahmaputra and Barak valley and the Imphal basin as well as the Tripura plains. The demographic reality coupled with tribal values and social customs create a new situation with these changes in the demographic structure overtaking the tribal areas in recent times. The present study aims at assessing the nature of demographic transition unfolding in these areas with regard to the process of aging.

The Region

The Northeast region is taken as the study area. All the seven states included in the region are taken into consideration while assessing the problems of the aged through a spatio-temporal study. The rationale for selecting the region has been the region's peculiarity of demographic reality unfolding in the region in sharp contrast to other regions of the country. The other most important consideration is the fact that the region has a very large concentration of scheduled tribes who have been exposed to urbanization in recent times only. Topographically, much of the region consists of hills and plateaus although some parts are located in plains notably, the Brahmaputra and Barak plains, the Manipur basin and the Tripura Plains. Economically the region continues to be characterized by subsistence agriculture and the Hills have the practice of shifting cultivation. Socially and culturally the region presents extreme diversity characterized by tribal cultures in the hills and peasant culture in much of the plains. The tribal culture extends to the plains too though in many cases the tribal people living in the plains have been assimilated to the peasant cultures in some very important ways.

The region presents the complexities of the sub-Himalayan ranges, the Indo-Burmese hills of Nagaland, Manipur and Mizoram and the eroded surfaces of the Meghalaya plateau, all encircling the Brahmaputra valley. The hills are sharply marked from the plains, physically as well as culturally, though so linked that to some extent they must be treated together (Spate and Learmonth: 1972). The boundary between the hills and the plains often present themselves as demographic boundaries too. The region presents itself as a replica of the subcontinent both physically as well as culturally, only on a much smaller scale. The northern mountains are in fact an extension of the Himalayan ranges with modification introduced in the erosional features due to much heavier rainfall. The Indo-Burmese hills are much less imposing as a relief feature. Parts of Tripura and Imphal valley represent area of low relief. The Assam valley is an alluvial expanse laid down by the mighty Brahmaputra and its numerous tributaries. The Meghalaya and Karbi Plateau, a fragment of the peninsular block, is a highly dissected tract.

The overall geographical setting of the region has provided an ideal habitat for a legion of tribal communities. "...the tribes of the Northeast India have a world of their own. Having lived in the marchland between India and China and in the triangle where the Indian and the Chinese worlds meet, they have picked up the impression that they belong to none" (Ahmad: 1983). The peculiarity of the geographical and historical conditions of this region has offered relative isolation to the culture groups who found their way into the region through passes from the north and the east. The northern and eastern mountain ranges and the southern plateau understandably provide more suitable tribal habitats compared to the Brahmaputra valley. However, the valley has not been totally averse to tribal people in providing them with a habitat. They have found suitable sites for settlement in the isolated hill features, forested portions of the valley and in marshy tracts. The northern bank of the river as well as the river islands still retains their predominantly tribal character. The area of the transition between the hills and the plains of Brahmaputra is also largely tribal in its ethnic composition. The plain tribals "generally represent the spill over communities from the hilly regions except for the Bodos who are a big tribal group largely confined to the plains (Sharma: 1984).

Aging in India

Incidentally, the growth rate of the elderly population is more rapid in developing countries like India compared many developed countries. The elderly population in India is the second largest in the world, next only to China and the older population has been steadily increasing in number and proportion. This segment numbered only 12.1 million in the year 1901 and it increased to 24.7 million by the year 1961. The 2001 Census recorded 77 million elderly people in India (7.5% of the total population) which is projected to reach around 137 million by the year 2021. In a country where bulk of the population lives in rural areas, 3 out of every 4 elderly persons actually lives in rural areas. The fact that the elderly population is growing at a phenomenal rate in India is borne out from their annual growth rate (3%) which far exceeds the growth rate of the total population (1.9%). The proportion of the elderly population is likely to exceed the proportion in the child age group by the year 2050 as projected by the UN. The population of India is aging in two ways: (i) aging at the base due to lower fertility and (ii) aging at the apex due to reduced mortality and dramatic increase in life expectancy. The index of aging (see Notes) has consequently increased from a mere 14.31 in the year 1901 to 22.7 in the year 2001. The analysis of historical patterns of mortality and fertility decline in India indicates that the process of population aging intensified only in the 1990's (Bose and Kapoor: 2004)

Looking at regional variations, Bose found that three states in India, namely Uttar Pradesh, Maharashtra and Bihar had more than 5 million persons in the 60+ category. It may be noted that in most of the states the population of 60+ males exceeded that of 60+ females, particularly in Bihar, Madhya Pradesh, Rajasthan and Uttar Pradesh. But in Kerala, Maharashtra, Andhra Pradesh, Karnataka and Gujarat, the 60+ female populations exceeded the 60+ male populations. Kerala had the highest proportion of 60+ population followed by Himachal Pradesh, Punjab, Haryana and Tamil Nadu. Among major states, the lowest proportion was in Assam followed by West Bengal, Bihar, Rajasthan, Gujarat, Madhya Pradesh, Andhra Pradesh and Uttar Pradesh.

Aging in the Northeast

The process of population aging, though less in magnitude than other states, has already begun in the Northeastern region. The population of persons aged 60 or over has almost doubled to 1.7 million persons by the year 1991. In some states like Manipur, Meghalaya and Mizoram, the growth rate of 60-plus persons has been faster than that of the overall population. Majority of the elderly persons in a great number of states are males. In terms of birth rate, total fertility rate (TFR), death rate, infant mortality (IMR) and life expectancy at birth, there have been welcome improvements over the years. It may thus be interesting to analyse the patterns in the process of aging in the region with respect to a few important indicators of aging. The indicators include (see Notes) the proportion of people in the age group of 60 and over, the aging index, the potential support ratio, old age dependency rate and the total dependency rate. The patterns have been identified by taking the districts which are dominantly inhabited by the tribal segment of the population. The ethnic divide in population admirably corresponds to a physical division of the region into the hilly and the plain areas, though with a few exceptions. The former category corresponds to the tribal areas while the latter is largely confined to the non-tribal population.

Overall Pattern

Inter-district variation in the process of aging in the Northeast region is analyzed below with the help of a series of tables for the region as a whole.

Table-1
Northeast: Distribution of districts in aged (60+) category, 1971-2001

% aged	*1971*		*1991*		*2001*	
	Males	*Females*	*Males*	*Females*	*Males*	*Females*
2-2.9	0 (00.0)	0 (00.0)	0 (00.0)	2 (02.8)	1 (01.4)	1 (01.4)
3-3.9	5 (06.9)	15 (20.8)	5 (06.9)	10 (13.8)	4 (05.5)	7 (09.7)
4-4.9	27 (37.5)	19 (26.4)	21 (29.2)	30 (41.7)	15 (20.8)	18 (25.0)
5-5.9	18 (25.0)	25 (34.7)	24 (33.3)	17 (23.7)	31 (43.1)	24 (33.3)
6-6.9	17 (23.7)	13 (18.1)	16 (22.2)	9 (12.5)	17 (23.7)	14 (19.4)
7-7.9	02 (02.8)	0 (00.0)	5 (06.9)	4 (05.5)	4 (05.5)	6 (08.4)
8-8.9	0 (00.0)	0 (00.0)	1 (01.4)	0 (00.0)	0 (00.0)	2 (02.8)
9-9.9	03 (04.2)	0 (00.0)	0 (00.0)	0 (00.0)	0 (00.0)	0 (00.0)
Total	72 (100)	72 (100)	72 (100)	72 (100)	72 (100)	72 (100)

Source: Census of India, 1971, 1991 and 2001
Figures in parentheses indicate the percentage of districts in each class.

Table-1 reveals the percentage of the aged (60+) for both males and females for the year 1971, 1991 and 2001. It is evident that the proportion of the aged in the population is less than 3 % only for females in the year 1991 in two districts whereas in the year 2001, one districts each contained a very low proportion of aged population, below three per cent. It is difficult to believe that there is a decline in the absolute old population in these districts over the years. The fall in the proportion of the aged in a few districts is due to excessive increase in child population in these districts characterized by a stable or relatively slow increase in the aged population. It is also evident from the table that in a larger number of districts the aged females constitute a smaller proportion compared to the males. For instance the aged males constituted less than 5 per cent of the population in about 45 per cent of the 72 districts in 1971 compared to a little over 46 per cent such districts in case of the females. The relative position in 1991 changed dramatically as only 36 per cent districts had less than 5 per cent aged population among the males compared to over 58 per cent districts in which aged females accounted for less than 5 per cent. Though the number of districts with a lower proportion of the aged declined overall, the male female disparity in aging however persisted. In a little over 27 per cent of all districts, the aged males constituted less than 5 per cent of the population in contrast to 37 per cent districts in which female aged were few. This shows that the gender gap in aging was lower up to 1971, then increased substantially by the year 1991 and shows a decline thereafter. In a large number of districts the female survival beyond 60 years of age was less compared to that of the males. The aged females constituted a very low proportion (below 8 per cent) in the year 1971. The situation marginally changed in the year 1991 as in some districts the proportion of the aged females increased to 9 per cent. By the year 2001 the aged female component increased in more districts. Interestingly there are no districts in 1971where the proportion of the aged for both the sexes falls below 2 per cent, but there are a few such districts in 1991 and 2001. These districts are mostly located in Arunachal Pradesh and Meghalaya. As many as 15 districts in 1971 contained a very low proportion of the aged females (4% or less). The number of such districts however came down to 10 only in 1991 and further reduced to 7 in 2001.These districts are mostly located in Assam, Nagaland, Arunachal Pradesh and Meghalaya. Most of the districts with a greater proportion of the aged are located in parts of Arunachal Pradesh, Mizoram, Nagaland, Assam and Meghalaya. Significantly number of districts with a greater proportion of aged females is more in the year 2001 compared to males. For example, there are 8 districts in which the proportion of aged females exceeds 7 per cent. However, in the case of males, the number of such districts is only 4. The extent of inter district variation in the proportion of the aged population has registered a phenomenal increase over the years and it is much more for the female segment than for the males.

Aged population, particularly among the women is very high, i.e. above 6 per cent in districts of Tripura along with some districts of Manipur, Arunachal Pradesh, Nagaland, Assam and parts of Meghalaya. It is significant that distribution of these districts are highly scattered in the region and hence do not indicate impact of regional factors for such changes in demographic structure.

Table-2

Northeast: Distribution of districts in aging index classes, 1971-2001

Ageing	*1971*		*1991*		*2001*	
Index (%)	*Males*	*Females*	*Males*	*Females*	*Males*	*Females*
4-7.9	15 (20.8)	13 (18.1)	12 (16.6)	22 (30.5)	2 (02.8)	3 (04.1)
8-11.9	42 (58.3)	48 (66.7)	54 (75.0)	44 (61.1)	16 (22.2)	21 (29.2)
12-15.9	12 (16.7)	11 (15.2)	6 (08.4)	6 (08.4)	26 (36.1)	21 (29.2)
16-19.9	3 (04.2)	0 (00.0)	0 (00.0)	0 (00.0)	20 (27.7)	21 (29.2)
20-23.9	0 (00.0)	0 (00.0)	0 (00.0)	0 (00.0)	7 (09.8)	4 (05.5)
24-27.9	0 (00.0)	0 (00.0)	0 (00.0)	0 (00.0)	1 (01.4)	2 (02.8)
Total	72 (100)	72 (100)	72 (100)	72 (100)	72 (100)	72 (100)

Source: Census of India, 1971, 1991 and 2001
Figures in parentheses indicate the percentage of districts in each class.

The aging index is calculated as the number of persons 60 years or over per hundred persons under age 15. The ageing index is a much more sensitive index of aging as it shows the proportion of the aged relative to the young age population. Table-2 clearly reveals a drastic fall in the number of districts with a lower aging index over the years. But the fall in the number of such districts in case of males is more uniform, but not in case of the females. The number of districts with lower ageing index indeed registered substantial increase by the year 1991 as far as the females are concerned, but fell significantly by the year 2001. Districts characterized by low aging index (4-7.9%) for both males and females in the year 1971 included nearly whole of Meghalaya; most of Arunachal Pradesh and few districts in Assam. Only a handful of districts in the year 2001 recorded very low aging index both for males and females. While none of the districts in the year 1971 had an aging index in excess of 20 per cent. Significantly none of the districts in the year 1991 had an aging index above 16 per cent indicating a decline in ageing index over 1971 and this is true for both the sexes. The situation underwent unprecedented changes in the year 2001 when the ageing index showed substantive improvement with over 11 and 8 per cent districts in the region recording an index of over 20 per cent for the males and females respectively. This index is close to the national average of 22.7 per cent in these districts.

Table-3
Distribution of districts in total dependency ratio classes, 1971-2001

Total Dependency Ratio	*1971*	*1991*	*2001*
50-50.9	0(00.0)	1(01.4)	3(04.2)
60-60.9	3(04.2)	5(06.9)	11(15.3)
70-70.9	11(15.3)	24(33.3)	23(31.9)
80-80.9	15(20.8)	29(40.3)	24(33.3)
90-90.9	19(26.4)	9(12.6)	9(12.5)
100-109.9	15(20.8)	4(05.5)	2(02.8)
110-119.9	9(12.5)	0(00.0)	0(00.0)
Total	72(100)	72(100)	72(100)

Source: Census of India, 1971, 1991 and 2001
Figures in parentheses indicate the percentage of districts in each class.

The total Dependency ratio is the number of persons under the age 15 plus persons aged 60 or older per one hundred persons in the age cohort of 15 to 60+. It is the sum of the youth and old-age dependency ratio.

Young Age Dependency Ratio is based on age group of 0-14 years and Old Age Dependency Ratio is based on age group of 60+ years. Hence, if the level of fertility is high, large proportion of the population will be in the non working age group 0-14 years resulting in higher dependency ratios. On the other hand if the life expectancy improves, a large proportion of the old age population will increase old age dependency. Thus the total dependency ratio generally indicates economic burden on the adult population which has to support these two dependent segments. Table-3 shows a generally declining number of districts over the years with higher dependency ratio. This means that in a large number of districts the overall dependence on the adult population is on the decline. In case the population is aging, overall dependence normally declines. This seems to be happening in a number of districts particularly after 1991. In 2001; total dependency ratio is below 80 per cent in over 50 per cent districts. The proportion of such districts was 41 per cent in 1991 and a meager 19.5 per cent in 1971. On the other hand the total dependency ratio continued to be exceedingly high (over 80) in as much as 48 per cent districts in 2001, though it declined from 58 per cent districts in 1991.

Table-4

Distribution of districts in different old age dependency ratio classes, 1971-2001

Old Age Dependence Ratio	*1971*	*1991*	*2001*
2-5.9	0(00.0)	0(00.0)	2(02.8)
6-9.9	17(23.7)	11(15.3)	50(69.4)
10-13.9	34(47.2)	35(48.6)	18(25.0)
14-17.9	18(25.0)	17(23.7)	2(02.8)
18-21.9	3(04.2)	8(23.7)	0(00.0)
22-25.9	0(00.0)	1(01.4)	0(00.0)
Total	72(100)	72(100)	72(100)

Source: Census of India, 1971, 1991 and 2001

Figures in parentheses indicate the percentage of districts in each class.

Old age Dependency Ratio is the ratio taken as the number of persons 60/65 years and over per one hundred persons in 15-60 years of age. Table 4 reveals a generally decreasing proportion of districts with higher old age dependence. This is contrary to what happens in a situation when the population is aging. Given that the total dependency is on the decline alongside declining old age dependency in a large number of districts poses an ironical situation with regard to the complex nature of ageing in this region. This is indicative of the fact that in many districts the adult population is growing at a much faster rate than the growth taking place in old age population. In 1971 there were a few districts with higher (over 18 per 100) old age dependency ratio. However, in 2001 no district shows such a high level of dependence.

Table-5
Northeast: Distribution of districts in potential support ratio classes, 1971-2001

Potential Support Ratio	*1971*	*1991*	*2001*
6-8.9	23(31.9)	13(18.2)	17(23.7)
9-11.9	25(34.7)	40(55.5)	40(55.5)
12-14.9	21(29.2)	14(19.4)	12(16.6)
15-17.9	3(04.2)	5(06.9)	2(02.8)
18-20.9	0(00.0)	0(00.0)	1(01.4)
Total	72(100)	72(100)	72(100)

Source: Census of India, 1971, 1991 and 2001
Figures in parentheses indicate the percentage of districts in each class.

The Potential Support Ratio is the number of persons aged 15-60 per every person aged 60 or older. This is exact opposite of old age dependency ratio. Table 5 reveals an increasing proportion of districts with lower potential support. In a great majority of districts (nearly 80%) the potential support ratio in 2001 is below 12 per aged. The proportion of such districts was lower at 74 per cent in 1991 and 67 per cent in 1971. Interestingly at least one district has experienced a large increase in potential support in the year 2001.

The Tribes

Needless to mention the hilly areas in the Northeast as also elsewhere in India comprise mostly of the tribal population. Thus the districts by and large located in the hills contain ethnically differentiated population as compared to the plains which contain a sizeable proportion of the non-tribal segment. There are 38 districts mostly located in the Arunachal, Naga, Mizo and Manipur hills, Meghalaya plateau, parts of Tripura and Assam containing over 50 per cent tribal population in their total.

Table-6

Northeast: Ageing in areas of tribal dominance: average for districts

	1971	*1991*	*2001*
% aged	5.3	4.8	5
Ageing Index	9.9	8.6	13.3
PSR	10.5	12.6	11.9
Old-age dependency	13.1	12.6	8.9
Total dependency	86.8	78.5	77.6

Source: Census of India, 1971, 1991 and 2001

As is evident from table-6, the tribal and hilly areas show the aging process to be highly muted owing largely to a very high fertility rate experienced in the tribal segment. The proportion of the aged in the year 1971, going by the districts average, was 5.3 per cent as against 5.1 percent in the non-tribal population (see Nayak: 2007) indicating a greater proportion of the aged population among the tribal segment. But the situation changed over the years and the proportion of the aged declined to 4.8 per cent by the year 1991 and marginally increased to 5 per cent of the total population by the turn of the present century. The aged among the males showed a decline over the years in terms of their proportion. So is the case with the females.

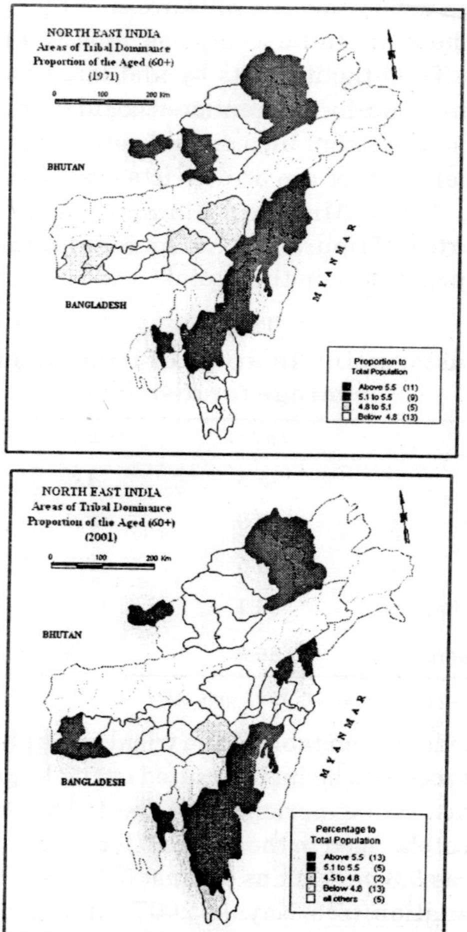

Fig 1: Changes in the Proportion of the Aged in Tribal Areas of the Northeast-1971-2001

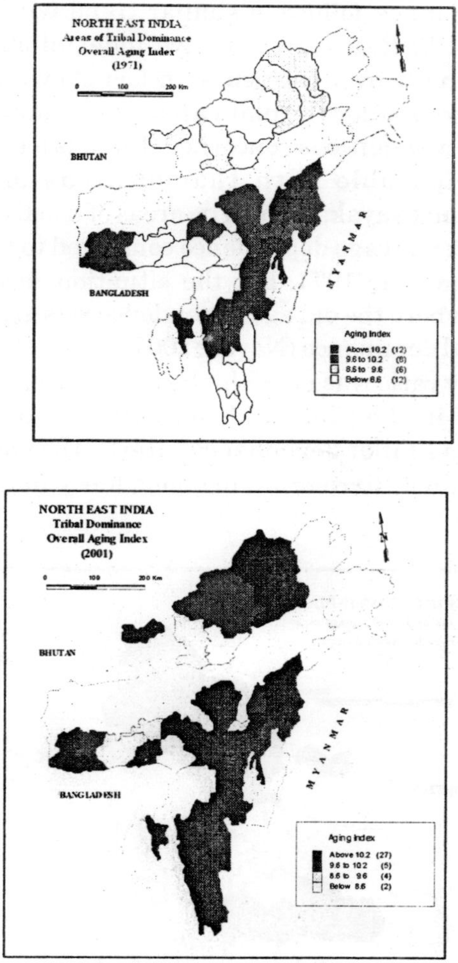

Fig. 2: Changes in the spatial Patterns in Ageing index in the Tribal Areas of the Northeast, 1971-2001

This situation is reflected in the aging index too which experienced a fall during the 1971-1991 period and increased marginally to 13.3 in the year 2001. The aging index of the females remains lower than that of the males in all the years though the index follows a similar trend with the overall. The overall PSR, a very sensitive index of aging changed only marginally over the years, in fact showing an upward trend unlike that for the plain areas. As regards the old age and total dependence is concerned, there is a general falling trend comparable with that of areas of non-tribal concentration (Nayak: 2007). The areas of tribal concentration had a greater old age dependence compared to the non-tribal areas in the year 1971, but the situation reversed by the year 2001 where the old age dependence was greater in areas of non-tribal dominance (Nayak: 2007). Interestingly the total dependency ratio was much higher in the areas of non-tribal dominance in the year 1971 but both the areas exhibited more or less similar dependency ratio by the year 2001. This reveals a much sharper fall in dependency in the non-tribal areas.

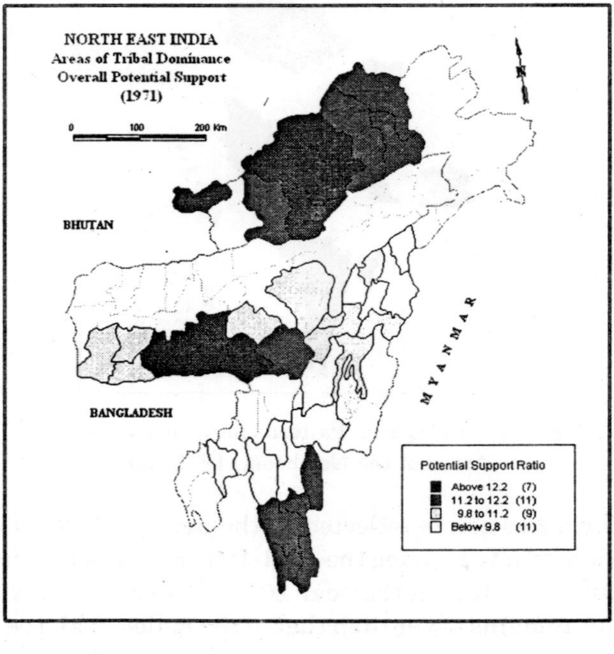

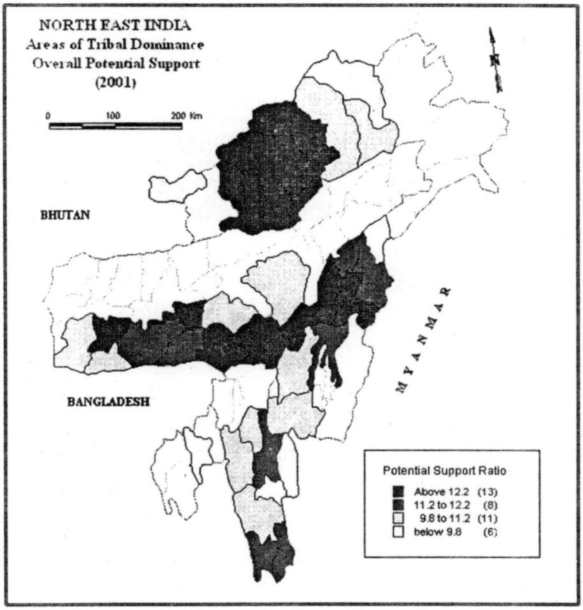

Fig.3 Changes in Potential Support Ratio in Tribal Areas of the Northeast, 1971-2001

Inter district variation in the proportion of the aged (figure-1) in the areas of tribal concentration shows a general fall in the percentage of the aged during 1971 and 2001. It ranges between 3.8 per cent in Lower Subansiri to a high of 8 per cent in Mon. By the year 2001, it ranged between 3.2 per cent in Dimapur to 7.8 per cent in Upper Siang. This is despite an increase in the number of the aged in all the districts. Such a situation has resulted from an increase in birth rate swelling up the proportion in the young age group. It is significant that the proportion of the aged remained stagnant or declined in a majority of 20 out of 38 districts. In fact the decline took place in over 40 per cent (16) districts.

Table-7
Tribal Areas: Distribution of Districts in Aged (60+) Category, 1971-2001

% aged	*1971*		*1991*		*2001*	
	Males	*Females*	*Males*	*Females*	*Males*	*Females*
2-2.9	0 (00.0)	0 (00.0)	0 (00.0)	2 (05.3)	1 (02.7)	2 (05.3)
3-3.9	3 (07.9)	6 (15.8)	2 (05.3)	8 (21.0)	4 (10.5)	6 (15.8)
4-4.9	15 (39.5)	11 (28.9)	18 (47.4)	16 (42.1)	12 (31.5)	13 (34.3)
5-5.9	8 (21.0)	14 (36.8)	10 (26.2)	8 (21.0)	15 (39.5)	11 (28.9)
6-6.9	8 (21.0)	7 (18.5)	5 (13.1)	2 (05.3)	5 (13.1)	4 (10.5)
7-7.9	1 (02.7)	0 (00.0)	2 (05.3)	2 (05.3)	6 (15.7)	2 (05.3)
8-8.9	0 (00.0)	0(00.0)	1(02.7)	0(00.0)	0(00.0)	0(00.0)
9-9.9	3 (07.9)	0 (00.0)	0 (00.0)	0 (00.0)	0 (00.0)	0 (00.0)
Total	38 (100)	38 (100)	38 (100)	38 (100)	38 (100)	38 (100)

Source: Census of India, 1971, 1991 and 2001
Figures in parentheses indicate the percentage of districts in each class.

Table-7 shows male female comparison in the distribution of districts with regard to the proportion of the aged in these districts. This reveals even a larger fall in the proportion of female aged in a great number of districts by the year 1991. The proportion of the aged in the year 2001 shows improvement in extremely few districts and is true for both males as well as females.

Going by aging index (fig-2), a simıլar trend and pattern becomes far too evident. The range of variation has indeed widened over the years. The ageing index in 1971 varied between 6.7 in Subansiri, upper Subansiri and Papum Pare to14.6 in Tuensang and Zuneboto. By the year 2001, the index ranged between 5.7 in Papum Pare to a high of 20.4 in Upper Siang. The index registered a decline in 6 districts mostly located in Naga Hills and a few districts of Arunachal Pradesh and Meghalaya. The remaining districts however recorded some increase in the aging index, the most spectacular increase being noticed in a few districts of Arunachal Pradesh and Mizoram.

Table-8
Tribal Areas: Distribution of Districts in Aging Index Classes, 1971-2001

Ageing	*1971*		*1991*		*2001*	
Index (%)	*Males*	*Females*	*Males*	*Females*	*Males*	*Females*
4-7.9	12 (31.5)	6 (15.8)	9 (23.7)	14 (36.8)	2 (05.4)	12 (31.5)
8-11.9	18 (47.5)	27 (71.1)	27 (71.0)	21 (55.3)	12 (31.5)	23 (60.6)
12-15.9	5 (13.1)	5 (13.1)	2 (05.3)	3 (07.9)	11 (28.9)	3 (07.9)
16-19.9	3 (07.9)	0 (00.0)	0 (00.0)	0 (00.0)	12 (31.5)	0 (00.0)
20-23.9	0 (00.0)	0 (00.0)	0 (00.0)	0 (00.0)	1 (02.7)	0 (0.00)
Total	38 (100)	38 (100)	38 (100)	38 (100)	38 (100)	38 (100)

Source: Census of India, 1971, 1991 and 2001

Figures in parentheses indicate the percentage of districts in each class.

Table-8 reveals that the aging index has increased for the males in a large number of districts by the year 2001, but has shown a decline in a majority of districts as far as females are concerned.

In terms of PSR (fig-3), the 1971 data reveals a range of 6.8 in Mon, Tuensang and Zuneboto to 14.8 in Lower Subansiri. In the year 2001 the PSR shows a general rise with a range of 6.9 in Upper Siang to a high of 25.7 in Papum Pare. Significantly the PSR index increased in 25 of the 38 districts and declined in the remaining 13 districts. Increase in PSR index in such a large number of districts is indicative of substantial rise in the proportion of the population in working age group in relation to the rise in old age population. The total dependency rate registered a fall in a vast majority of districts numbering 27 whereas nearly all the districts barring three registered an increase in the old age dependency.

Discussion and Conclusion

Demographic parameters in the Northeastern region of India have improved remarkably reflecting interesting patterns over space. Population ageing has slowly but surely manifested itself against a background of continued high fertility in the region. However, the patterns are highly varied within different sub regions and among different ethnic categories making it a highly complex phenomenon not lending itself to an easy explanation.

In terms of the proportion of the elderly population the entire region lags behind the country average of 7.6 per cent. The areas of tribal concentration show a very low proportion of elderly population in the total. The most significant aspect of aging in the hilly and tribal areas refers to the fact of a declining trend in the proportion of elderly population over the three decades, which is surely linked to continued high fertility among the tribal segment. There is only a marginal increase in the proportion of the tribal elderly population since 1991.

Unlike the all India average, the proportion of the aged among the female segment is lower than that of their male counterpart in the Northeast. The elderly among the tribal males constitutes a higher proportion than their female counterparts in all the years. The gap however is reducing over the years.

If one goes by the most sensitive index of aging, i.e. aging index, it is significant to note that the aging process seems to have picked up momentum since the year 1991 in the country as a whole, but is weak in the case of the areas of tribal concentration as evident in such areas of the Northeastern region of the country. There has been indeed a fall in the aging index till the year 1991.

In terms of PSR, the areas of tribal concentration show a reverse situation of increasing PSR over the years. This is indicative of an increasingly larger proportion of adult population compared to the aged in the areas of tribal concentration. In terms of dependency, there has been a general decline in both the indicators over the years.

Going by international standards and comparing with the developed countries which have a longer history of aging it is expected that countries /regions beginning to age should experience an increase in the proportion of the aged, in aging index and in old age dependency ratio, while there should be a fall in potential support ratio and total dependency ratio. The patterns observed in the Northeast, particularly in the areas of tribal concentration do not conform to these parameters with equal vigour. The hilly and tribal areas experience an increase in aging index only. The proportion of the aged in the total population is showing signs of an increase in recent years only and the PSR too is showing some signs of falling in most recent years. All these indicators only suggest the beginning of the aging process in hilly and tribal areas. This is supported by a drastic fall in total dependency ratio, but contradicted by equally drastic fall in old age dependency ratio. These features are perhaps common to a population that has just begun to experience aging.

NOTES

Elderly Population = 60/64+ years Aging Index (AI):=(Elderly Population/ Youth Population)* 100

Old age Dependency Ratio (OADR):= (Elderly Population/Working Population)*100

Potential Support Ratio (PSR):=(Working Population/Elderly Population)

Total Dependency Ratio (TDR):=(Young Population+ Elderly Population)/ Working Population * 100

REFERENCES

Ahmad, A. (1983) "Education of the Scheduled Tribes: Some Aspects of Inequality", *Workshop on Indicators of Equity in Education,* October 24-28, NIEPA, New Delhi (mimeo)

Bagchi, K. (ed) (1997) *Elderly Females in India.* Society for Gerontological Research and HelpAge India, New Delhi.

Bagchi, K. (1998) "Some important areas of Gerontological Research in India", *Research and Development Journal,* 4, (2)3, HelpAge India.

Bali, A. (1997) "Elderly females: an ignored silent majority" in Bagchi, K. (ed), *Elderly Females in India,* Society for Gerontological Research and HelpAge India, New Delhi, Chapter 2.

Bali, A. (ed). (1999*a*). *Understanding Greying People of India,* ICSSR, Inter-India Publications, New Delhi.

Bali, A. (1999*b*) "Introduction" in Bali, A. (ed). *Understanding Greying People of India,* ICSSR, Inter-India Publications, New Delhi,

Bhat, Anitha Kumari and Dhruvarajan, Raj (2001) "Ageing In India: Drifting Intergenerational Relations, Challenges and Options" *Ageing and Society* 21, 2001, 621±640.

Bose, Ashis (2000) "Demographic Transition" Paper presented in *Ageing: a Symposium on the graying of our society* Downloaded from website *http://www.india-seminar.com/2000/488.htm*

Bose, Ashish and Shankardass Mala Kapur (2002) *Growing Old in India: Voices Reveal, Statistics Speak*, B. R. Publishing Corporation, New Delhi.

Dhar Chakraborty, Rajagopal. 2004. *The Greying of India*. New Delhi: Sage.

International Moneytary Fund (IMF) (2004) *IMF World Economic Outlook*, Downloaded from website www.imf.org/external/pubs/ft/weo/2004/02/

Lee, Ronald (2007) *The Economic Implications of Changing Age-Structure* Downloaded from website www.un.org/esa/population/cpd2007/presentations/lee.hz.shr.ppt

Leete, R. and Jacobs, T (2002) "The Older Poor and the Excluded in the Developing World" in *Situation and Voice: The Older Poor and Excluded in South Africa and Indias*, United Nations Population Fund, Population and Development Strategies Series No.2. New York.

Nayak, D.K. (2007) *A Geographical Perspective on the Trends and Patterns in Ageing in India with a Special Reference to the Northeastern Region*. Research Monograph No. GE/UGC/DKN/7. Department of Geography, North Eastern Hill University, Shillong.

National Institutes of Health, Washington, DC (2007) *Why Population Ageing Matters: A Global Perspective* downloaded from website http://www.state.gov/g/oes/rls/or/81537.htm#over

Robyn Stone, "The Feminization of Poverty Among the Elderly", in *Women The New York Times* (13 October 1998), pp. A1 and A8.(quoted in U.N. Economic and Social Council, 1999, *Gender and Ageing: prôblems, perceptions and policies* Commission on the Status of Women (Report of the Secretary-General). Downloaded from website http://www.un.org/womenwatch/daw/csw/ageing.htm

Sharma, B.D. (1984) *Planning for Tribal Development*, Prachi, New Delhi

Spate, O.H.K. and Learmonth, A.T.A. (1972) *India and Pakistan*, B.I.Publications, New Delhi

U.N. *Economic and Social Council* (1999) *Gender and ageing: problems, perceptions and policies* Commission on the Status of Women (Report of the Secretary-General). Downloaded from website http://www.un.org/womenwatch/daw/csw/ageing.htm

UNFPA (1998) *The State of World Population*, New York.

United Nations (2001) *World Population Prospects: The 2000 Revision* Department of Economic and Social Affairs, Population Division, New York, Population Database. Downloaded from website www.unpopulation.org

UNPFA (2002) *Population Ageing and Development: Operational Challenges in Developing Countries*, Population and Development Strategies Series, No. 5, New York

11

Indian Rural Elderly: Problems and Interventions

K.L. Sharma

Very little attention has been given to the plight of the elderly population in rural areas of India. Field studies pertaining to the problems of aged in rural India reveal that deteriorating health and economic insecurity are the most pressing problems facing the elderly population in the villages (Kumar 2003). It does not mean that the condition of urban elderly is satisfactory. There is a huge proportion of elderly also whose living circumstances, specially the economic state pose great challenge to the society. The studies related to socio-economic conditions, dependency ratio, living arrangements, health problems and physical disabilities in rural elderly, are rare and scarce (K. Viswesara Rao, 2004, Kumudani Dandekar 1996).

The paper aims to present the urban- rural divide of the Indian demographic scenario, its consequences and suggests improvements. It also highlights the various problems of rural elderly and the steps to be taken by Government agencies (both Central and States) and NGO's to render improved services to rural elderly in India.[1]

The Phenomenon of Demographic Transition

The rise in the proportion of aging population is one of the major challenges of the 21st century. The percentage of older people in the world population has increased rapidly from 8.6 per cent in 1980, 9.2 per cent in 1990, 9.9 per cent in 2000, and is expected to further increase to 10.8 per cent 2010 and 12. 9 per cent in 2020. In other words, the world's elderly population, which was 484.7 million in 1990 and 608.7 million in 2000 in expected to increase to 1011.6 million by 2020. These figures also show that there were 87 million people in 80 plus age group in 2005. Their number is expected to rise to 320 million in 2050.

In India, since 1961 sharp decline in the overall death rate and also in mortality levels in the older age groups initiated a process of ageing. This has accelerated after 1971 when the fertility level also started declining. The elderly population from 12.06 million in 1901 to 19.61 million in 1951 shows an increase of about 63 percent. Between 1951 and 1971 the number of elderly increased by about 67 percent, reaching 32.70 million by 1971. During 1971-81, the increase in the aged population was about 32 percent as against the increase of 24.7 per cent recorded for the total population during this period. During the decade 1981-91 the old age population increased by 13.5 million with a decadal growth rate of 31 per cent. It has been projected that the likely number of the elderly by the year 2020 will be around 149.7 millions. The data clearly reveals that the absolute number of elderly population (60 years and above) is increasing rapidly. The growth of old-old and very-old more or less remains same over time, but other age groups between 69 to 80 years shows an increasing trend over the decades. (See table 1).

Table 1
Worldwide trend of population of 60 years and above : 1980-2020

Region / Country	*1980*	*1990*	*2000*	*2010*	*2020*
A. Population Aged 60 and Over (in Million)					
World	381.2	484.7	608.7	754.2	1011.6
Developed	173.3	203.6	234.6	232.4	308.2
Developing	207.9	281.8	374.1	491.8	703.4
Africa	23.4	30.9	41.8	57.0	82.0
Latin America	23.4	31.7	41.9	56.4	80.7
Asia (excluding Japan)	160.0	218.2	290.0	377.7	539.9
China	73.6	101.2	131.7	167.9	238.9
India	44.6	60.2	81.4	107.0	149.7
B. Proportion of Aged 60 and Over Population (in Per cent)					
World	8.6	9.2	9.9	10.8	12.9
Developed	15.2	16.8	18.4	19.7	22.4
Developing	6.3	7.0	7.7	8.7	10.9
Africa	4.9	4.8	4.8	4.9	5.6
Latin America	6.5	7.0	7.7	8.8	11.0
Asia(excluding Japan)	6.5	7.4	8.5	9.8	12.8
China	7.4	9.0	10.5	12.4	16.6
India	6.5	7.3	8.4	9.9	12.6

Source: United Nations,World Demographic Estimate and Projections,1950-2025 United Nations, New York Population Aged 60 and Over (in Million).

Practically all sections of the world have experienced continuous improvements in life expectancy and India is no exception to this phenomenon. Life expectancy in India has shown a steady increase over the years. It was 39.4 years for males and 38 years for females in 1950; 62.1 years for males and 63.7 for females in 1998. It is likely to increase to 67 years by 2016. The life expectancy at 60 years was 16.2 years for men and 17.1 for women in 1991-95.In Indian context, men out-number women. This phenomenon is also true in the young-old (60-70 years) age groups. But as age increases, the sex ratio is in favour of women in the old-old and very-old age groups. Another important feature that can be mentioned here is the men's life expectancy; at this age level is uniformly, lower than women's. Life expectancy and healthy life expectancy (disability flee) has been differentiated and it was found that healthy life expectancy is more for females than males. That is, two-thirds of the life expectancy at 60 is the disability free life expectancy for females (Roy, 1991). Therefore, the quality of life in the older years should be the major concern of policymakers and the caring families. If the disability free share of life expectancy can be increased, the burden on the caring families can be reduced. Also the elderly can be a source of help to the family and community in various ways.

The other consequence of such phenomenon is reflected in rural-urban living. In India, like in other developing countries, the number of rural elderly have increased from 683,140 thousand in the year 1995, 699,951 thousands in 1997, 725,508 thousands in 2000 and projected to 783,594 thousands in 2020. (See Table 2)

Table 2

Percentage of elderly population by place of residence (2001)

India/	*Rural%*	*Urban%*	*States*	*Rural%*	*Urban%*
India	72.22	27.78	W.B.	71.97	28.08
J&K	75.12	24.88	Jharkhand	77.75	22.25
Himachal	90.21	9.79	Orissa	85.03	14.97
Punjab	66.05	33.95	Chhatisgarh	79.32	20.68
Chandigrah	10.22	89.78	M.P.	73.33	26.67
Uttarakhand	74.41	25.59	Gujarat	62.65	37.35
Haryana	7100	2900	Daman & Diu	63.74	36.26
Delhi	6.99	93.01	Dadar Nagar		
Rajasthan	76.62	23.38	Haveli	77.11	22.89
Uttar Pradesh	79.22	20.78	Maharashtra	57.6	42.4
Bihar	89.53	10.47	A.P.	72.92	27.08
Sikkim	88.9	11.1	Karnataka	67.02	33.98
Arunachal	79.59	20.41	Goa	51.23	49.77
Nagaland	82.26	17.74	Lakshadweep	55.53	44.47
Manipu	76.17	23.83	Kerala	74.03	25.97
Mizoram	50.5	49.5	T.N.	56.14	43.86
Tripura	82.98	17.02	Pondichery	33.43	66.57
Meghalaya	80.37	19.63	Andaman Nicobar		
Assam	87.28	12.72	Island	67.33	32.67

Census of India, National Commission on Population 2001
Total elderly population of India is 1,027,015,247;
Rural population is 741,660,293 and Urban population is 285,354,954).

Dependency Ratio

India being an agrarian country, three fourth of the aged person approximately are residents of rural areas. As a consequence of which the effect of aging of population is more severe in the rural areas than it is in the urban areas. In rural areas out of one thousand 320 male are fully dependent on others and 513 are not dependent on others. On the other hand 720 females in rural area are fully dependent on others and 139 are not dependent on others. The dependency ratio for elderly living in urban areas is quite different. 555 male are not dependent on others and 301 are fully dependent on others. Only 170 urban females are not dependent on others and 721 are dependent on others. It means that more numbers of elderly will need support from their family in the coming years. The increased life span with added fragility will mean that more elderly will have to depend on the younger and productive age groups of the future. Thus such increases in dependency in absolute terms have implications for social, economic and health needs and many other services. (See Table 4 and 4C).

Table 4
Per 1000 distribution of aged persons in India by state of economic independence/dependence in rural and urban areas

	State of Economic Dependence				
Gender	*Not Dependent*	*Partially Dependent*	*Fully Dependent*	*No response*	*Total*
		Rural			
Male	513	152	320	15	1000
Female	139	124	720	15	1000
Person	326	138	520	16	1000
		Urban			
Male	555	134	301	10	1000
Female	170	95	721	14	1000
Person	326	138	520	16	1000

(2.) *Source :* The National Sample Survey of India 60th Round , January 2004 - June 2004
(some persons did not give their responses)

Table 4 C
Per 1000 distribution of economically independent aged persons by their dependents

India	*Number of Dependents*					
Gender	*Nil*	*1*	*2*	*3 - 5*	*6 or above*	*Total*
				Rural		
Male	35	348	150	266	201	1000
Female	157	242	102	162	337	1000
Person	52	332	144	251	221	1000
				Urban		
Male	32	434	181	218	135	1000
Female	175	303	101	91	330	1000
Person	51	416	170	201	162	1000

Source: National Sample Survey 52nd Round Survey, 1995-96.

The main occupations of the rural elderly are agriculture and non-agricultural or unorganised labour (Table 5). Induction of mechanization in recent years in agriculture and industry has adversely affected the work participation of the elderly in both the sectors. Little census data is available on incomes and economic characteristics of the aged population. Since existing self-employment schemes are all youth oriented, there is less scope for many elderly to work and get financial assistance to be self-reliant in their older years. The gradual decrease in jobs for the rural elderly of unorganised sector, the dependency ratios is also expected to increase significantly in rural India. It will raise the issues of possible future vulnerability of rural elderly as a group in view of the pressures which will be placed on the family and community institutions. The migration of rural youth to towns, cities and metros in search of jobs leaving elderly parents in villages, is also enhancing the problems of rural elderly and in a general devaluating their status in rural areas.

Table 5
Per 1000 distribution of usual (principal) activity status of aged

India	Usual Activity Status				
Sex	*Self employed in Agriculture*	*Non-agrculture*	*Regular Employees*	*Casual*	*Total Labour*
			Rural		
Male	662	111	12	215	1000
Female	509	92	29	370	1000
Person	627	106	16	251	1000
			Urban		
Male	176	567	147	110	1000
Female	203	354	152	291	1000
Person	182	523	150	145	1000

Source: National Sample Survey 52nd Round Survey

Although the traditional family resources and norms of assistance to and integration of elderly are not too eroded as yet, but the increase in dependency burden will contribute to erosion of family values and will increase elder abuse and neglect. It is also true that in Indian society, cultural values and traditional practices emphasize that the elderly members of the family be treated with honour and respect. The families of the aged persons are expected to ensure the needed care and support for the aged.

But, the positive views about the values of traditional rural families should not hide, the often, harsh realities the rural elderly face due to major changes in social structure brought about by modernization, urbanisation, industrialization and migration of rural youth(resulting in breaking up of joint family system and increased tendency of individualism in younger generation) be used as a pretext for inaction where required. The main issue of concern for the *rural* elderly is that the projected numbers of *urban* elderly are expected to increase dramatically. It is feared that the increase in number of elderly may results in the fact that there is a danger that efforts to answer their needs would be directed mostly to the urban elderly.

Living Arrangements

By living arrangements we understand the family type in which the elderly live, the headship of the house holds the elderly enjoy the place where they stay and people with whom they stay the kind of relationships they adjust to the changing environment. (Rajan and et al.,). It is true that the family is still the key unit that provides social and economic support to the individual at different stages of life. In India, the family structure is even now horizontal with children and fewer generations above. The extended family system is the dominant form of family. Very high percentages of the aged person are still living in family with spouse and sons or kin. In such a system, the aged who have lost their spouses, depend on their children for living, a true reflection of Indian tradition. The rural-urban difference is negligible in this respect. Very few percentage of the aged have no surviving children. Regarding living arrangement, one distressing observation is that while majority of the aged males are living with their spouses, majority of their counterparts are living either alone or with their surviving children or live with other relations and non-relations. This pattern is observable due to the impact of the higher incidence of widowhood generated by difference in age at marriage and longer life expectancy of elderly females. The other important phenomenon is the care-giving role of the family. But this role also has undergone many a changes due to the impact of urbanization and industrialization as said earlier. The consequence of which is the relinquishment of traditional role and status by the elderly. Thus the family can neither fulfil their needs nor is to give them physical, material and emotional supports. This is the reason that elderly feel alienated at this age of their life.

Many factors have contributed to the change in the family structures and alienation of elderly:

- Migration of young couples from the rural areas to cities in search of better employment opportunities to fend for themselves.
- Elders who have been in control of the household for a long time are unwilling to give up the responsibility to their children.
- Youngsters on their part are sometimes resentful of the attitude of their parents.
- Many youngsters have moved to places far away from their native homes and in the recent past to many countries abroad. So even if they want to they cannot accommodate their parents in their own homes.
- Elders are sometimes too incapacitated or unwell to look after themselves or get medical care especially in an emergency.

The Indian elderly living in rural areas show wide variations in health status. They are vulnerable to greater socio-economic and health marginalization mainly due to inadequate provisions of services and economic deprivation. As with the urban elderly, locomotors, visual and hearing disabilities, as well as life threatening conditions of coronary heart disease, diabetes and hypertension are common among rural elders also. The primary health centres are the only source for health care for them. They can not afford tertiary health care or private nursing care due to financial constraints. Infections and smoking are also important causes of mortality in rural areas. (Tables 6, 7 and 9)

Table 6
Living arrangements (percentages) for elderly people by sex and residence for the year 2004 (Total)

Living Arrangement	*Rural*		*Urban*		*Sub Total*
	Male	*Female*	*Male*	*Female*	*of R &U*
Alone	2.8	7.6	2.1	6.5	5.2 (R), 4.3(U)
With Spouse only	16.2	8.7	13.3	7.5	12.4(R), 10.4(U)
With Spouse & Other Members	59.7	28.4	64.9	29.4	44.1 (R) 47.1(U)
With Children	16.8	47.5	5.4	48.2	32.1(R) 31.8(U)
With Other Relations & Non-relations	4.5	7.8	4.3	8.4	6.1 (R) 6.3(U)

Source: National Sample Survey 6oth Round Survey, January 2004 – June 2004.

Table 7
Per 1000 distribution of aged persons having chronic diseases by gender

India *Type of Chronic Disease*	*Rural*		*Urban*	
	Male	*Female*	*Male*	*Female*
Cough	250	1958	179	142
Piles	33	16	32	18
Problems of Joints	363	404	285	393
High / Low Blood Pressure	108	105	200	251
Heart Disease	34	27	68	53
Urinary Problem	38	23	49	24
Diabetes	36	28	85	66
Cancer	2	3	2	4
Any of the Above	527	514	528	560

Source: National Sample Survey 52nd Round Survey, 1995-96
Note: Multiple Responses Occurred

Table 8
Per 1000 distribution of aged persons having type of physical disability by sex

India *Type of Physical Disability*	*Rural*		*Urban*	
	Male	*Female*	*Male*	*Female*
Visual	249	291	225	260
Hearing	139	156	111	132
Speech	32	38	29	3
Locomotor	107	115	80	94
Amnesia / Senility	96	113	61	80
Any Disability	380	425	333	367

Source: National Sample Survey 52nd Round Survey
Note: Multiple Responses Occurred

Table 9
Per 1000 distribution of care provider of economically dependent aged

India	*Economic Care Provider*				
Gender	*Spouse*	*Own Children*	*Grand Children*	*Others*	*Total*
			Rural		
Male	113	766	50	71	1000
Female	159	717	52	72	1000
Person	142	735	52	71	1000
			Urban		
Male	105	792	54	49	1000
Female	182	695	56	67	1000
Person	156	728	55	61	1000

Source: National Sample Survey 52nd Round Survey, 1995-96

The positive association of well-being and health with variables such as living with family, having children and community involvement support the usefulness of joint family systems and life long social and physical activity. These things foster healthy ageing. Therefore, the time honoured value of joint family system needs to be pressed and strengthened. Effective geriatric health care services need to stress a community approach to primary health care with provision of support and training for both family care givers and professionals. Government should give emphasis on health promotion, cost effective indigenous system of Medicare and gender sensitive programmes.

The demographic, health and psycho-social implications of ageing of population in the Indian context raises some important policy issues, which will create newer problems to the aged during the immediate as well as in distant future. It is also a fact that the ageing process is immensely influenced by the socio-economic development of the society. So, if we are late in thinking about socio-economic implications of population ageing, there will be more issues and questions than answers. It is proper time to seek appropriate and positive solutions to meet the challenges of aging. The most who suffer of ageing (rise in the number of age and increment in life span) are the aged living in villages.

The Policy Initiative of India

Government of India and states governments have started some schemes to provide care and support for the aged. Also, there are some NGOs who have under taken the various types of activities related to the welfare of the senior citizens.

In 1999 Government of India announced National Policy on Older Persons. This policy emphasizes various useful services to the aged. In the December 2007 Government of India has passed an act named as The Maintenance and Welfare of Parents and Senior Citizens Act, 2007.

Under Clause 5(1) of the act, a senior citizen or a parent may apply for maintenance under Clause 4 of the bill. (A senior citizen is an Indian citizen who is at least 60 years old. A parent could be father or mother, whether biological, adoptive or step father or step mother, whether or not the father or the mother is a senior citizen). If the senior citizen or parent is incapable, any other person or a voluntary organization authorized by the senior citizen or parent can apply for maintenance on their behalf. The Tribunal may take cognizance suo motu (that is, it can act on its own cognizance). These two provisions are welcome since most senior citizens or parents do not have the energy (they do not have the money anyway) to apply for maintenance.

The said Tribunal may, when a proceeding regarding monthly allowance for the maintenance under this section is pending, order such children or relative to pay a monthly allowance for the interim maintenance of the senior citizen including parent. The State government is required to constitute within a period of 6 months from the date of commencement of the law (Act), Tribunals for the purpose of adjudicating and deciding upon the order for maintenance under Clause 5.

According to Clause 4(1), the senior citizen including parent is entitled to apply for maintenance under Clause 5 if he is unable to maintain himself from his own earnings or out of the property owned by him. A parent or grand-parent can make an application for maintenance against one or more of his children who are majors ('children' includes son, daughter, grandson and grand-daughter). The obligation of the children to maintain his or her parent extends to the needs of such parent either father or mother or both, as the case may be, so that such parent may lead a normal life. A childless senior citizen, on the other hand, can make an application against his relative ("relative" means any legal heir of the childless senior citizen who is a major and is in possession of or would inherit the property after the childless senior citizen's death; property means property of any kind, whether movable or immovable, ancestral or self-acquired, tangible or intangible and includes rights or interests in such property).

Thus Clause 4 makes a reference to grand-parent while Clause 5 does not. In other words, Clause 5 is silent about how the application for maintenance should be made by a grand-parent (who is not yet 60) under Clause 4. I wish the learned law-makers took notice of this inconsistency lest vested interests should exploit this well-intended provision.

If the senior citizen has transferred by way of gift or otherwise, his property, subject to the condition that the relative shall provide the basic amenities and basic physical needs to the senior citizen and such relative refuses or fails to provide such amenities and physical needs, Clause 23 (1) says the said transfer of property shall be declared void by the Tribunal, if the senior citizen so desires. This is a welcome provision since it protects naïve senior citizens from exploitation by relatives who intend to renege on their promise subsequently.

The State governments are also required to prescribe a comprehensive action plan for the senior citizens so that these schemes should percolate to the majority of elderly living in villages.

Therefore, the decision makers need to be alerted to the relative vulnerability of the rural elderly so that they may see that a large percentage of the future rural elderly might not suffer from any significant facilities such as pension, health insurance, social security support and other facilities which are being planned for senior citizens be limited mostly to urban elderly. There are many reasons to be concerned about the effectiveness of present social support mechanisms and institutions in meeting the needs of the elderly in view of future pressure on them.

From such a perspective, the problems of the old-old (80+) and of the increasing sex ratio in favour of elderly women should not be ignored. The sex ratio is in favour of males in rural areas (even up to 80 years) while it is the opposite in urban areas. However, the issues are not just issues for elderly women; they have a broader gender dimension. The gender ascribed roles for each sex vary through the life cycle and the status of elderly men and women can be different from that ascribed at younger ages. More importantly, from a rural perspective, is the modification of gender roles due to declining activities of husband and/or wife and to widowhood at older age. More precisely, what happens to issues such as land property or tenure and to other assets of widows or single elderly women? The situations need to be analyzed and efforts should be made so that their rights are assured.

On the other hand, the ageing of rural populations should not be viewed purely negatively. Elderly may be useful in promoting sustainable development of rural society. However, little attention has been paid until now to such issues. The real value and potential or wisdom of the elderly need to be promoted by the agencies working for elderly. Just to give one example, rural elderly, including women, have considerable knowledge and experience about the agriculture, and also about plants and their various uses (medicinal, nutritional, etc.). In order to protect biodiversity, which is an essential element of sustainable agriculture, such knowledge should not be lost. Rural elderly are also crucial in the inter-generational transmission of culture and of societal identity and cohesion.

As an intervention to help elderly to lead quality living two essential steps should be taken.

Development of Proper Health Care System

One of the key components of healthy aging is a working health system, with its roots firmly grounded in the villages of India. With the increasing life expectancy, changing family structure and role of elderly, the stage is set to usher an era where the elderly would find themselves alone and much more vulnerable than before. The non-communicable diseases (NCDs) are now the major cause of morbidity and mortality in the ageing population. The morbidity due to these has a crucial effect on the quality of life. The health system should be thus directed to address this critical issue of confining the impact of NCDs. The western countries which have had geriatrics as a sub-speciality for a long time now, have been able to provide their ageing citizens lead a enjoyable life by developing and implementing guidelines to treat NCDs and other significant ailments like cataracts, osteoporosis, hearing loss, falls, syncope and alike. They have a multi-disciplinary approach with the expertise from physiotherapist, social-worker, dietician, pharmacist, occupational therapist along with the treating doctor.

Where do we start? How do we go about putting a system in place which gives our elderly population good health, both mental and physical? The health system (including the state and the policy- makers) will need to re-organise itself to the needs of the elderly. A national health policy dedicated to the specific needs of the elderly population (akin to RCH for child and reproductive age females) should be brought forth. This policy, like any other would be based on information, accessibility, targets and constant review. This should happen at all the levels starting from the villages. The medical fraternity at the primary health centres should have outpatient clinics only for elderly. They should find ways which are viable in their setup or according to the needs of the population. Like, somewhere community visits by the doctor may be needed, whereas at other places a trained nurse can educate the elderly population about healthy living and common NCDs. There should be measures in place to provide for the care at an affordable price, though ideally should be free. The medicines for the elderly may be made available free/subsidised price. At a tertiary level more doctors should be trained in geriatrics as a sub-speciality.

It is important to realise that geriatrics is a capital intensive field. We cannot sustain the care without the help and support from the family. Our culture and tradition of revering our elderly members of the family has been the pillar of hope and support towards healthy ageing. We cannot do without this.

Ensuring Economic and Social Security

Majority of rural elderly are not aware of facilities such as pension schemes, concession in railways and bus fares etc. provided to them by the State and Central Governments. The number of Old Age Homes, Day Care Centres and Mobile Medicare Units in India are not sufficient looking at the size of senior citizens. These facilities unfortunately are not available for rural elderly. The recently passed bill by Government of India (now known as Maintenance of Parents and Senior Citizens Act-2007) has a provision to construct one old age home in each district of India, but the implementation of this provision will take time and how it will be beneficial for rural elderly is also a big question. At the time of draughts, floods and other natural calamities the elderly are ignored. They need special attention in such situations. Village panchayats at their level should have meeting places for elderly and should organise activities for the recreation of elderly from their own budget.

How to achieve these goals is an issue? It is suggested here that if we mobilise Panchayti Raj system as envisaged in the National Policy on Older Persons[3] of Government of India.

Therefore, the Panchayti Raj system, as emphasized in the National Policy on Older Persons, should be strengthened to address the issues and needs of rural aged. Panchayat Raj institutions need to be conveyed in very strong terms that considerable space is available for them to act in the area of empowerment of elderly people through information sharing. For this the elected members of Pachayats should be sensitized by giving them information and training about ageing population, its challenges and the strategies to meet the challenges. The village Pachayats should take lead in informing to rural elderly about the various schemes of government and help them to utilize the benefits of these schemes. This would help people to protect themselves from exploitation by forces within the government and outside, and exert pressure on officials and institutions which are mandated to deliver specified services to be responsive to their needs and changes. The area of interventions is indeed very large, ranging from information about preventive aspects of public health and personal hygiene, linkage between nutrition and health, skill development opportunities, availability of Welfare Services and benefits accruing from education and strengthening of ties between intergenerational relations. Panchayats themselves should also develop programmes such as income generating activities, day care centres and leisure time activities at their level to make the quality of life better for the rural elderly. The Panchayti Raj system will help in the implementation of the programmes by utilizing the talents and skills of rural elderly for community's development by organising various activities at Panchayat, block and district levels.

Indian Gerontological Association conducted a pilot study to involve and sensitize a selected group of ward members of four Panchayat samitis in Rajasthan to the cause of elderly of their area. According to Census of India, 2001 the total population of Rajasthan is 66.47 million (urban population is 13.20 million 23.4% and rural population is 43.27 million that is 76.6%). Out of 40,97,856 total number of older people(60+) in Rajasthan 32,53,116 live in rural area and 8,44,740 urban areas. Rajasthan state has 32 districts and 88,516 ward members in all the panchayat samitis.

The Pilot Project

The purpose of this pilot project was:

- To find out the living conditions, economic status and social and personal problems (or real situation) of elderly living in villages
- To promote the rights and social welfare of rural elderly and to advocate the minimum standard of living guarantee for them.
- To emphasize on the importance of land assets for elder rural citizens (specially single or widows)
- To highlight the traditional values, family support, disputes and the role of law in the light of recent act of maintenance of parents and senior citizens 2007 in gaining social status in the society.
- To sensitize the ward members of villages about the problems generated due to ageing of population so that they may properly address the problems (economic, health related and socio-psychological problems) of senior citizens living in rural areas of Rajasthan.
- To involve the senior citizens in to the developmental activities at village level so that they may lead better quality of life in their remaining period of life.

Method

In this pilot project 31 ward members of four Panchayat Samitis of Jaipur district viz. Govind garh (Chomu), Dudu, Sanganer and Bassi were invited to participate in the two workshops organized in the months of April and May, 2008.

The first workshop was organized in Govan Garth village panchayat samiti's office in which 32 persons (17 ward members and other villagers) attended the workshop.

The second workshop was organized in Jaipur. In this workshop total 14 ward members from three pachayat samitis viz. Dudo (5), Sanganer (4) and Bassi (5) participated.

The purpose of these workshops was to sensitize these ward members of different panchayat samitis about the problems (generated due to the ageing of population) of senior citizens living in rural areas.

Training Module of the Workshops

These selected ward members were given demographic information about the elderly people in India and especially about Rajasthan. Information regarding the schemes of central and state Governments for the welfare of senior citizens, National Policy on Older Persons, and detailed information about the recently passed ACT (Maintenance of Parents and Senior Citizens Act 2007) and its operation and implications was also shared with them.

The participants were also asked to go their wards and collect information about the senior citizens living in their respective areas and collect information about them in the Performa prepared for the purpose. These ward members were also asked to give their views about the problems of elderly persons on the basis of their own experiences.

The content of the data (information related to elderly persons living in these areas) provided by the ward members, was analysed.

The Findings

Out of 550 total respondents 49 per cent were male and 51 per cent were female. In terms of age classification 67 percent were in the age group of 60 and above, 25 per cent and 8 per cent were in the groups of 70 and above and 80 and above age groups respectively. 32 per cent females were widows and 7 per cent were widowers and remaining 61 per cent were married.

Three per cent respondents are getting old age pension because they come under BPL (below poverty line) category. 4 per cent were retired from government jobs and getting pension from the government.6 per cent respondents live alone, 2 per cent live with their spouses and remaining 92 percent live with their sons.

Most of the respondents reported that they badly need financial assistance because they are living in poor conditions and are the burden on their children. Due to the certain rules of government they can not avail the benefit of old age pension scheme. The sons who are looking after their parents should be given some incentives (as suggested in National Policy on Older Persons 1999) so that they may not find economic hardships in maintaining their parents.

Most of the respondents reported that their health is satisfactory and simultaneously they also complained about some disabilities such as bad eyesight, difficulty in hearing, weakness and pains in joints.

Conclusions

This pilot project, based on very small sample, highlights the situation of Indian rural elderly. The rural elderly are remembered by Indian politicians only at the time of elections, otherwise they are the most neglected lot of society. It is being suggested here that the rural ageing is important because approximately 75 per cent elderly live in rural India. By the effective planning and policy development we can allow the communities to tap the resources of older citizens. By this process rural elderly will be perceived as contributors to society and not simply consumers of services. It is the time to address these issues now with the help of Panchayti Raj system. The in this can cause the lives of millions of rural elderly to be more difficult. NGO's and other agencies should take lead in this project and attract the attention of political leaders to promote the concept of healthy rural elderly.

NOTES

1. The distinction between Urban and Rural is arbitrary and differs from country to country. The characteristics of rural to be low population density, remoteness from large towns and cities, extensive agricultural lands and forests or mountain regions. Rural inhabitants enjoyed few to no modern facilities (water, sanitation and roads), few to no social services (schools, hospitals, transport) and their subsistence economy offered limited opportunities to young people. Rural population is perceived as being conservative and having a traditional way of life with larger extended families and closer social ties and inter action than urban populations. There occupations are seen as those traditional to rural areas (e.g. farming with little or no industry).

   The contrasts between rural and urban vary in intensity according to multiple factors : social, economic, environmental, cultural, historical and demographic—International Rural Project 1997 – 2001

2. The Ministry of Statistics and Programme Implementation, government of India set up the National Survey organisation (NSSO) in 1950 in order to collect data on various features of the India economy. The NSSO classifies the information through sample surveys across the nation and intends to assists the government in socio-economic planning and policy making.

3. Panchayati Raj institutions will be encouraged to participate in the implementation of the National Policy, address local level issues and needs of the ageing and implement programmes for them. They will provide Forums for discussing concerns of older persons and activities that need to be taken. Such forums will be encouraged at Panchayat, block and

district level. They will have adequate representation of older women. Panchayats will mobilize the talents and skills of older persons and draw up plans for utilizing these at the local level. Amongst others, the help of the Social Justice Committees of the village panchayats will be taken to advocate different measures for giving effect to the Policy."

REFERENCES

K.Viswesware Rao (2007), *Ageing in Rural India,* The Association of Publishers.

Kumar, S. Vijay (2003) "Rural Ageing: Ageing in Poverty" in A. B. Dey (ed.), *Ageing in India : Situational Analysis and Planning for the Future*, New Delhi, AIIMS, 103-108.

Kumudini Dandekar (1996), *The Elderly in India*, Vedams Books, Delhi.

Roy, G. (1991). "Perspectives on population ageing in India", in Indira Jai Prakash (ed.). *Quality Ageing: Collected Papers.* Varanasi: Association of Gerontology (India).

12

Psychological Well-being and Elderly

G.S. Saun

Grow old with me the best is yet to be,
The last of life, for which the first was made.
Our times are on his hand,
Who said "A whole and Planned, Youth shows but half;
Trust God, see all nor be afraid".
(Excerpts from '*Rabbi Ben Ezra*' by Robert Browning).

In this poem the poet wants us to look forward to old age. He thinks that old age is summation of our life. This is a vantage point from which we look back and get proper perspectives of our life. So the poet recommends trust God, see all, nor be afraid because the best is yet to be.

But a very few people look forward to it with joy and expectation. Most of the people are inclined to be pessimist about their old age. Most of the people rather believe with Shakespeare that old age is:

Last scent of all,
That ends this strange eventful history,

Is second childhood and more oblivion,
Sans teeth, sans eyes, sans taste, sans everything.
(*'As You Like It'*, Act II, Scene VIII. William Shakespeare).

Most of us are scared of becoming old because of the sufferings and infirmities of old age.

Infancy, childhood and youth are the period of development. During the middle ages we reach a period of maximum capacity and thereafter our various capacities may show a slow but sure decline. And, therefore, we would rather avoid this stage of ready decline which is but nothingness. What an inglorious end to our glorious hopes and expectation in our youth. Is, then, our life worth living? No, says the pessimist. (Desai, K.G. Naik).

So we have the extreme views of optimism and pessimism about old age. Perhaps the middle approach is the right path to proceed towards the old age and also to know more about our elderlies. No doubt the problems at old age are more but we should try to understand and minimize them.

Health problem of aged needs much more attention because of speedy growth of the aged all over the world and India is no exception to it. In India, according to 2001 census, they are approx 7.4 % of the total population. This percentage in 1991 was 6.49%, and 5.96% in 1981 census report. According to the census estimates, by 2021 A.D. the population of our elderly is going to touch the landmark of approximately 10%. At the same time life expectancy of an average Indian has increased.

These figures put a big challenge before our Gerontologists, Government and organizations involved in the welfare activities of aged, particularly in health.

Besides all other problems Psychological problems of old age are also very complex and they need to be understood more deeply by us.

Concept of Aging

The term aging has three different, but interrelated dimensions, viz. biological aging, social aging and psychological aging.

The physiological changes that occur in an individual in later part of his life comprise biological aging.

Through the process of socialization, as an individual moves from one-grade to the next he acquires new roles and privileges in accordance with the prevailing practices of the society, it is known social aging. Psychological aging consists of a general decline in the mental abilities that accompany old age. Generally physical aging preceeds mental aging, though this is not always the case. According to *Parker* psychological aging is not to be measured in terms of capabilities alone but in the use to which they have been applied from early age through all the years of maturity: Some of the psychological changes in respect of an individual's conception of the self, his ideas about the world as an individual and as a member of social groups, his feelings about the attitudes and behaviour of others towards him and his general view of life and world, play significant role in the process of psychological aging.

Some scholars like Pratha N. Mukherji (1972) distinguished between biological and sociological or psychological age. They say biologically a person may be old but if he possesses a youthful mentality, sociologically and Psychologically speaking he should be included in younger generation. To illustrate this distinction he gives the example of such leaders as Pandit Jawaharlal Nehru, Subash Chandra Bose etc. who in their middle age inspired the youth movement before the second world war. This distinction is valid only in theoretical context as majority of the empirical studies reveal that both seem to coincide.

Concept of Well-being

Physical and psychological well-being are matters of great social as well as personal concern because health and illness affect an individual's performance of basic personal tasks, of daily living, and of expected social roles. Impairment and disability increase the probability of failure in carrying out personal tasks and social roles; and such failures in turn increase dependency which, particularly for adults, challenges for independence. Moreover, loss of autonomy tends to have negative effect on self evaluation and life satisfaction (Ethel & George 1976). Health is thus both a key personal resource for any individual and a social concern.

The exclusive concern with the remembering self is a notable feature of well-being. The vast body of literature devoted to subjective well-being is dominated by the questions, 'How satisfied are you with your life as a whole?' and 'How happy are you these days?'

The hybrid concept of well-being distinguishes two components, which are labeled 'experienced well-being' and 'evaluated well-being'. Both are subjective, and both refer to a period of time that may be measured in days or months. The first component includes the statistics of the momentary affective states experienced during the reference period. The second component includes global subjective evaluations of one's life during the same period. The two components are not independent and are therefore expected to be correlated, but they are distinct, empirically as well as conceptually.

With a rapid increase in the population all over the world aging and aged need to be given greater recognition by the biological scientists, social scientists, government agencies and social workers.

All societies have been confronting the problem of old age all times. The industrialized countries, after empirical documentation of the health and other related problems, have been able to provide sufficiently community interventions for the total well being of their elderly, the adequate attention to the problems of their' aged people. A problem is considered social when difficulties met by a group of people, (a) result from the functioning, organization and structure of society (b) may endanger society at large and (c) can and should be solved through social policies and political initiative (Philibert, 1968; 23). The problem of old age is no doubt emerging as a social one, but it cannot be looked in isolation. Study of psychological factors is equally necessary to understand the problems of elderly it should be studied in the form of a socio-psychological problem.

The change brought out in our society due to modernization and industrialization, the breaking norms of joint family system has drastically changed the fate and status of our geriatric group of people. In the pre-industrial agrarian set-up. Most of the old people remained financially independent throughout their lives. The traditional social and cultural value also did not permit grown-up children to leave their financially and physically insecure old parents alone. Moreover, the prevailing economic, political and value systems of the pre-industrial social order which were based on the preseververation of inherited in-equality, enabled old people to enjoy leadership roles and powerful positions of decision makers and advisers, in the joint family, caste group and community (D. Souza, 1971).

The changing social structure in the new industrial social order, based on egalitarian ideals, has resulted in old people being dislodged from leadership positions in the family, caste group and the community.

The individualistic and materialistic values that perforce develop in the new socio-economic conditions prompt sons to adopt for their own freedom and improve their own standard of living. They tend to absolve themselves of the responsibility of looking after their parents. Consequently, either married son and parents get separated while living in the same town or conflicts between the two generation members of the family take place quite often, if they are forced by the circumstances to live together (Mishra 1989).

Since the knowledge and experience of aged people are not considered necessary for the rapidly changing society, the older start feeling neglected, isolated and dissatisfied with life. Their socio--psychological needs are neglected. Under these circumstances it becomes more essential to understand more deeply the problems of this neglected class of our society and to suggest ways and means for their solution within the approachable means. Thus aging is not a smooth process, but a painful one, in which the old are exposed to the vulnerability of the aging process. They have to depend on their own resources for leading satisfactory life in their later years.

Conflicts arise when the sick and tired mind and body cannot cope with physical, psychological and emotional stresses (Chadha, 1990). In other words, the interaction among personal and environmental factors makes the elderly vulnerable to serious consequences of brain disorders as well as psychological conditions in which the role of organic factors is less clearly defined. The latter include depression, anxiety helplessness, alienation, schizophrenia, paranoia, hypochondria, and insomania. Thus, living a longer age may also mean greater liability of senile psychosis/dementia and other degenerative disorders (Venkaba Rao, 1979, 1988-89).

The first serious effort in India in systematic psychological gerontology was made at Sri Venkateswara University (Ramamurti & Jamuna, 1984). Psychological wellbeing is somewhat a malleable concept, which is to do with people's feelings about their every day life activities and refers to the way specific life concerns and their evaluations fit together in people's thinking. Such feelings may range from negative mental states (e.g., *depression, anxiety, unhappiness, cognitive, disorientations, lower self-esteem, general dissatisfaction*) to a more positive out - look which extends beyond the mere absence of these negative states (as health is something beyond the mere absence of illness) into a state which has been identified as positive mental health (Jahoda 1958, Wanse, 1978).

In India research on the aged has not only considered negative indices of psychological well being, but also has taken into account the positive indices of psychological well being/ mental health such as *adjustment, self esteem and life satisfaction.* The role of socio--demographic variable like family and institution-alised care has also been taken into account vis-à-vis each of the indices of mental ill health or lower psychological well-being.

Let us discuss first the positive indices of psychological well-being.

Adjustment

The term adjustment is simply a process, involving both mental and behavioural responses by which individual strives to cope with inner needs, tensions, frustrations, conflicts and to bring harmony between these inner demands and those imposed upon him by the external world (Shaffer & Shoben 1956). It can be defined as a process by which an individual maintains balance between his inner needs outer circumstances and by which the gratification of inner needs is effected. In brief, adjustment is an individual's ability to harmonize with environment.

Man is a social animal. He lives in a community and not in isolation. He grows with those of his age and generation and interacts with them. His life and living is intricately interwoven in the rubric of familial and community life. As a member of the community and family he has to play certain roles appropriate, to his self. These roles are the expectations in the behaviour of positions that an individual occupies in the society and which are of meaning both to the community and to himself. They give a direction to his behaviour and determine the quality of his relationships with others. The role thus plays and important part in determining the adjustment and happiness of an individual. The roles a person occupies and plays depend upon various factors such as his age, physical condition and developmental status, socio-economic, marital and familial position etc.

There may be primary role such as parent and spouse, secondary roles such as that of a friend and third order roles such member of a community. With onset of old age many of these roles change drastically and some even disappear. This change and reduction of roles has immense effect on the adjustment and happiness of an older person. A number of studies have examined adjustment problems of the elderly with regard to socio--economic/educational status, the elderly from lower socio-economic class and/or with lower educational status showed poorer level of personal and social adjustment (Ananthraman, 1979 'b', Bhatnagar and Randhaawa, 1987, Chandrika and Ananthraman, 1981, Ramamurti, 1970).

The data on the adjustment, life satisfaction and quality of life of the widows show that generally the widows were less adjusted than widower or single women. The situational and socio-familial factors largely determined the nature, of adjustment. Also the widows were less satisfied with their lives and had a poorer quality *frought* as it is with negative changes in the psychological and socio-economic status of the individual, it is difficult to isolate age as a factor in the causation of any increase in observed maladjustment. (Ramamurti). It is worth while to note that it is not age *perse* that is important variable in the determination of age changes but what happens to the individual during the lapse of time that is of significance.

The effect of work on adjustment is such that it contributes to positive self-feeling (Kleemier, 1951). Retirement appears to have a negative effect on personal adjustment in so far as there is economic deprivation and attendent feelings of difficulty in keeping oneself occupied (Thanson Streits & Kosa, 1960). Those who have favourable pre-retirement attitude and a accurate conception of retirement, and have made definite plans 'for retirement, adjust with care to retirement, (Moffatt & Rich, 1957 Thamson, 1958).

Study 'A' by Litwin

In an interesting study H. Litwin, (2007) after studying retirement age and longer life found that medium level education and being employed at baseline were associated with lesser mortality risk. Nevertheless, the timing of retirement, viz. early versus normative exit from the workforce, was not related to survival.

The relationship of retirement to adjustment was reported in an extensive study by Richard, Livson and Peterson (1962). The non--retired were found more anxious about retirement than the retired. Retirement not only removes the definitive functions of work as a means of warding off anxiety but the need to work is also reduced. Further, idleness, loneliness, feelings of worthless-ness and fear of physical and mental deterioration are greater immediately before retirement than after retirement. *The older retired individuals are found to have a tendency to relinquish unrealized aspirations and accept them realistically with greater ego-strength.*

Study 'B'

In yet another study on the age and the timing of retirement David De Vaus and others, (2007) found that retiring gradually allows time for people to make changes to their lifestyle, but having control over the timing and manner of leaving work had a greater positive impact on psychological and social well being, and this persisted three year after retirement.The findings suggest that policies and employment practices that promote employees control of their retirement decisions will enhance well-being in later life and facilitate longer workforce participation.

Interview data from a sub sample of respondents to the 1979 National Health Interview Survey, showed that non-married females who live alone had better health status and less illness behaviour than their widowed peers who live with others. These differences were more pronounced among the older age group widows who lived alone. (Ofra, 1988).

Adjustment or the lack of it results from person's use of his or her creativity or otherwise, Thus it seems that by activating the creative potential among the aged their potential for adjustment can been enhanced. Only a non-creative person lacks adjustment and the use of creative thinking and problem solving enlarges one's scope for better adjustment. A positive relation between creativity and adjustment has been found.

Some of the methods that can be used for developing the creativity among the aged are suggested below:

(a) Development of ideational fluency

(b) Brain storming technique

(c) Use of visualization/fantasy/playful thinking etc.

(d) Development of the sense of humour.

Self-esteem

The self is a inner core of personality. Self has many dimensions such as self-concept, self-esteem, self-evaluation, self-disclosure, self-acceptance etc.

Self-esteem means how much a person is conscious about his ego and how much he feels his self respect in deciding any act in the social environment.

The personal and social adjustments are influenced by the self--esteem and self acceptance of an individual (Ananthraman-1980©; S, Sharma, 1970). They have documented the deterioration of self esteem in old age. Apart from other reasons, the negative attitudes of the younger generation towards the elderly contribute to the loss of self esteem (Deb, 1988; Joseph 1986).

In a study Balakrishna, Thilagam etc. (1991) found that there are significant sex differences is masculinity, feminity, and *androgyyng* but no significant sex differences in either self- esteem and social desirability related to masculinity among male pensioners. Self esteem is positively and significantly related only to Androgyny.

In another study Chadha (1991:) observed larger perceived self ideal discrepancy (lower self-esteem) among older people from institutionalized groups than their non-institutionalization (old Age Homes) can represent a majore discontinuity in the life of an aged individual, and thus can be expected to result in *concomitant* changes in the self esteem.

Self-concept

Self-concept is a composite of person'a thoughts and feelings, strivings and hopes, fears and fantasies, his view of what he is, what he has been, what he might become and his attitudes pertaining to his worth.

In view of the general social stigma attached to both old age as well as widowhood, one would expect that the elderly and widows would have negative self feelings. In other words it is the self concept that gets influenced and gets affected as a result of aging and widowhood.

Ramamurti (1990) in his study found that there is worsening of the self-concept with increasing age. Also widows exhibit more negative self-concept than non-widows, the forward class widows appear to have more negative self-feeling than backward class and schedule caste widows.

Life Satisfaction

A person's satisfaction with present life is a sort of a barometer of the impact of life stresses and the extent to which a person is able to circumvent them and find satisfaction. Mainly it may be said to reflect the mood of the person with regard to satisfaction with his present life conditions. Life satisfaction may be perceived as a strong indicator of total well being. For the measurement of life satisfaction most of the Indian studies have used the index of life satisfaction that emphasizes the individual's own evaluation of his present and/or past life, his satisfaction or his happiness.

Recent psychological view of happiness is based on Martin Seligman's new movement of Positive Psychology. In his highly valued and quoted book- "Authentic Happiness" (2002), he commented that truly happy people have a full life which is fulfilling at three levels: the pleasant life, the good life and the meaningful life. Thus he identified three forms of happiness.

Seligman observed that "People who are impoverished, depressed, or suicidal care about much more than just the relief of their suffering. These persons care-sometimes desperately-about virtue, about purpose, about integrity, and about meaning. Experiences that induce positive emotions cause negative emotions to dissipate rapidly. The strengths and virtues function to buffer against misfortune and against the psychological disorders, and that may be the key to building resilience.

In most of the studies it is found that a perceived social support and leisure activities led to better life satisfaction.

Chadha (1991) also observed that married older people, regardless of gender, had higher life satisfaction than their widow or widower counter parts. These studies showed that the non--institutionalized elderly were more satisfied with their life as compared to their institutionalized counter-parts.

Negative Indices of Psychological Well-being are as following:

Depression

It is an emotional state of dejection, gloomy "ruminations guilt, inappropriate thought patterns that generalizes every event as a calamity. Depression is the most common psychopathologic syndrome of the aged (Gupta & Vohra 1987). Depression alone contributed sixty seven percent of the total psychiatric morbidity in a large community survey.

In another study Venkoba Rao (1986 b) attempted to make the compassion of relative frequency of different symptoms in depressives from two age, groups (60 plus years and below 40 years). The commenest symptoms in the elderly were sadness, depressive mood, somatic symptoms.

Suicidal ideas, lack of energy, tension, inability to fall a sleep, psychomotor restlessness and joylessness/inability to enjoy. He concluded that the depressive symptomatology in the elderly tends to be more bland while variety marks the younger generation, otherwise the symptoms of depression do not significantly differ.

Cognitive Disorientation

Such disorientations of the aged include feeling of hopelessness, helplessness, self rated inferiority, alienation from self or from others, and death anxiety. Jindal (1987) studied the nature and intensity alienation of aged males. Alienation was defined as a state of powerlessness, normlessness, isolation and meaning-lessness. All the aged were found to suffer from one or another component of alienation. Feelings of powerlessness and normlessness were stronger among non-functioning heads. With regard to marital status the feelings of isolation and meaninglessness were more prevalent among widowers than the ones having a living spouse.

With regard to death anxiety Rai and Thakur (1968) found that the elderly with negative attitude toward aging tend to be higher on death anxiety than their counter parts with positive attitudes.

Stressful Life Events

A life event is defined as stressful if it causes changes in and demands readjustment of an average person's normal routine. As indicated earlier, a number of life changes occur in old age like retirement, widowhood, anticipated death, abundant, leisure, lack of social interaction, reduced income etc. The study of the nature of strategies adopted by the aged to cope with their unique life stresses has now emerged as an important area of concern for researchers and health workers.

Emotion

Positive emotions are essential elements of optimal functioning, and therefore an essential topic within the science of well-being. The theory, together with the research reviewed here, suggests that positive emotions: (1) broaden people's attention and thinking; (2) undo lingering negative emotional arousal; (3) fuel psychological resilience; (4) build consequential personal resources; (5) trigger upward spirals towards greater well-being in the future; and (6) seed human flourishing. People should cultivate positive emotions in their own lives and in the lives of those around them, not just because doing so makes them feel good in the moment, but also because doing so transforms people for the better and sets them on paths toward flourishing and healthy longevity.

When positive emotions are in short supply, people get stuck. They lose their degrees of behavioural freedom and become painfully predictable. But when positive emotions are in ample supply, people take off. They become generative, creative, resilient, ripe with possibility, and beautifully complex.

Functional and Organic Mental Disorders

Functional disorders/psychoses have no demonstrable organic basis but involve mental disorders attributed primarily to psychological stresses. Organic mental disorders are basically physical disorders that have psychological symptoms associated with them. These involve brain dysfunction based on either aging or the ingestion of *substance* that affect brain activity. This dysfunction could be both temporary and permanent.

Jhingan et al. (1986) found organic depressive psychosis as the commonest disorder in the aged followed by schizophrenia and organic brain syndromes. They further observed that the frequency of organic brain syndromes shot up after the age of sixty.

Suicidal Behaviour

Depression has been shown to be associated with enhanced risk of suicidal behaviour. Despite the fact that the orderly constitute a high risk group which is vulnerable to self destruction; very few studies have examined this issue. However, a low and varied incidence of suicidal behaviour in the aged has been observed.

The studies have shown that more suicide attempts end totally in the old people, particularly those who are depressed. Relatively lower incidence of suicide by the aged in India, as observed, vis-à-vis their western counter parts, besides other factors can be attributed to the paucity of the guilt feelings among the depressed aged in India.

Motivation and Activity

1. Locomotor activity tends to decrease with advancing age after sexual maturity, but a significant decrepet does not usually occur until serenity
2. It is not yet clear as to whether aversive stimuli are equally motivating for all ages.
3. Over- involvement or over arousal resulting in a heightened drive state may impair performance for the elderly relative to the young.
4. Sexual activity continues among a majority of healthy men in their seventies.
5. Sexual competence and interest continues for many older persons long after sexual activity ceases. Loss of spouse or willingness or ability of spouse to perform sexually is the major reason given for cessation of sexual activity especially among women.
6. Age differences in a variety of activities may be more related to changes in motivation than to intellectual or physical comptence.

Memory

1. Age differences in short term memory are minimal, provided that the items have been fully perceived and that no reorganisation is required.
2. Long term memory tends to decline with age. This is contrary to the previous general belief that memory for remote events is unimpaired by aging.
3. Recognition memory (recongnising items when they are presented) shows less age related decline than recall memory (recalling n item on demand)

Learning

1. In verbal learning tasks, older individuals are particularly disadvantaged when time to respond is short.
2. Older people tend not to use encoding strategies as often or as well as younger individuals.
3. At ages beyond 65, longitudinal studies show decrease in learning abilities.

Perception

In general, most researchers agree that all five senses (vision, hearing, taste, touch and smell) tend to decline with age. More specifically there tend to be declines on the average in all perceptual abilities.

Intellectual Abilities

1. There are general declines in intellectual abilities post age 65.
2. Longitudinal studies may minimize the extend of decline because of practice effects and because of selective dropout.
3. People who perform relatively well when younger will perform relatively well when older.

In summary, research in the United States has tended to be numerous declines in all areas of psychological functions with age.

Major Theories of Social Gerontology

1. ***Modernization Theory***

It is only through the development of human culture that the aged have been able to achieve any security. In most primitive societies the aged's status has remained fairly low because of the constant struggle to survive and relative inability of the aged to contribute their share for the survival. The condition of aged was best in the stable agricultural societies. Due to industrialization it deterioted a recent development in this theory suggests that this decline is beginning to level out and may even swing back up in post industrial societies.

2. *Minority Group Theory*

Some Gerontologists are of the view that the aged should be considered as a emerging minority group. They agree that the aged are different from social and ethnic minority groups in several respect, such as not having been born that way (Streib, 1965). Others feel that such recognition may result into the development of inferiority feeling and group consciousness among aged. It is observed that many elders seem ashamed of their age and are unwilling to identify themselves as aged.

3. *Disengagement v/s Activity theory*

The basic level of the disengagement theory are that the process of mutual with-drawal of aging persons and of society from each other is typical of most aging persons: This process is biologically and psychologically intrinsic and inevitable; and disengagement process contribute to healthy, satisfying adjustment in old age (Cuming & Henry, 1961).

In contrast, activity theory holds that majority of normal aging persons maintain stable levels of activity and engagement; the actual amount of engagement on disengagement is more influenced by past life - styles and the culture than by any intrinsic process; and maintaining substantial level of physical, mental and social activity is usually necessary for successful aging. (Palmore, E. 1980).

The engagement theory, therefore, propounds that successful aging means the maintenance and creation of social climate as far and as long as possible of the activities and attitudes of middle age, while disengagement theory implies the acceptance of process of disengagement from active life.

Most of the methodologically sound theories tends to support engagement theory.

Under the circumstances only well equipped aged, having higher socio-economic and health status and variety of alternative activities to participate in, can enjoy life while the ill equipped unfortunate ones, lead their lives in miserable conditions, unable to solve their problems and look towards society to rescue them from the threatening environment (Mishra. S. 1991).

Most of the studies indicate that the aged do not prefer institutionalized care and most of the cases they accept it as a last resource for their rehabilitation. Institutionalization adversely affects the emotional adjustment. Institutional arrangement should be made available only for those who neither can look after their selves nor can get family support.

In order to maintain better psychological health efforts should be made to create a congenial atmosphere for the expression and channelization of aged's emotions .and feelings. In the family, no doubt, their psychological needs can be met much more easily. But in this direction the members of the family should not take them as a burden. Younger generation should .be taught to give due respect to the elderly which will be helpful in building self-confidence, reduce the sense of dejection and inferiority feeling among them. Efforts should be made to narrow down the generation gap.

It is true that adequate mental health services are not available for majority of the elderly, still most of the mental health problems of aged could often be prevented or reduced by means that do not require placement of the affected in institutions. These measures include training of the *practitioners,* training and supporting the family and students of human care professions in principles and skill in relevant areas of gerontology, psychogeriatrics and geriatric nursing (Bakshi; 1987 Doshi 1989). Besides the development of officious intervention packages for the aged from different backgrounds, comparative studies are required regarding the achievement of objectives of different care delivering systems and relative cost effectiveness for achieving optimum intervention effectiveness (Nair 1991) .

Thus we may say that the older people who have once enjoyed a position of authority, it is never easy for them to step down in a subsidiary role. They can remain content only if they feel loved and appreciated and if their position and security within the family and society is assured. Old people need to be needed and this is easier if they can be of some service, however small to others. They usually do not parade their grief in any dramatic way but withdraw themselves from life. This withdrawal can be prevented by understanding their mental health problems from cultural, social, familial, economic, physical, philosophical and spiritual point of views. This approach may help to keep our' geriatric group more healthy, happy and valuable source of inspiration, particularly for the younger generation and the society in general.

REFERENCES

Ananthraman, R.N., [1979 (b)], Adjustment and its correlates in *Indian Journals of Clinical Psychology,* vol. 6, no.2, September pp.165-188.

Ananthraman, R.N., [1979 (c)], Self Concept and Adjustment in Old Age, *Journal of Psychological Researches,* vol. 24, no.1-2, January -May pp.59-61.

Balakrishnan, R., Thilagam, N. Rajkumar S. & Lakshmi Narayanan, T.R., (1991), Self-esteem in Relation to Sex Role

Identity among Male and Female Pensioners, *National Seminar on Aging*, 23-24 December, Coimbatore.

Bakshi, H.S., (1987), "A Approach to Support Services for the Elderly, Aging in India" *Challenges for the Society, Delhi*, Ajanta pp.220-231.

Bhatnagar G.S. & Randhawa M., (1987), "Social Adjustment among Retired Persons, Aging in India", *Challenge for the Society, Delhi*, Ajanta pp.152-160.

Chadha, N.K. & others, [(1991) (a)], Hopelessness Alienation and Life Satisfaction among Aged, *National Seminar on Aging Souvenir* PSS College of Arts and Science, Coimbatore.

Chandrika P & Anatharaman R.N., [(1982) (b)], Life Changes and Adjustment in Old Age, *Journals of Psychological Research*, vol. 26, no.3, September pp 137-141.

Cuming E. & Henry W., [(1961) (c)], *Growing Old* New York, Basic Books.

Chadha, N.K., (1991), Self Concept and Life Satisfaction among Aged, *Indian Journal of Gerontology*, vol.5, no.1-2, pp 47-54.

Desai, K.G. & Naik, R.D., (1990), *Problems of Retired People in Greater Bombay*, A Study sponsored by Research Programme Committee of Planning Commission, Govt. of India, New Delhi.

De Souza, Alfred, (1982), *The Social Organization of the Aging among the Urban Poor*, New Delhi, Indian Social Institute pp. 7-8.

Deb, M., (1988), Younger Generation's Perception of the Old Members of Rural and Urban Families, *Indian Psychological Review* vol 33, no.3, March pp. 24-31.

Dutt, S.K., (1986), Aging and Nutrition, *The Hindustan Times*, Saturday, September 27, New Delhi, vol. LX-III no.247, p.8.

Ethel, Shanes & George M.L. (1976), Aging Health and organization of Health Resources, *Hand Book of Aging and the Social Sciences* by Robert H. Bislock & Ethel Shanas. pp.592.

Gupta, P. & Vohra. A., (1987), "Patterns of Psychiatric Morbidity in Sharma," M. L. & Dak T.M. (eds) *Aging in India; Challenge for the Society*, Delhi, Ajanta, pp.241-221.

Joseph, J., (1986), A Study of the Problems and Personality of the Aged in Kerala, *Ph.D. Thesis*, Unit of Kerala, Trivandrum

Jindal, B.L., (1987), Alienation Among the Aging Males in Sharma M.L. & Dak T.M. (eds) *Aging in India; Challenge for the Society*, Delhi, Ajanta, pp.103-134.

Jhingan, H.P., Singh, R.K., Srivastava P .K. & Munjal, G.C. (1988), Psychiatric Morbidity Amongst Elderly in a Referral of Personality and Clinical Studies, vol 4,no. 2, September pp.157-160.

Litwin, Howard, (2007), Does Early Retirement Lead to Longer Life? *Aging and Society*, 27, pp.739-754.

Kay D.W.K., (1972), Epidemiological Aspect of Organic Brain Disease in the Aged, In C.M. Goitz (ed.) *Aging and the Brain*, New York, Plenum.

Mahadevan, K., (1986), A System of Policy for Welfare of the Elderly Citizen, *Indian Journal of Social Work*, vol XLVI, no.4, pp. 497-505.

Mathur, D. and Sen A., (1989), Depression in the Elderly and Some of its Psychogical Concomitants Only; A Study of the Efficacy of Age Care Center, *Indian Journal of Community Guidance Service*, vol.6, no.1, January pp.27-39.

Mishra, S., (1989), *Problems and Social Adjustment in Old Age*, Delhi, Gian Publishing House.

Motwani J. K., (1986), An Exploration of Activity Theory of Optional Aging in India; A Cross Cultural Perspective, New York, *Ph. D. Thesis*, Fordham University (Mimeograph).

Mukerji, Pantha, N., (1972), Conflict of Generation Social Change, *Journal of the Council for Social Development*, vol.-II, no.-2, pp. 9-11.

Nair, K.T., (1991), Community Care of the Elderly: A Study of the Family and Community Based Services for the Elderly in Madras, *Ph. D. Thesis*, Hyderabad University.

Ofra, A., (1988), Evidence that Elderly Women Living Alone May be in Better Health than Their Counter Parts, *Journal of Sociology and Social Research*, 72 (2), 114-117.

Oberoi, K and Deys., (1991), Satisfaction Level of Rural Aged and Urban Aged Persons for Various needs in Samastipur -District, *Indian Psychological Review*, vol.37, no.7-8, July-Aug. pp.6-10.

Parker, E.,(1961), The Seven Ages of Women, Balaimore Johu Hopkins, quoted in E.B. Hunlock, 1968, *Developmental Psychology*, p.85 (TMH Edition), New Delhi, Tata Me Grow Hill.

Palmore, E, (1980), *International Hand Book on Aging*, Macmillan Press Ltd. p.451.

Ramamurti, P.V., (1979), A Study of Certain Socio-Economic Variables Related to Adjustment in Aging, *Journals of Psychological Research*, vol. 14, no.3, September pp.91-94.

Ramamurti, P.V., (1979), The Status, Psychological Adjustment and Mental Health of Middle Aged Older Widows, *ICSSR Project* 1990, p.25.

Rai R.N. & Thakur G.P., (1988), Death Anxiety and Attitudes towards Old age, *Indian Psychological Review*, vol.33, no.1, January pp.11-15.

Reddy, B.S.K. & Ramamurti, P.V., (1990), Stress and Coping Strategies of the Rural Aged, *Journal of Personality and Clinical Studies*, vol.6, no.2, September p.171-175.

Seligman, M., (2004), Authentic Happiness: Using the New Positive Psychology to Realise your Potential for Lasting Fulfillment, New York: Free Press.

Shaffen L.F. & Shoben, E.J., The Psychology of Adjustment (II Edn.) Boston: Houghten, Mifflin Coy.

Streib, G., (1965), Are the Age a Minority Group? in A Gouldner and S. Miller, (eds), *Applied Sociology*, New York, Free Press.

Sharam, S., (1970), Self Concept and Adjustment, *Indian Psychological Review*, vol.6, no.2 February, pp.71-76.

Van Zant, S. Mau, R & Abbatt, D., (1989), Mental and Physical Health of Rural Elderly and Non-Widow, *Proceedings of XIV International Congress of Gerontology*, Mexico, June 18-23, p.339.

Vaus, David D. et al., (2007), Does Gradual Retirement Have Better Outcomes than Abrupt Retirement? *Aging and Society*, 27, pp. 667-682.

Venkoba Rao & Madhvan, T., (1982), Geropsychiatric Mobility in a Semiuran Area Near Madural, *Indian Journals of Psychatry*, vol.24,no.3, pp. 258-267.

World Health Organization, Regional Office for Europe (1959), *The Public Health Aspects of the Aging of the Population*, Report of an Advisory Group.

Section-III
Socioeconomic Aspects of Ageism

13

Socioeconomic Implications of Aging Population in India

K.K. Lakshmanan

"We can not heal old age, but let us protect it, promote it and prolong it".

—*Sir J. Ross*

Introduction

Aging is defined as, "a progressive decline in the physiological capacity leading to a decreased ability to adapt to stressors" or "the loss of adaptability of an individual organism over time". Becker defines as "those changes occurring in an individual as a result of the passage of time". Stieglit describes "aging is a part of living" It begins with conception and terminates with death. Old age is also called "later childhood". Fifty years is the end of youth but the birth of old age. Robert Butler, in late 60s, coined the term AGEISM. Paul Wallace, (1999) added the term AGEQUAKE to gerentological vocabulary.

Let us look at "elderliness' in various dimensions: *Biological* process of aging begins as early as puberty and is a continuous process through adult life; *Socially*, the characteristics of the members of the society respecting them as "Light of the JFS" or put them in orphanage; *Economically* remains as dependent on their merciful children or possibly after much struggle from the government; *Chronologically,* the numeric age is used in defining the term, "elderly" (Kasthuri, 2007).

Observations

Age of the Elders

United Nations recognize 60 years as the age of the old. Some psychologists state that it begins at the age of fifty one. India fixed 55 years as age to retire from service, now raised to 58, in some sectors such as the Universities it is 60 and in judiciary furthermore, and those who decide the destiny of the country never becomes old. States of Assam, Mizoram, Orissa, Chandigarh, Gujarat, Karnataka and Kerala, in line with the Centre, recognize 65 years as the old age.

Status of Elders - Community - Countries

People above 60 are called as senior citizens, aged people and so on. Indian tradition recognizes them as Elders, blessed with wisdom, experience and vision. They are considered as respectful aged. As a Chinese saying

"There is nothing more beautiful in this world than a healthy, wise old man" - Un - U- Tang.

It is a symbol of Joint Family System (JFS). They are national asset so long as they are mentally alert and physically sound and utilized by the country. A country like India can tap this enormous wealth of experience, unbiased expression on national policies and involve them in various welfare schemes.

In countries with JFS there was much scope for saving. In JFS countries like Japan the saving percentage is 3.2, South Korea 4.4, Spain 4.6, Netherland 7.1, Italy 11.6, China

35.0 and in India it is 28.0%. At the time of 1930 economic depression the United States could recover soon because joint family savings were quite high.

In contrast, in Individualised Income System (IIS) there is no saving and loans, credit cards and every family is with debts. Savings in the US was minus 0.4%, Canada -0.2%, Australia - 2.6%, 7 New Zealand - 148% and in the UK - 0.5%.

With the dawn of the new Indian economic policy, 1991, coupled with liberalization and privatization human value has been pushed to the back burner. The strong fabrics of JFS start shredding. The grandparents guiding, helping the young in household duties, sharing their experience on health, family budgeting, children education and all such activities became commercialized. As a result more income is required and the younger generations start leaving home for work with elders left alone.

Elders in India are not homogeneous. People in lower social classes (nearly 75% of elders) are biologically older than those of that age in higher status.

The Western experts analysed key pieces of DNA called telomers (Srinivasan, 2008) which correlate to biological ages. Telomeres are repeated sequences of DNA situated at the ends of the chromosome protecting them from damages.

Professor Tim Spector, St. Thomas Hospital, London, opine "Not only does social class affect health and age-related diseases but seems to have an impact on the ageing process itself'. Ageing reflects on national economy as well.

In 1981 people BPL (Below Poverty Line) earning less than 1.25 USD/Day was 1.9 b. It will turn to be half the global population by 2015. In South Asia which was 60% in 1981 has been reduced to 40% (600 m elders) in 2005. In China it has come down to 18% (207m) from 80% distinctly with industrial revolution of 1991 BPL in India has increased from 420m to 455m. Nearly 90% of Indian elders are from the unorganized sector denied any specialized health and social services. As the younger generation moves to cities the physical and mental strength of the elders are affected. About 22m are widows, a majority are destitutes with no income or support.

About 30% of elderly deaths are on account of lack of government care. No pension (now about 10% of elders receive) no provident fund (mostly worked in unorganized sector), and no medical facility. Healthcare system for elders do not move further beyond filing and publicity.

Grand Parents Boom

Extensive research is on to study the possibility of attenuating the deleterious effects of age-dependent disorders including neurodegenerative - Alzheimer, Parkinson, Huntington, Stroke etc.

It has been shown that the genes where mutated extend or shorten the life span of species of *Drosophia,* mice and humans. While science and technology can create human cells, can they not modify by molecular mechanism this fascinating, yet undesirable process "oldness"?

Aging is Unnatural

As we are seriously discussing about aging Bharat Savur, co-author of the book "Fitness for Life" argues aging is unnatural!

Proteins, neutrons, DNA, electricity all that constitute and run the body do not age. Why then the body? According to Ayurveda all the changes with the age are due to *Pragya aparadh* (Erroneous thinking). Leading an uncomplicated lifestyle makes one's life stronger and longer (Bhat, 2007). Buddha warned, "The mind is everything what you think, you become". Be peaceful, cheerful, contented thoughts preserve and stimulate memory of wholeness cheer, and readiness materialise qualitatively in our cells as elasticity, strength, vitality, alertness. In other words one should be stress-free.

Secondingly exercise according to the age at least for 30-45 mts. It initiates the beautiful process of purifying the system. Walking or cycling is a cardiovascular exercise that floods oxygen into the cells, burns the dross and enliven's the cells. Bends and stretches restore the memory of flexibility to the special and joint tissue.

Next step is dietary regulation to elevate the body, mind the sprit. Plant or animal food with less fat, oil, salt and spread over 5 to 6 times what normally taken in 3 sittings.

The overall glow and vitality of youth on face and body language come from fresh fruits, vegetables and, dry fruit are also rich in vitamins. Rice and wheat, maize promote serene vitality, sprouted pulses build muscles, figs, detoxify. Need not go for apple and almond, but orange, wood apple, guava are quite good.

Meditation relieves from stress enables the mind to relax, releases the rush of fear.

Cheerful attitude exercise, regulated, limited diet, meditation are the four steps to agelessness.

Demography

Globally the present population of elders and the projected one of 2040 portray a grim picture. The number of elders per 100 people of working age will be in Britain 34 to become 65, France 36 as 69, Germany 37 will rise to 72, and the climax in Italy with 103 of the present 40. Almost all of them are from organized sector.

The demographic analysis is presented in a table (Table 1).

In developed countries various deductions are made from the salaries towards health, pension and other social programmes. The government is bound to take care of every citizen.

In Italy people retire at 57 years. The pension is so liberal showing 36 b USD pension deficit in the annual budget. So it has been proposed to raise the retirement age as 60 by 2010 and three fly as 62.

In Germany the problem is tackled by raising the retirement age to 67 and increasing the pension contribution by 2.5% not allowing any to retire before 64 years.

Table 1

Global Demographic Trends 2005

I. Life expectancy	
World	**India**
USA: 78.0	1970 - 49.3
UK: 78.8	2011-16 - 67
France: 80.0	2021 - 70.2
II. Population of elders	
1980 - 8.6%	1991 - 56 m elders
1990 - 9.2% - 484.7m	2001 - 71 m
2000 - 9.9% - 608.7	72.22% rural (741660293)
2010 - 10.8 %	27.78% urban (285354954)
2020 - 12.9% - 1011.6	2016 - 113
	2030 - UN 198 m
	2050 - UN 326 m

Elders above 85+
2005 - 87m
2050 - 320 m

The birth rate is far low. Italy offers incentives to "make more babies" offering "Baby bonus" for every new-born child, a sum of 800 USD and in France child benefit of 140 USD is offered every month for first three years. In Japan the government comes out with all incentives to have more children.

Among the developing countries, China, has remarkably controlled its population explosion. In India although child birth is reduced by:

I. Extensive awareness programmes to have not more than one child a family.

II. Can marry one only.

III. Early mortality of the babies, before age 3, due to malnutrition and undernutrition. Governments offering funds to have healthy pregnant women, part of it is snatched away while paying every month.

IV. Due to pollution and poisoning of the groundwater with industrial effluents the fertility potentcy is reduced in several parts of the country as in Kongunadu area of TN. The fertility 6% in 1971, became 4.8 in 1981,3.6 in 1991 and expected to be 2.6 in 2021.

V. About 30% of death of elders is due to poverty either because government welfare funds are far less or do not reach the elders in the rural areas.

Regionwise, peninsular India will have 8% of aged in contrast with 5.6% in North-East region of India. Similarly old age dependence ratio is high (13.2%) as against 9.5% in NE. In the latter sex ratio shows more females (1139 men 1000 woman) an against 954 men for every thousand.

The statistical jugglary in population numbers is due to lapses in data collection. It should be made mandatory that every elder is registered. Registration, besides by the authority, can be carried out by others such as, NGOs, social organizations and individual agents. They can be provided with incentive in registering the elders and welfare schemes may be operated through them, as envisaged in the National Policy.

Some of the Government Welfare Programmes

1. ***Maintenance and Welfare Parents and Senior Citizens Act, 2007***

"Welfare" means provision for food, healthcare, recreation centres and other amenities necessary for elders (60+).

State governments by notification in the Official Gazette make rules for carrying out the purposes of this Act.

2. ***National Old Age Pension Schemes***

65+ offered a pension of Rs.200/months, that is 66 p/couple /day (Ministry of Rural Development) Recipients of the pension in UP are 1576481, Bihar 904916, Tamil Nadu (TN) 494996. Is it justified that our record showing the elders in TN are just 5 lakhs. The state has 1.8 crores of ration cards for families BPL of which at least 60% will have 1 elder in each family.

Fourteen states offer Rs.75-150 from 60+. Gujarat, Rajasthan, Punjab, Haryana, Bengal, Delhi and Chandigarh offer Rs.200-300 (65+) while TN offers Rs.400.

3. ***National Family Benefit Scheme***

On death of family head (64+) is given Rs.10,000/-, however, Tamil Nadu Government has increased it to Rs.15,000/--

4. ***Annapurna Scheme***

The scheme operated by the States offer 10 kg of free food grains / person / month. Tamil Nadu offers 20 kg per ration card. In ration a kilo a rupee is mostly welcomed.

5. ***Free Legal Aid - Ministry of Law***

6. ***Health facilities - Ministry of Health and Family Welfare***

   - separate queues in hospital OPD - out of turn at the registration counters, consultancy
   - AIIMS, Safdarjury Hospital on specific days offering Geriatric clinics.

Health care in Gujarat, Kerala, Maharashtra. However they do not meet the needs of the elders.

Han Seangsoo (2002) President, UN General Assembly observed, "Older persons must be seen as an asset, not a burden. A million men and women turn 60 every month, 75% of them in the developing world.

In India 25.6 m of elders of 1961 will touch 340 m in 2061. Dunng that span of the century, population will climb five times but the elders soar 13 times, with the prevailing economy, healthcare and fertility potential. Most of the elders are from villages. According to the Census of India 2001 rural elders are (741660293) as against (285354954) of urban sector (Rural 72-22% urban 27.78%) Total 1,02701527).

In 2050, 70% of global elders will be in China (194m). India with 119 million (India 21.0%) which according to UN will be 326m. The Registrar General of India and National Commission on population 173.18m (2001) states that the 83.58 m elders of 2006 will turn to be 173 m in 2026 (NISD 2008).

In Japan people living in Okinawa eat 20% less food than in Tokyo. They have high number of people living longer than 105 years, called supercentenarians - mild climate, unique eating habits and active lifestyle are the basis (Willcox *et al.* 2006) to *add* years to life; Add life to years, add quality to added life.

The existing elder care institutions take care of less than 1 % of the elders. The community care institutions and geriatric nursing homes for chronically and terminally ill are very few (Jamuna, 2003).

The country should rise to enact "Active ageing" policies and programmes that enhance health, independence and productivity of the elders (WHO, 2001).

Health Care

The elderly segment facing risks with respect to their health or socio-economic status, such as "High risks" are very old (80+), living alone or merely as couple, elderly women single, elderly couple chronically ill one or both and those living in elders Homes, Orphanage, (Kasturi, 2007).

India can not afford modern medical system to the rural elders although attractive programmes are published. Therefore Indian Systems of Medicine can be better utilized.

The structural, functional, mental and emotional status of the elders are so different that they need special health needs. Illness can neither be predicted nor assessing its manifestation is easy. Their physical illness is associated with depression, mental loneliness and other causes (Shaji, 2003).

The elders are prone to chronic and non-communicable disease, as well as disabilities. The top four illness are visual, arthritis, insomnia and stress.

They should be immunized just like the tots for polio, with pneumococcal vaccination to prevent infection which can cause pneumonia, septicaemia (blood poisoning), meningitis (inflammation around the brain). Physical handicap in chewing and swallowing due to dental decay, immobility, mental restrictions are common. Some general geriatric problems of the elders are - anxiety, stress, osteoporosis, urinary incontinence, stroke, dementia

(Paraswani *et al.*, 2005) (spectre of Alzheimer's disease) (Paraswani *et al., 2005).*

As the rural elders are in poverty sufficient vitamins and minerals are needed to protect against cancer, cataract, rheumatoid arthritis and cardiovascular diseases. Primary Health Centres, Hospitals and their subsidiaries can provide medication and substitutes for nutrition.

WHO recognized the limits of providing disease specific interventions. So a Commission on Macroeconomics and Health (2002) was erected which advocates the use of a "close-to client" system, including outreach services, health centres and local hospitals more accessable to the poor.

1. Primary care at community level,
2. specialized care by an internist or geriatrician and
3. specific intervention by a specialist physician or surgeon.

Health is a function, not only of medical care but also of an overall integrated development of society — cultural, economic, literacy, social and political.

General medical care of elders is concerned with clinical, preventive, remedial and social aspects of illness.

Specialised geriatric care are available hardly in 5,6 medical colleges among 170 institutions (Jamuna, 2003).

It may not be possible to enhance the capacity of dhathus but they can be protected and rejuvenated. Ayurveda offers several therapies for prolongation of life boosting of memory and intelligence, immunomodulatory effects against diseases (Bhat, 2007).

"Good health at low cost" published by Rockfeller Foundation (1980s) recognizes China, Costa Rica, Sri Lanka and Kerela State in India as having achieved affordable and effective health systems. However the most desired, "Health for All - 2000" is yet to be achieved in the country

Geriatric centres should be in all hospitals. Geriatric research centre be established in every medical college. Geriatric wards are reported to function in Chennai and Madurai and by Lions Club in Coimbatore.

Dr. V.S. Natarajan, Geriatric expert, who did yeomen service in establishing the Geriatric division, Madras Medical College, Chennai offers some suggestions to the elders. He insists on confidence, exercise, meditation instead of feeling lonely, an unavoidable event, keep a dog, cat, parrot or fish tank, observe and relax if human do not care.

To avoid (insomnia) sleeplessness, go to bed at a regular time, slight exercise in the evening, bath, few minutes meditation, a little milk. Never feel you have become aged. Keep dried grapes ready and take few whenever you feel lonely, depressed. Have medical check up annually if below 65 or six months once still older.

Palliative care aims to provide coordinated medical, nursing and allied services for those who are terminally ill, delivered wherever possible in the environment of the choice of the patient. Palliative care involves not only the specialists, general practitioners, and nursing staff but also involves friends and relatives, to be prepared for terminal eventuality and offer love. In short it affirms life, provides relief from pain and other distressing systems, integrates psychological, emotional and spiritual aspects of that elders and brings a sense of calm and final acceptance of their coming demise.

Discussion

Caring for the Disadvantaged Elders

The society and the governments should evolve active aging approach based on human rights of the older people and the UN principles of independence, participation, dignity, care and self fulfillment. Constitution of India, Article 41 direct the states to improve the quality of life of elders.

The National Policy visualizes that the State will extend support for financial security, healthcare, shelter, welfare and other needs of the elders, provide protection against abuse and exploitation. The policy recognizes that the elders are a resource.

Indian life is based on the political environment. The elders in India accounts for 12% of the vote bank. A political party wins hardly with 28% of votes. So elders can change the wind of the political system. Unfortunately the retired elders are unconcerned with the problems. Most of the Indian elders are in rural areas and are susceptible to petty gift for their votes due to poverty making democracy a mockery.

In such an environment one should analyse the problems and possible solutions to make their life worth living.

Problems of the Elders

1. Poverty - Nearly 70% of illiterate, unskilled elderly workers are in dire poverty. About 30% death of elders is due to poverty.
2. Nearly 20 m women are widows, living alone or destitutes.
3. World Health Organisation speaks about active aging determined by (i) social factors such as literacy, rights and social support (ii) physical environment with assured shelter and basic social protection (iii) economic factors such as income, work (iv) personal factors adaptability and hereditary (v) Healthcare (vi) Behavioural factors such as physical activity, nutrition, appropriate medication, free from abuse. All the above are to be addressed for prevention, intervention and rehabilitation.

4. Lack of adequate healthcare.It is a multitude of services rendered to indivividuals, families or communities by the agent of health services for promoting, maintatining monitoring and restoring health. Under pressure from the World Bank, Primary Health Centres were established - remaining without expansion under staff and poorly equipped. Even the eight key components of the Alma - Ata Declaration (1978) did not offer special care for the elders.

   A separate aged health care be established in every PHC and hospital (Dey, 2003) proposed a model for healthcare. Health care staff at PHC level may not be able to offer gerontological care. However PHCs strengthened, number increased to address rural health problems.

5. Protection under law. Instead of the government taking upon itself in protecting the elders, by Maintenance and Welfare Parents and Senior citizen Act 2007 force the children or close relatives to take care of the elders what can not be done by love can not be forced by law. Moreover nearly 32% of rural unorganized labourers live on seven rupees a day. In Tamil Nadu 25% of population exist with Rs.571/- mensem and 20% with Rs.2000/- with such earning, members can not to take care of their elders.

6. The existing facilities offered by the government can hardly address 1 % of the elders.

7. The younger generations leaving their elders in the village move to cities. Even well educated children going abroad can provide financial assistance but can not help in their loneliness, domestic assistance.

8. Ill health is more due to depression, mental torture.

9. Joint family system is fast eroding.
10. The governments are in a fix. The administration has never met with such a problem as elder care. The machinery is also averse to visit rural areas to focus the needs of the elders effectively. As D'souza (1990) described :" the simmering problems of the elderly - will burst into flames"
11. The lonely elders in urban areas are often exposed to robbery, murder.

The remedial measures to treat the elders with respect, comfort and utilize their wealth of experience new programmes are to be evolved taking voluntary organizations and institutions into confidence.

1. A massive drive is to be made to enroll all the elders. The elders in rural and backward areas can be linked with ICDS programmes (Prakash 1991).
2. Care homes can be established by public organizations with various motives - shelter, food, recreation, nursing, dementia, mental disorders, physical disability drug / alcohol addiction
3. Cultural contacts. The government should plan to interact with people to avoid starving in loneliness. "Neighbours clubs" can be organized by private sector.
4. Arrange periodical tours to peaceful green environment, bird sanctuaries, places of worship.
5. Knowledge care - To keep the brain alert, facilities be provided to visit local fund libraries, library can move to houses, to attend to religious, musical programmes
6. Personal Security: All the elders be provided with addresses and telephone contacts in cases of emergency -looting, attempts to murder.

7. Working facilitates: Villagers can not sit idle. They can be provided with some work what their mind and body can permit. The experienced rural elders illiterates can guide younger generations in honeybee keeping, preparation of various compost knitting, rural handicrafts, fine arts, narrate events to inculcate patriotism in young minds.

8. Health care for the elders

"Ageing is a boon but not a bane"

Awareness and acceptance of the fact that aging has physiological, psychological and social determinants would make the aging process - not a disease - acceptable, cheerful, perhaps even desirable by making living meaningful.

Use your time purposefully continue your hobby, social activities, maintain old contacts exchange ideas. Maintain cordial relationship understand and tolerate younger generations. Do not thrust you views on any. Plan your way of life - to be socially active, to maintain good health (Dietary programme, exercise, meditation). To keep mental health accept life as it comes. Practice pet therapy (have a dog, cat, aquarium) or garden (green therapy) to ignore loneliness. To maintain peace of made attend religious discourses, visit libraries.

The governments offer several welfare schemes, health programmes but lack a body to review periodically how far they have reached the elders.

Some sort of Health Management Organisations (HMO) be established. All private practitioners can serve the society. Private hospitals can also register. A package will take care of medical check up, another the management of chronic ailments, yet nother on symptom - based cases and so on.

National Rural Health Mission (NRHM) should proceed towards assuring the health rights of the people: New Deal for Disabled People (NDDP) and RSVD (Retired on Senior Voluntary Programmes may also take care of elders). The government hospitals can provide elders' ward, geriatric wards in every district.

The health care and free hospital facilities will not be utilized by the urban pensioners where they are available.

Palliative care is needed to provide coordinated medical, nursing and allied services for those who are terminally ill. It involves not only the specialists, general practitioners, and nursing staff but also involve friends to be prepared for terminal eventually offering love, help and support.

> "You matter because you are you and you matter to the last moment of your life. We will do all we can, not only to help you die peacefully, but to live until you die".
>
> - Dame Cicely Saunders

Today's youth are tomorrows' elders.

REFERENCES

Bhat, S., (2007), Greying with grace, *Health Action* (6), p.15-17

Dey, A.B., (2003), A Model Healthcare for Older People in India, in A.B. Dey (ed.), *Ageing in India Situation Analysis and Planning for the Future*, Ministry of Health and Family Welfare and WHO, New Delhi, pp.269-274.

D'Souza, V., (1990), *The Simmering Problems of Aging in India*, Bold (UN) 1(1); pp.17-21

Jamuna, D., (2003), Issues of Elder Case and Elder Abuse in the Indian Context, in Liebig, PS. and Rajan, I.S. (ed.), *Aging in India Perspectives, Prospects and Policies*. The Haworth Press, Inc. NY, pp.125-142

Kasturi, A., (2007), Travails of a Greying Nation, *Health Action* (6), pp. 4,5,19

Age Care in India: National Initiative on Care for Elderly. National Institute of Social Defence, Ministry of Social Justice and Empowerment, Government of India, Jan 2008. pp. 95.

Paraswani, M.J., Sharma, M. P. and Bharath, S., 2005, Care Givers Distress, Mobidity and burden in Dementia: Rationale for Intervention, in I.J. Prakash (ed), *Aging in India: Retrospect and Prospect,* Bangalore University, Bangalore pp.123-132.

Shafi, S., (2003), Health Need of the Elderly, *Health Action* (7), pp. 34-35

Wallace, P., (1999), *Agequake: Riding The Demographic Roller Coaster, Shaking Business, Finance and Our World,* Nicholas Brealey Publication Ltd., London.

WHO, (2001), *Health and Ageing: A Discussion Paper,* World Health Organisation, Geneva.

14

Socioeconomic Condition of the Assamese Elderly of Guwahati

Chandana Sarmah

Aging is a biological process that begins with birth and ends with death of an individual. The process of aging, as is now generally known, consists of progressive changes that take place in a cell, an organ or the total individual. The changes relating to aging begin after the attainment of maturity and they are mostly degenerative and irreversible. As a result there is gradual impairment in the structure and functional ability of an individual with advancement of age.

In the last century, two demographic changes occurred which brought about a significant change in the age structure of the world population. The first is the increase in the average life expectancy and the other is decline in fertility rate. The average life expectancy of population is the average age at which people born in a particular year die. The increase in the average age at which people die brings about an increase in both the average age and the life expectancy of the population. Moreover, the average number of children born to each woman has come down. As a result the proportion of children to the total population has gone down, resulting in a higher average age. These two features of increase in life expectancy and decline in fertility have occurred in the twentieth century primarily due to social advancements and achievements made in the fields of medical science and public health. The outcome of these features is that the proportion of elderly population to the total population has gone up. This pattern of change in the age distribution of the population is called population ageing. Thus, population ageing, is defined in terms of the ratio of the aged population to the total population. According to the United Nations (1956), a population is called an aging population if more than 7% of the total population belongs to the aged category.

The developed countries of the world have witnessed this change in the age structure of their population much earlier, i.e. before the World War II. In the developing countries, the process of change in the age structure has begun much later. However, in these countries the number of elderly is growing at a phenomenal rate. In 1990, the population of 60 years and above in the developing countries exceeded that of the developed countries. By 2030, the world elderly population is expected to be around 1.4 billion which would be almost triple the 1990 figure. Most of this growth will take place in the developing countries and over half of it in Asia (World Bank, 1994). The two major population giants of Asia, namely China and India will contribute significantly to the growth of this figure (Rajan, Misra and Sarma, 2000).

In India, the proportion of elderly in 1961 was 5.6%. This rose to 6.6% in1991 and according to a projections of a study by the Centre for Development Studies, Thiruvanthapuram, it is expected to rise to 7.1% in 2001 (Rajan, Misra, Sarma 2000). The actual figure according to 2001 census is 7.4%, which is slightly higher than the estimated proportion. The proportion appears to be small because of the large population base the country has. But in actual figures, the number is quite high. Demographers predict that by the year 2015, India is going to have the third largest aging population after China and Japan.

The present study is on the aged in Assamese society in the urban context of Guwahati. Guwahati is one of the oldest townships of the northeastern region. The city because of its geographic location acts as a connecting link to the other states of northeastern part of India with the rest of the country. With the gain of importance as the link, the city is soon responding to the needs of urbanisation and modernisation. The people of the city, however, appear to be in a state of transition. It is the younger generation who is rapidly adapting to the changes whereas the elders still adhere to the old social morals and values.

The elderly in the Assamese society occupies a very respectable position. In the rural areas of Assam agriculture is the main occupation. The knowledge and experience of the elderly people are sought after in an agrarian society and as such the status of the elderly people is quite high. However, in the urban areas of Guwahati, the occupational pattern is completely different from that of rural areas of Assam. As a result aging has emerged as a problem in Guwahati just as in any other urban centre of India. Some of the factors which are mainly responsible for the growth of the ageing problem in Guwahati are the rapid rate of urbanisation, urban migration, adoption of the urban way of life, education and employment of women in the service sector and the subsequent change of role of women in the family structure, etc. The problem of aging is not specific to the aged alone but to the society in general, as the presence of the elderly and their problems affect the functioning of the society.

A large majority of the people currently residing in the city is of rural origin. They have come here either in connection with their occupation and have settled down here or have accompanied their children to the latter's home at much later stage of their life. In case of the second category of people they are forced to move to the city by circumstances of not having anyone to look after them in their own homes. In both the cases feelings of nostalgia and longing for their former home is found to exist. The people who migrate to an urban area later in life have to adjust with a completely new situation beginning at the very household level. In such circumstances the problems of the elderly become evident. In addition to coping with their own biological process of ageing, they have to deal with a social difference and adapt to a situation with which they are unfamiliar. Even the original residents of Guwahati have witnessed a sea change in the place. Changes have occurred in all spheres of life ranging from the structure and functioning of the family to the society. Earlier, it was the women in the household who used to take care of the elderly within their homes. With the employment of women in service outside their homes, a change has occurred in the care giving role. Women are no longer able to devote as much time to their traditional role. Moreover the joint family system is breaking down. In a traditional joint family, the elderly are surrounded by a number of kinship relations. This type of family in a way has been able to provide emotional as well as physical security to the elderly. The changing family situation has led to the emergence of a number of conflict situations both from the caregiver and care receiver's point of view. Even where joint families are present, it appears to be impossible to provide the care and attention necessary for the elderly due to pressures created by the demands of a modern urban life style. It is in these situations that the problems of the elderly emerge.

Material and Methodology

The study, as the title suggests, is among the elderly from the Assamese community living in the city of Guwahati.

People who are sixty years and above are categorised as 'aged' in the present study. It is a cross-sectional study consisting of both male and female respondents. Mainly the snowballing technique has been applied to locate the respondents which proved to be most effective as the elderly are sparsely distributed. The sample consists of respondents from three income groups i.e. the high-income group, the middle income group and the low-income group. The model designed by the National Council of Applied Economic Research has been used in classifying the income groups.

The sample consists of 280 respondents, of which, 100 each belong to the high and middle income group and 80 belong to the low income group. The hundred respondents from the high and middle income group comprise of 50 male and 50 female respondents. The low income group comprises of 50 female and 30 male respondents. Structured schedules were used for collecting data and the field work was conducted during parts of 2003 and 2004.

Socioeconomic Condition of the Assamese Elderly

The social and economic changes taking place in the society are important from the point of view of the elderly as they have serious implication in their life. Some of the factors which have a considerable influence on the life of an elderly person are breakdown of the joint family structure, lesser number of children per couple, greater longevity, physical separation of parents from children due to age selective migration, changing attitude of the younger generation against the older ones, elderly migration to urban areas at a later stage in life to stay with children, etc. Some of the social conditions of the elderly of the Assamese community living in Guwahati are discussed below.

Age-Sex Distribution of the Sample

There are fifty male and fifty female respondents from

the high and middle income group. In the low income group there are thirty male and fifty female respondents. The sample is further categorised into young old (60-69 years), middle old (70-79 years) and old old (80+years) after the classification of Burnside (1979). The highest concentration of males (43%) is in the middle old category and that of females in the young old category (58.67%). If the age-sex distribution of the respondents is examined against income group (Table 1), it is seen that the respondents from the old old category are from the high and middle income group. In the low income group there are only 4.35% males and no females in the old old category. On the whole, there is a gradual decline in the number of female respondents from the young old to the old old category. Among males, on the other hand, the decline in number with increase in age is observed from the middle old age category.

Marital Status

Marital status is an important demographic feature of any population. Among the elderly especially, it plays a significant role in their life satisfaction level. Married couples are able to face the social and emotional crisis in life in a better way than single ones. In the Assamese society, women are generally younger than men at the time of marriage. Moreover, life expectancy in women on an average is higher than men. In the study, it has been found (Table 2) that the proportion of elderly women who no longer have a surviving spouse is high (62%). The number of women who currently have a surviving spouse is high in the young old age category and the number gradually declines with increase in age. With increase in age the number of widows gradually increases. The proportion of men, on the other hand, who no longer have a surviving spouse, is much lower than women (11.54%). Only a very small number of elderly men and women of the study are found to have remained unmarried or are separated from their spouse.

Living Arrangement

The joint family is the characteristic feature in a traditional Assamese society. This type of family embraces the members in a web of relationships, providing the much needed emotional and physical security to the elders. As there are many members in a joint family, one or the other member can take care of the needs of the elderly. Some of the factors which have currently emerged as problems for the elderly, used to be taken care of in the traditional joint family system.

Till some decades ago, the urban life was more or less a reflection of the traditional rural atmosphere. However, in recent years the family structure is undergoing rapid change under the impact of urbanisation and modernisation. Certain features emerging out of these two aspects and which are seen to directly influence the family structure are as follows:

1. The changing value system of the younger generation.
2. Migration of the younger generation for education or employment, leaving their parents alone.
3. The profession of the males in an urban setting demands them to be very busy with their occupation, where they have very little time to attend to other family members.
4. More employment of women in the service sector, which compels them to remain away from home for quite sometime, leaving the elderly alone at home. It subsequently also brings about a change in the traditional care giving role of women.
5. Even when the women are not employed, the urban lifestyle demands them to be busy with different outdoor activities relating to their children, social occasions, functions, or sometimes in their own recreational activities. They no longer remain confined to their homes.

As a result, a change is taking place in the role of the women towards the elderly and home.The younger generation can adapt to these changes quite well. But these aspects are new to the elderly and have a bearing on their life. Thus, the study of living arrangement has emerged as an important feature in gerontology or the study of aging.

Some of the other factors which commonly influence the living arrangement are age, sex, marital status, economic condition, the number of children the elderly has, etc. A very old, economically or physically dependent person cannot stay alone. A change in marital status also brings about a change in the structure of the family. When the children after marriage continue to live with parents, a joint family emerges. On the other hand, if the children set up independent homes, the elderly parents, in the absence of another child may have to stay alone. In case of an elderly couple staying alone, the death of one of the spouse brings about a drastic change in the family structure. The surviving elderly, in such a situation may have to either stay alone or may be forced to move in with their children. The elderly generally do not like to give up their home, but sometimes they are left with not much choice. Relocating in a new place at a later stage in life is difficult for the elderly as it requires adjustment to a totally new physical as well as social environment.

Joint family is still found to be the predominant type of family in the study (51.07%). But what has emerged to be significant (Table 3) is that it is followed by the type of family where an elderly couple lives alone (18.93%). The proportion of such families appears to be increasing and this reflects the changing pattern of family in the Assamese society. Nuclear families are found predominantly among the elderly of the young old age category. In such families, it has been found that the children are still dependent on their parents, or are in the process of completing their studies or are unmarried. The pattern of these families may change in the event of any change of social and economic status of any family member. 7.86% of the elderly stay with alone. Higher proportion of elderly women than men are found to be living alone. Most of the women who live alone are widows or are unmarried. 7.14% of the elderly of the study live with relatives, mostly married daughters. They either do not have a son or their son lives in a place where the elderly do not want to emigrate to. They are forced to move in with relatives because of their age or their physical condition, which no longer permit them to live alone. A very small number of elderly, mostly women are found to be living in the only old age home in Guwahati.

Past and Present Occupation

As the sample of the study consists of elderly who are sixty years and above, most of them have retired from their professional occupation. The past occupation of the elderly male varies from wage earners and petty traders to professionals like doctors and lawyers, depending on their income group. Many of them were also employed in government service. Women, on the other hand, were predominantly housewives. Only a very few of them were employed as school teachers, government servants or professionals (Table 4).

The objective of looking into the present occupation is to understand how the elderly spend their time. The past occupation to a large extent plays a determining role in their present occupation. 27.69% male and 12% of the female elderly continue to be involved in economically gainful activity. People from the high income group, especially professionals and retired government servants take up employment as a means of keeping themselves engaged. Whereas the people of the lower income group continue to do so as it is their only means of sustenance. Women were mostly housewives and they continue to be actively involved in household activities. They are found to remain active up to the young old age category, but with increase in age and deteriorating physical condition, they become unable to remain active for long (Table 5). Then there is a shift to being occasional workers i.e. they do housework only when their health conditions permit. There is yet another group of elderly who are unable to do any work, within or outside their house anymore. Some of them can only perform the activities relating to their daily personal care, while others need assistance even in such activities. This group of elderly for the purpose of the study has been placed in the retired category.

In the 60-69 years age category, the proportion of active and occasional workers among elderly women is more or less the same. However, in the next decade, i.e. 70-79 years the proportion of occasional workers rises significantly and active workers declines markedly. The same trend is seen even among elderly men, but it is not so marked as in women. Men continue to remain active for more number of years than women. But in the 80+ age category almost all women and a very high proportion of men belong to the retired category i.e. they are no longer able to do any work. Thus, it can be said that retirement from active work is much earlier in females than in males, as is found from the higher number of retired females from the 70-79 age category.

Current Source of Income

The past and present occupation of a person plays a role in determining the economic condition of an elderly. Economic conditions in turn determine the role and behavior of an elderly within the family or society. Economic independence gives greater satisfaction, security as well as deciding power to the elderly.

It is observed that both past and present occupation pattern of the elderly varies according to age and sex. As a result, the variation in the economic conditions between the two sexes in different age groups is quite apparent among the elderly of the present study. The economic condition of the elderly individual has been determined from their current means of subsistence. Some elderly have their own source of income or are economically independent and others do not have any and are economically dependent. The independent elderly have earnings from different sources like earnings from current occupation, past savings, pensions and rent of property. Those who do not have any income source become dependent on their children.

51.79% of the elderly in the sample are independent and the remaining 48.21% are dependent (Table 6). There is significant gender variation among the independent elderly having some income source, with more men (61.54%) having an income than women (29.33%). Among the elderly who have their own income, past savings and pension (26.15%) are the major source. 24.62% of elderly men have earnings from current occupation and 10.77% have earnings from rent of property in addition to their pension.

As women are predominantly housewives, their husband's income or pension is one of their major means of subsistence. Only 4.67% of the women have their own pension or have earnings from current work, 10.67% have additional benefit of family pension and earnings from rent of property, 18.67% of the women depend on current income or pension of spouse.

Those elderly who are entirely supported by their children are referred to as fully dependent and those who derive some pension but also need the support of their children are referred to as partially dependent in the present study. Dependency among women (56.67%) is found to be greater than men (38.46%), mainly because of their past occupational pattern. There are some elderly who do not have any source of income and are completely dependent on their children. Total dependency is greater in women (34%) than men (14.62%).

Problems of the Elderly

The biological decline with aging brings about a limitation in the functioning of their social roles and also the roles within the family. This eventually gives rise to problems of another nature among the elderly. Other than their health problem, the main problems that are found to be prevalent among the elderly are that of loneliness, utilisation of time and financial problems. Declining health is found to be the most prominent problem among elderly. The other problems like loneliness, utilisation of time, financial, etc. may sometimes arise out of health problem or sometimes these problems may ultimately give rise to health problems.

The distribution of the elderly by their problems is shown in table 7. 7.69% of the male and 2.67% of the female elderly reportedly do not have any problem. The elderly who do not have any problem belong to the young old and middle old age category.

Health as has already been mentioned is the most prominent problem. 19.23% of the elderly men have only health problem. This is followed by the prevalence of health problems along with other problems like loneliness (16.92%), utilisation of time (16.92%) and finance (16.15%). Loneliness and utilisation of time together is found to occur among 16.92% of elderly men. The proportion of elderly having these problems increases with age. Among elderly women health problem along with loneliness are found to occur most frequently (34.00%). The number of women who have these two problems together is found to be much higher than men and from the young old age category onwards. Health problem along with financial problem is the second most (23.33%) prominent problem among elderly women. As has already been discussed most women do not have their own source of income and as a result are facing financial problems in their later life. In case of women also declining health is a major problem and this is generally found to occur along with other problems. Loneliness and utilisation of time without any major health problem is found to be prevalent among 12% of elderly women.

Loneliness and utilisation of time have emerged as major social problems in the study area, in spite of the fact that the largest portion of elderly are living in extended families. With the increasing employment of women outside the household, the elderly are mostly left to themselves during the day. There are certain other associated implications of this factor. Women generally like to transfer some of the household responsibilities to their daughters-in-law. Such transfer of responsibilities becomes impossible in cases where the daughter-in-law is a working woman. In such a situation the elderly women are forced to manage their home even with not very good health condition. Sometimes they are to look after their young grandchildren as well. Grandparents usually like to spend time with their grandchildren but looking after grandchildren at the infant stage and attending to their every need, without any extra help, becomes difficult for the elderly.

Discussion and Conclusion

The Assamese society is undergoing a lot of socio-economic and cultural changes. The social factors in aging in this society are found to be aggravated by the changing cultural and socio-economic conditions. The social structure is undergoing change due to change in the traditional occupational pattern. There is heavy migration of the younger generation to places outside the state for education and employment. This brings about a change in their value system as well as in the family structure. Moreover with the increase in the level of women education, the number of women employed outside their home has gone up considerably creating a void in the traditional care giving role in the family.

Life expectancy as a whole has gone up, especially women's life expectancy. Due to greater life expectancy, women are found to live for more number of years and mostly as widows in their later par of life. Moreover, family structures are changing. Traditional joint families are giving way to nuclear families. The younger generation is very mobile, moving to places outside the state for education and occupational purpose. This is further fragmenting the nuclear families from the point of view of residence. Elderly people try to remain active as long as physically possible but ultimately have to succumb to their declining health condition. Some elderly people continue to be employed in economically gainful activity to remain active. However, there are others who have to do the same for their sustenance. They do not have anyone to support and look after them in their old age. Men continue to remain active for more number of years than women, but with increasing age the gender variation is no longer found to exist. Women have in earlier times mostly remained within the house. As a result they do not have financial independence. They were either dependent on their spouse and after their spouse are dependent on their children. Financial dependence in old age can greatly hinder life satisfaction level in elderly people.

Declining health has emerged as the most prominent problem among the elderly of the Assamese society. The other problems that are found to be prevalent among the elderly are that of loneliness and problem of utilising their time. Both these problems are more or less the result of social disability created out of declining health. In case of elderly people, one problem may become the cause of another problem. For example, health problem which lead to social disability may give rise to problem of utilising their time and subsequently to loneliness. The reverse may also be true when loneliness and not having any other person to interact with may give rise to health problems. In an urban situation, people mostly remain busy and are unable to give the elderly the necessary time and attention. The most important thing that needs consideration in dealing with the elderly is that the emotional needs of the elderly change with age. The family members need to understand the special nature of needs of the elderly. The solution to the problems of the elderly lies in their remaining integrated in the family.

REFERENCES

Burnside, I.M., P. Ebersole, H.E.Monea(edited). (1979). *Psychological Caring Throughout the Life Cycle*, New York; McGraw-Hill.

Rajan, S.I., U.S. Misra, P.S. Sarma. (2000). Ageing in India: Retrospect and Prospect, *Indian Social Science Review*, 2.1, 1-47.

United Nations. (1956). c.f. *Aging in India with Special Reference to North East India,* P.B. Das memorial lecture delivered by Deepak Tyagi in the Department of Anthropology, Gauhati University 2000.

World Bank. (1994). Averting the Income Crisis for the Old in *World Bank Policy Research, Bulletin,* 5: 4.

Table 1

Distribution of elderly by age, sex and income group

Age(years)	*Sex*	*Income Group*							
		High Income group		*Middle Income group*		*Low Income Group*		*Total*	
		No.	*%*	*No.*	*%*	*No.*	*%*	*No.*	*%*
60 – 69	Male	14	29.78	16	34.00	17	36.17	47	36.15
	Female	21	23.86	29	32.95	38	43.18	88	58.67
70 – 79	Male	23	41.06	21	37.50	12	21.43	56	43.08
	Female	17	36.17	18	38.30	12	25.53	47	31.33
80 +	Male	13	48.15	13	48.15	1	3.70	27	20.76
	Female	12	80.00	3	20.00			15	10.00
Total	Male	50	38.46	50	38.46	30	23.08	130	46.43
	Female	50	33.33	50	33.33	50	33.33	150	53.57

Table – 2

Distribution of elderly by marital status

Age(years)	*Sex*	*Marital Status*									
		Never married		*Currently married*		*Widowed*		*Separated*		*Total*	
		No.	*%*	*No.*	*%*	*No.*	*%*	*No.*	*%*	*No.*	*%*
60 – 69	Male	2	4.26	41	87.23	4	8.51			47	100
	Female	4	4.55	39	44.32	43	48.86	2	2.27	88	100
70 – 79	Male	1	1.79	51	91.07	4	7.14			56	100
	Female			11	23.40	36	76.60			47	100
80 +	Male			20	74.07	7	25.93			27	100
	Female			1	6.67	14	93.33			15	100
Total	Male	3	2.31	112	86.15	15	11.54			130	100
	Female	4	2.67	51	34.00	93	62.00	2	1.33	150	100
Grand total		7	2.50	163	58.21	108	38.57	2	0.71	280	100

Table 3
Distribution of elderly by their living arrangement

Age(years)	*Sex*	*Living arrangement*											
		Living alone		*Living with only spouse*		*Nuclear family*		*Joint family*		*Living with relatives*		*Institutions and homeless*	
		No	*%*	*No*	*%*	*No*	*%*	*No*	*%*	*No*	*%*	*No*	*%*
60 – 69	Male	1	2.13	7	14.89	17	36.17	19	40.43	2	4.26	1	2.13
	Female	12	13.64	15	17.05	10	11.36	46	52.27	4	4.55	1	1.14
70 – 79	Male	1	1.79	20	35.71	3	5.36	29	51.79	2	3.57	1	1.79
	Female	7	14.89	5	10.64	4	8.51	24	51.06	5	10.64	2	4.26
80 +	Male	1	3.70	6	22.22	3	11.11	15	55.55	2	7.41		
	Female							10	66.67	5	33.33		
Total	Male	3	2.31	33	25.38	23	17.69	63	48.46	6	4.61	2	1.54
	Female	19	12.67	20	13.33	14	9.33	80	53.33	14	9.33	3	2

Table 4
Distribution of elderly by past occupation

Age (years)	*Sex*	*Past Occupation*													
		Wage earner & Petty trader		*School teacher*		*Non-gazetted Govt. servant*		*Gazetted Govt. servant*		*Profess-ional*		*House wife*		*Busine-ssman*	
		No	*%*	*No*	*%*	*No*	*%*	*No*	*%*	*No*	*%*	*No*	*%*	*No*	*%*
60 – 69	Male	11	23.40	1	2.13	12	25.53	19	40.43	2	4.26			2	4.26
	Female	10	11.36	4	4.55	1	1.14			1	1.14	72	81.82		
70 – 79	Male	10	17.86			6	10.71	31	55.35	8	14.29			1	1.79
	Female	3	6.38	1	2.13							43	91.49		
80 +	Male			4	14.81	7	25.93	12	44.44	4	14.81				
	Female			1	6.67					1	6.67	13	86.67		
Total	Male	21	16.15	5	3.85	25	19.23	62	47.69	14	10.77			3	2.31
	Female	13	8.67	6	4	1	0.67			2	1.33	128	85.33		

Table 5
Distribution of elderly by present occupation

Age(years)	*Sex*	*Present Occupation*									
		Involved in economic activity		*Social work*		*Active housework*		*Occasional housework*		*Retired*	
		No	*%*	*No*	*%*	*No*	*%*	*No*	*%*	*No*	*%*
60 – 69	Male	15	31.91			9	19.15	19	40.43	4	8.51
	Female	14	15.91			33	37.5	35	39.77	6	6.82
70 – 79	Male	17	30.36			4	7.14	22	39.29	13	23.21
	Female	4	8.52	2	4.26	5	10.64	22	46.81	14	29.79
80 yrs	Male	4	14.81	1	3.70	1	3.70	3	11.11	18	66.67
and above	Female			1	6.67					14	93.33
Total	Male	36	27.69	1	0.77	14	10.77	44	33.85	35	26.92
	Female	18	12	3	2	38	25.33	57	38	34	22.67

Table 6

Distribution of elderly by means of subsistence

Age(years)	*Sex*	*Independent*								*Dependent*			
		Income from current work		*Past savings and pension*		*Pension and rent of property*		*Current earnings or pensions of spouse*		*Support of children*		*Pension and Support of children*	
		No	*%*	*No*	*%*	*No*	*%*	*No*	*%*	*No*	*%*	*No*	*%*
60 – 69	Male	14	29.79	17	36.17	6	12.77			5	10.64	5	10.64
	Female	12	13.64	4	4.55	10	11.36	22	25	22	25	18	20.45
70 – 79	Male	14	25	12	21.43	6	10.71			8	14.29	16	28.57
	Female	2	4.26	3	6.38	6	12.77	6	12.77	16	34.04	14	29.79
80 years	Male	4	14.81	5	18.52	2	7.41			6	22.22	10	37.04
and above	Female									13	86.67	2	13.33
Total	Male	32	24.62	34	26.15	14	10.77			19	14.62	31	23.85
	Female	14	9.33	7	4.67	16	10.67	28	18.67	51	34	34	22.67

Table 7
Distribution of elderly by their self identified prevailing problems

	Problems among Elderly							
Age and sex	*Elderly having no problem*	*Health problem*	*Loneliness, Utilisation of time*	*Financial Problem*	*Health, loneliness*	*Health, finance*	*Health, Utilisation of time*	*Financial, loneliness*
Male								
60-69	6(12.77)	6(12.77)	12(25.53)	5(10.64)	1(2.13)	10(21.28)	6(12.77)	1(2.13)
70-79	4(7.14)	13(23.21)	9(16.07)		10(17.86)	7(12.5)	11(19.64)	2(3.57)
80+		6(22.22)	1(3.70)		11(40.74)	4(14.81)	5(18.52)	
Total	10(7.69)	25(19.23)	22(16.92)	5(3.84)	22(16.92)	21(16.15)	22(16.92)	3(2.31)
Female								
60-69	2(2.27)	9(10.23)	12(13.64)		30(34.09)	22(25.0)	9(10.23)	4(4.55)
70-79	1(2.13)	7(14.89)	6(12.77)		16(34.04)	13(27.66)	4(8.51)	
80+	1(6.67)	8(53.33)			5(33.33)		1(6.67)	
Total	4(2.67)	24(16.0)	18(12.0)		51(34.0)	35(23.33)	14(9.33)	4(2.67)

(Figures in parentheses indicate percentage)

15

The Aging Scenario Among the Tribes of Manipur

Linus Neli

"Live long, live healthy, live wealthy, and live smart!"

– 21st Century slogan

Introduction

The people of Manipur are popularly classified into "valley people" (*tammi*) and "hill people" (*chingmi*)[1] largely due to anthropological and topographical reasons. The Meiteis and the Meitei Pangals are the main inhabitants in the valley, while the two generic groups of the Nagas and the Kuki-Chin Mizos populate the hills. These tribes fall into the category of Scheduled Tribes of the Indian Constitution and there is no caste system. Besides, every tribe follows patriarchal system.

The entire hill region has been divided into five administrative districts of Senapati, Ukhrul, Chandel, Tamenglong and Churachandpur. For over a hundred years, the majority of the hill people have embraced Christianity, but adhering to different Churches or denominations.[2] The original religion of the hill tribes is animism and it survives even today by a few adherents from every tribe. Due to urbanization many hill people have migrated to the valleys.

Scope of the Study

The paper is limited to the aging scenario of the hill people. The study was conducted on 997 elders (male 516 female 481) selected randomly from five hill districts situated in rural areas. All the respondents were above 60 years of age. The economic status is determined on the basis of total assets and monthly income. Whereas the social status is determined on the basis of several parameters: sex, education, occupation, health condition, family, and lifestyle.

The data was consolidated from a broad questionnaire that was circulated among various village leaders and teachers situated in the hill districts. This was supplemented by interviews and informal discussions with the respondents and with some of the active pastors and educated leaders.

Background of the People

The Nagas occupy the northern, north-eastern, and north-western hills of Manipur. The sub-tribes of the Nagas in Manipur are: *Aimol, Anal, Chiru, Chothe, Kharem, Khoirao, Koireng, Kom, Lamkang, Liangmei, Mao, Maram, Maring, Mayong, Monsang, Poumai, Puimei, Rongmei, Tangkhul, Tarao, Thangal, Zeliang, Zemei, etc.* The communities of Zeliang, Liangmei, Rongmei (Puimei) converge themeselves into a single community known as Zeliangrong. There are many more Naga tribes in Nagaland, Arunachal Pradesh and Myanmar.

The Kuki-Chin Mizos are distributed widely in Manipur, occupying mostly the south-western, south and south-eastern hills consisting of Churachandpur, Tengnoupal (a sub-division of Chandel District), and Sadar Hills in north Manipur. The sub-tribes of the Kuki-Chins are: *Gangte, Hmar, Paite, Purum, Ralte, Salhte, Simte, Sukte, Thadou,*

Vaiphei, Zou, etc. The people who migrated from Mizoram are called Mizos and are educationally advanced. All the Kuki-Chin Mizo tribes have a lot of common elements in their dialects and cultural affiliations. Likewise, some tribes among the Nagas have linguistic similarities with Kuki-Chins but culturally they are affiliated to the Nagas.

Table 1
Population of the hill tribes

Sl. No.	*Hill Districts*	*2001 Census*	*Percentage*
1	Churachandpur	2,28,707	9.57
2	Tamenglong	1,11,493	4.67
3	Chandel	1,22,714	5.14
4	Ukhrul	1,40,946	5.90
5	Senapati	379214	15.87
	Total	9,83,074	41.15
	Valley Population	14,05,560	58.85
	Total State Population	23,88,634	100

Age determination

It is difficult to ascertain the exact age of the elderly people among the hill tribes of Manipur, because decades ago most of their parents were either illiterate or they did not have the habit of recording their bio-data. Apart from the traditional birth ceremonies, there has been hardly any customary practice where the birth anniversaries were celebrated. When asked about their age, these elderly people would begin with the phrase: "When the *Japan War* broke out (meaning WW II), I was ..."[3] The Second World War had had a deep impact on the elderly people as they came into direct contact with the Allied Forces and the Japanese troops marching past their villages, occasionally slaughtering their pigs and chickens for 'fast-food' or plundering their gardens. Even today they have collections of the bombshells (some of which are now used as Church bells) and ruined arms and ammunitions, although most of them had been confiscated by the Indian security forces in 1960's. Depending on the descriptions of what they did at that time, one has to calculate their approximate age. With a few exceptions, majority of the old people range from 70-80 years of age.

Economic Condition

The Kuki-Chins follow the chief system and the ownership of the land rests on him. The Chief allots land to the villagers for cultivation. Unlike the Kuki-Chins, the Nagas own land individually and it is handed down to posterity through patriarchal line. Every Naga clan also owns a considerable plot of land held in common used either for cultivation or for timber and firewood. The poor and landless are preferred to the use of such land. Economically the tribal society is self-sufficient to meet its simple and daily needs.

The respondents pointed out several sources of income. They are cultured crops, forest produces, cane works, livestock, government pension, old age pension, rent from property, financial support from children and miscellaneous. None of the respondents had assets from the bank saving accounts or reserve gold and silver. A factor that is presumed by all the respondents is the immoveable land (homestead, fields, etc) owned by them or utilized with the permission of family members or clan without having to pay any rent. Their income is not constant. It varies according to season and health condition.

Table 2
Sources of income

Sl.No.	*Particulars*	*Male*	*Female*	*Total (p.c.)*
1	cultured crops	102	177	279 (27.98)
2	forest produces	60	39	99 (9.94)
3	cane works, handicrafts, etc	35	14	49 (4.91)
4	livestock	90	109	199 (19.97)
5	government pension	74	5	79 (7.92)
6	old age pension	8	11	19 (1.9)
7	rent from property	16	13	29 (2.91)
8	financial help from children	40	61	101 (10.13)
9	miscellaneous	91	52	143 (14.34)
	Total	516	481	997 (100)

There have been instances that the recent ethnic clashes had a traumatic impact on the elderly people. Apart from the economic instability, the sudden displacement and new adjustment have brought about psychological depression and long-term social concerns. The communities are not equipped to address such type of issues that require professional counseling and assisted accompaniment to get well adjusted in the new situation.

Social Status and Lifestyle

In early days the elders played a significant role in moral and social affairs. They exercised discretionary powers in decision making, particularly over traditions and customary practices. They were highly respected citizens. Today, with the rapid change of lifestyle and governance, their role has considerably diminished in many respects.

The concept of retirement does not exist among the tribals. As long as physical strength endures, the elders are enlisted in the working class. There are some lucky senior citizens who are more secured due to the support of their children. Among the respondents only 6 per cent had access to television. Even those who could afford were living in the interior areas where there is no electricity and where no radio transmission reaches them.[4] Their only leisure time is to bask in the sun and their normal recreation is to be with their grandchildren. Some of the respondents observed that they were missing the rhythm of the youth in their villages, because most of them stay away in towns and cities in search of education and jobs. They come home during vacation, especially in winter - a season of festivals (Christmas, New Year, weddings and conventions). Even then, the elders are deprived of their share of participation and due attention. They grieve to see the 'rock n roll' lifestyle of the youth and the permissive moral standard which once was under their command and control.

Educational Status

For the purpose of the study, the respondents are classified as illiterate, those who read classes I-VIII, matriculate, secondary, graduate, and post-graduate. The number of illiterate elders is considerably high and the female category is higher than the male category. Fifty years ago, tribal women were socially tabooed to go to school, thinking that education would lead them to a life of promiscuity and bring shame and curse to the family and to the clan. Some communities never allowed their girls to grow long hair for fear of natural disasters on their crops. The female beauty was neglected because the paddy fields demanded intensive supply of human labour and care.[5] Today, the women of yesterday are categorized as senior citizens. After a long span of toil and suffering, they remain totally illiterate having worked as the burden of the beast. In their old age and ill health, and bent as they are at the sunset of their lives, they now deserve every respect and consideration as the unsung heroines of their respective tribes.

Table 3
Educational status

Sl.No.	*Particulars*	*Male*	*Female*	*Total (p.c.)*
1	Illiterate	201	397	598 (59.98)
2	Classes I-VIII	179	40	219 (21.97)
3	Matriculate	83	23	106 (10.63)
4	Secondary	32	14	46 (4.61)
5	Graduate	12	7	19 (1.91)
6	Post-Graduate	9	-	9 (.9)
	Total	516	481	997 (100)

Dietary Habits

The National Policy on Older Persons seeks to assure the elderly people with - among others - financial security, health care and nutrition, shelter, provision of appropriate concessions, rebates and discounts. Nothing of these seems to percolate among the respondents. The respondents came up with an amazing source of food and nutrition, often taken for granted in the tribal world. That is, the natural sanctuary (wild animals, birds, fish, insects, creatures, green leaves, etc) that nurtured them for centuries.

The hill people do not have much sense of low or high calories in food habits. They go for availability and good taste. Certain food items are associated with health or sickness. The methods of preserving food items (such as meat, fish and certain vegetables) are simple and natural – normally dried (in the sun or over the fireplace), fermented (in pots or bamboo pipes), and buried with straw or with certain preservative leaves. They consume an unadvisable amount of salt and hot pepper (*chillies*). The cooking is simple with hardly any condiments and processed ingredients. The use of spices and edible oil is a recent phenomenon and it has not yet reached the poor and interior villagers. The traditional drink of the people is rice beer. It contains a high degree of starch and it is considered to be the principal food of the elderly people (if not banned by social and religious disciplinary measures). Remarkably, the widely distributed presence of the Indian security forces in the hills has made the 'Indian made foreign liquor' easily available to the public. It has become a matter of serious concern due to its harmful effects caused to individuals as well as family life and economy.

Health Scenario

The elders are normally shy to expose their problems and anxieties, largely due to poverty, ignorance and customary beliefs. As a whole the health condition of the respondents does not indicate a positive trend. The salient features of general health complaints are: visual impairment, locomotive disorders, respiratory problems, digestive problems, gastroenterology, dental diseases, bones, joints and muscles, numbness, impaired hearing, cardiovascular diseases, genito-urinary disorders, skin diseases, diabetes mellitus, neurological disorders, psychiatric cases, etc. Only 3 per cent of the respondents did not have major health problems. Several of the respondents were aware of the new phenomenon of HIV/AIDS, because they had seen young people dying of this disease, and the same wave is affecting even in the interior areas. The present statistics show that 28 per cent of the affected population in the State comes from the hill districts.[6]

A good number of the respondents acknowledged the assistance rendered by Church communities, especially those institutions that regularly run dispensaries in various parts of the hills. Some of them claimed that they were still alive, because of the goodness of the missionaries who took them to the hospitals for major interventions and who gave them financial assistance.

Some of the respondents pointed out their difficulty in seeking health care services in the district hospitals as they would have to spend great fortunes against their low income. For instance, if a person from Choithar village went to Ukhrul district hospital (9km), it would cost him a minimum amount of Rs. 2500/- by hiring taxi, lodging in hotels and bearing minimum cost of basic investigations. Similarly, the respondents from Sajitampak village of Chandel district and Senvon village of Churachandpur district lamented the absence (or not in operation) of health care centres in their locality.[7] They appreciated the medical services of the Army camps recently established in view of containing the militants. To resort to medical service the people from Sajitampak village would have to go to Sugnu (20km, requiring 1 hr 15 mts journey by jeep at a fare of Rs. 50/- per head) where a Government primary health centre is set up. But most of the time the medical officers would not be found on duty. Senvon village has its nearest primary health centre (19km) which, they said, is not functioning. So they would have to go to Churachandpur district hospital (150km). Now the Indian armed forces have come as a relief as they have encamped 20km away from their village. Still the great problem remains as good pharmacies are not within their reach. Since the people cannot afford expensive treatment, they bear up their problems and illnesses patiently; or turn to local herbs, faith healers and even black magicians.[8] To meet the medical expenses, the respondents gave different answers. The majority expressed that they had to convert their property into money by selling land, paddy, domestic animals, firewood and others.

The respondents manifested a problem peculiar to the inhabitants of the hills and mountains. They faced locomotive syndrome in ascending and descending the rugged terrain. The moment the hill people get old, their movement is curtailed to a tiny part of their village – at home in a smoky hut.

Automobile services do not exist in the interior villages. Their desire to visit their dear and near ones, to go to Church (normally built on top of the village not for any theological reason but for aesthetic view) and to witness social activities is but a wishful thinking.

Societal Response to the Old People

The first and foremost response to the problems of aging comes from family circles. Traditionally, the immediate responsibility of looking after the aged parents falls on the youngest son as he inherits the family property. Nevertheless, it is not strictly confined to him alone. The moral responsibility extends to all the children, clan members and to society at large. The call to humanitarian service is deeply embedded in the tribal traditions. The bond of oneness of family, clan and tribe has been one of the primordial ingredients of tribal social system. We focus on five agents that act as organized institutions to address various social issues, including the ageing people.

1. *Government*

The government is the principal agent to promote the welfare of the people. It builds infrastructure, generates resources and makes policy to accomplish its goals. The National policy on senior citizens (e.g. "The Maintenance and Welfare of Parents and Senior Citizens bill 2007", "Old age pension schemes", etc) addresses different needs of the aged population. The setting up of district hospitals and primary health centres in every district has eased the public to have access to health care services. The government is yet to develop a systematic geriatric care network in the State. There are several developmental projects and schemes implemented by various departments that would considerably enhance the economy and living standards of the people. Currently, the government has been implementing the Indira Gandhi National Old Age Pension Scheme, launched on 19th

November 2007, for the elders below poverty line. These beneficiaries get a sum of Rs. 200/- per month. A total number of 11,889 beneficiaries has been recorded in the hill districts: Churachandpur (2,765), Tamenglong (1,349), Chandel (1,485), Ukhrul (1,705) and Senapati (4,585). It is unfortunate that the benefits of most of these welfare and developmental programmes do not percolate to the public due to corruption and lack of public probity on the one hand, and due to lack of social commitment and growth of anti-social movements on the other.

2. ***Christian Churches***

The Christian idea of service is derived from the commandment of Jesus Christ: "Love the Lord your God with all your heart, with all your soul, with all your strength, and with all your mind; and love your neighbour as yourself".[9] Jesus Christ further exhorts his followers to "love one another as I have loved you ...and by this sign all will know that you are my disciples".[10] A Christian, therefore, is not merely given the concept of service but actually called by God to respond personally and to take swift and spontaneous service to the poor and needy. This is a special mandate from Jesus Christ to his followers.

The introduction of Christianity brought a qualitative change in the tribal world. To become a Christian meant to enter into a worldwide (Catholic or Universal) community and solidarity. Through Christian missionaries, the tribal life, culture and tribal Churches came into direct contact with the international community.

The role of the Church or Churches in promoting health care and solidarity is expressed in diversified activities. The Church as a community takes much pain to pay proper attention to the elderly people. Today, almost in every district, there are considerable number of Christian institutions running hospitals (3) and dispensaries (25). The respondents felt that adherence to a particular Church community made them feel more comfortable and secure. Several respondents expressed deep appreciation for Christian fellowship and regular family visits. A few of them admitted that they embraced Christianity in their old age as they feared that there would not be anybody to bury them if they died as animists (tribal religion).

3. *Non-Governmental Organizations*

The growing interventions of the various Non-Governmental Organizations (NGOs) in developmental programmes, self-help groups and humanitarian services have brought about a considerable change in the economy of the hill people. The present interventions of the NGO's are mainly related to agriculture, awareness programmes, orphanages, rehabilitation centres, HIV/AIDS patients and education. There is no direct intervention concerning the care of elderly people like setting up old aged homes, geriatric care centres, old age security arrangement, etc. Hence, the magnitude of the problems faced by the ageing people has not been addressed even today by the principal agents of social workers.

There is a wide scope in which the NGOs can play a catalyst role: conduct a scientific survey of demographic change and quantify ageing pattern among the hill tribes, do a need-based research of the elders, conduct social awareness camps, medical camps, and periodically recommend to the Government in matters of policy direction in the interest of ageing population.

4. *Military yeoman service*

The humanitarian service rendered by the Indian security forces operating in the Northeast cannot go unnoticed. Due to the increasing number of insurgency, militancy, and extortion groups in Manipur, hundreds of military and paramilitary forces have pitched their camps in the strategic hill areas. In almost every camp there is a medical centre and a canteen opened to the civilians. Through its Fraternity Fund and other civil oriented programmes, the security forces have displayed national sympathy to the people. The setting up of community halls, construction of roads, installation of small hydro-electric power stations, students' hostels, computer education centres, stadium, supply of provisions and man power during public conventions – all these are some of the tangible services extended by the armed forces to the hill people. However, it must be admitted that there is no direct gerontological intervention even from this institution.

Major Findings

The survey has revealed various dimensions of the problem of elderly persons among the hill tribes of Manipur.

- *Elderly population:* The number of elderly population in the hills is increasing. Most of the respondents do not know their age accurately as their parents were illiterate and, besides, there was no culture of recording bio-data in their time. About 59.98 per cent of the respondents themselves were illiterate. This explains why they did not have active participation in social life and they were no longer wielding authority as they used to in their respective villages.

- *Psychological dimension:* about 65 per cent expressed different types of fear, anxiety, depression, and other psychological symptoms. Several reasons made the elders feel left out in their living context. One such example is the experience of being isolated as animists (tribal religion) as most of the younger generations have embraced Christianity. They had the fear of dying as animists, which meant being isolated as a minority in the village and there would not be people to bury them in their traditional custom. These elders were practicing varied ways of dispelling their fear and they were using ingenious tactics to combat the evil spirits (e.g., use of spears, knives, scented leaves, certain sacrifices, reading aloud the *Holy Bible*, prayers to God, wearing religious articles, holy water, etc). The study indicated that those who had higher education had lower level of individual's anxiety. The illiterate group suffered more from irrational fears and anxieties.

- *Financial problem*: about 85 per cent of the respondents reported their helplessness in getting financial assistance from any quarter. The worst affected group being the illiterate adults who did not have children to support them. Their deep relationship with the tillable land gave them sustenance and their only periodical chance of holding some cash in hand was when they sold something of their livestock. Since most of the respondents had their own homestead and other plots of land, they did not feel the threat of insecurity and rejection on account of homelessness and house rent harassment.
- *Displacement*: The recent ethnic clashes and dam constructions had had a significant impact on some 5 per cent of the respondents as they had problems in adjusting to new environment due to sudden displacement. Some respondents were unwilling to move to towns and cities to live with their children.
- *The spirit of endurance:* The study has recorded the uniqueness of the enduring spirit of the elders among the tribal world. There is no concept of retirement among the tribals. They do not give up their struggle nor do they curse anyone for their plight of aging amidst hardships and wants.
- *Elders grieve on youth*: There are three main factors that cause the elders to lament on youth. First, many

people are dying young (age between 20-40) due to ethnic conflicts, militancy, and HIV/AIDS. Second, the elders miss the rhythm of the youth in villages as (most part of the year) they are settled in towns and cities in pursuit of studies and works and seldom they came home for holidays. The social life in the village was totally different in their time. As of today, the village tends to be guarded by cultivators, elders and poor children. Third, looking somewhat at the permissive lifestyle of the youngsters, the elders are greatly displeased to see the decadence of their social and moral order. The sexual behaviour and the moral code of the village once considered to be sacred have been overturned by the post-modern values and lifestyle.

- *Health condition:* The respondents pointed out that the degree of health problems varied with the change of season. The old people were worst affected during monsoon season (from July to September), while children suffered more in cold and dry season (diarrhoea, measles, etc. between December-April). The elders found sunshine immensely conducive to their health. They would bask in the sunshine for hours. A prolonged stay at the fireplace would burn their skins and they would develop skin diseases on their legs. The study also pointed out that health, religion and spirituality are closely interconnected. The respondents who had strict discipline according to the teachings of their religion (like prohibition of alcohol, tobacco, betal nuts, etc) suffered less from related diseases than those who had been more liberal in their habits. It also ascertained that health and spirituality are integral components of the well-being of an individual and indirectly it affects the family economy.
- *Sources of nutrition*: about 90 per cent of the respondents were not aware of the National Policy on

older persons for financial support, health care, nutrition, shelter, etc. The study has revealed an amazing source of nutrition for the elderly persons living in the interior villages. That is, the natural resources from fields and forests (wildlife, creatures, edible insects, etc).

- *Transport and communication:* The respondents expressed the dire need for four-wheeler transport services at a reasonable cost. Often they had been carried on pole-chairs to the hospitals. At times youngsters offered their bike services but the elders were not expert as pillion riders and that, too, on rough roads.

- *General impression:* The study does not find the respondents living in abject poverty. Instead, about 45 per cent of them were staying in unhygienic condition (coohabitation with domestic animals, improper ventilation, food preparation, etc). As human beings they needed more care, someone to listen to their sentiments, to be respected and valued as old coins, and not to discard them when they are unable to eat and go for their needs on their own. When they have meals they would require at least a small piece of meat or fish or edible insects or chillies in their plate to stimulate their appetite (palatable to old and toothless persons with various health complaints). The elders do not mind dying early, if God wills, but as long as they live they expect minimum care, acceptance and respect. During interviews these elders were happy to share their stories, especially the folklores of the days of yore and the listener would be moved to heart when their meanings are applied to human lives. For these elders the tribal world is their paradise. Even if they die, their spirit lives on.

Conclusion

Today's senior citizens are different from their predecessors. They have to be more active if they have to live long, healthy, and wealthy with dignity and respect. It is our duty to maintain their lives and make them fit and agile with good health so that they can live in society decently and with dignity. Old people are becoming increasingly vulnerable during and after humanitarian crises, due to their physical frailty and lack of mobility. Aging is a challenge that cannot be addressed by the public or private sectors in isolation. A new era has come for us, an era of qualitative literacy – to learn, unlearn, and relearn the science of aging. The purpose of this paper is to lead to further research studies on senior citizens and to solicit all governmental and non-governmental institutions for immediate gerontological social work intervention. We are all called to be compassionate and faithful to humanity, especially to our times.

NOTES

1. The nomenclatures "*chingmi* (hill people) and *tammi* "(valley people) are two Manipuri words which became popular since some centuries. Often they signify the contrasting difference between the two groups of people in terms of religion, culture, language, food habits, dress, methods of cultivation and governance. The "chingmi" people basically come under the Indian Constitution recognized as Scheduled Tribes (ST), while the "tammi" people come under the General Race and Scheduled Castes (SC). While there is no restriction for the hill people to come down and own land in the valleys, their counterparts from the valleys are not legally permitted to own land in the hills. Hence the study of demography will show significant difference in size, composition and distribution of population between the hills and the valleys.

2. Christianity was founded by Jesus Christ in the 1st century. Jesus Christ drew some followers and built up a believing

community. This visible body of believers is known as the Church and is sustained by God, the Living Spirit. Christianity has its background from the Jewish tradition but eventually the new Christian way of life was opened to the whole world with the principal message to love God and one 's neighbour. In course of time, due to socio-political reasons, the followers split up into churches (Catholic, Orthodox, Protestants) and denominations (divisions from among the Protestant groups which came into being during the Reformation period, and further leading to an ongoing reformulation of the concept of the Church).

3. The Battle of Kohima was fought between the British and Indian Forces and the Japanese Troops from April 4 to June 22, 1944 around the town of Kohima in Nagaland, India. Aftermath, the British and Indian Forces had lost around 4,000 men, dead, missing and wounded. The Japanese had lost more than 5,000 men in the Kohima area fighting. Cf. http://en.wikipedia.org/wiki/Battle_of_Kohima.

4. Currently the A.I.R. Imphal transmits its programmes through MW (882 KHz/340.16m), SW (4775 Khz/60m) and FM (7150 Khz/41m). With the poor reception in the hills and a pair of dying, a villager in the remote areas cannot enjoy this media service of the government. Efforts are in progress to erect FM towers in strategic hill areas of every District.

5. This reality once reflected among the Meitei society as they have a saying: "It is better to marry a tribal girl than to buy two bulls to plough the fields."

6. The first HIV+ case in Manipur was reported in February 1990 from a blood sample collected in October 1989 from among a cluster of Injecting Drug Users (IDU). On 3rd October 1996, Manipur became the first State in India to have State AIDS Policy. As of now many old people are not affected by HIV/AIDS as the HIV positive categories belong to the following: Injecting Drug Users (IDU) 19.8%, Female Sex Workers (FSW) 11.6%, Men Having Sex with Men (MSM) 12.4%, Pregnant Women (ANC) 1.4% and STD Patients 4.8%. It is reported that, in the State of Manipur, there are 29,602 (7821 females) with HIV+ and 4,363 suffering from AIDS. These are mostly

between 0-40 years of age. Cf. *Epidemiological Analysis of HIV/AIDS in Manipur*, Report of the Manipur AIDS Control Society (MACS) 2008, published in *The Sangai Express*, Imphal, September 6, 2008.

7. As of now Churachandpur has the best health care infrastructure in the hill districts: District Hospital (1), Sietmal Christian Hospital (1), Primary Health Centres (9), Community Health Centres (64), Urban Health Centres (1), Private Clinic Maternity (1), NGO Rehab Centres (9), NGO Medical support clinics for HIV/AIDS (5) and Dispensaries (3). The great lamentation of the people is that these are not functioning properly.

8. In the practice of black magic, an individual who is endowed with spiritual power would diagnose and spell healing power on the sick. This exercise is accompanied by sacrifice of chickens, dog, white cocks, etc to appease the spirits.

9. See *The Gospel of Luke* 10:27; *The Gospel of Matthew* 22:34-40; *The Gospel of Mark* 12:28-31.

10. See *The Gospel of John* 13:34-35. Jesus also exhorts forgiveness and reconciliation in times of failure.

16

Aging in Manipur: The Social and Moral Issues

Ch. Priyoranjan Singh

Aging in the world has been accelerating in a rather fast pace because of the increase in longevity in the developing countries. If the rate of aging at present continues, the world is likely to have above 13 per cent of its total population belonging to the category of the elderly above 65 years of age by 2030. This is then likely to confront the poorer nations of the world with administrative, financial and moral problems, the magnitude of which these nations are not likely to be able to face in a responsible manner. The seriousness of the impending problem has been put in perspective by comparing the effects of aging on the world to the effects of the wave of globalization that is worrying the developing nations in the recent past. Faster demographic transitions in developing countries means that these countries are going to face the risks and opportunities of ageing within a short period of time. Unlike the developed countries, however, the developing countries are growing old before getting rich. This has opened up the larger issue of the capabilities of many nations to manage the risks and disadvantage of aging populations. Are the developing nations physically, socially and psychologically prepared to meet the demands of aging national populations? Do they have the experience or the expertise to handle the situation in the right manner or are they going to address the situation on the basis of learning by doing, with grave consequences on the well being of the elderly?

The international call for better policy making for aging societies is 'to integrate an aging perspective for all realms of social and economic perspective instead of having aging specific policy, programmes and budget. This paper is a preliminary inquiry into issues of aging in Manipur with a focus on the rural dynamics and how society is coping with the problem and how new problems related to the elderly are giving rise to ethical as well as social issues that are new to the people of the state and alien to their cultural experiences and value systems. The paper also touches upon how structural changes in the economy has led to fragmentation and loss of family values and undermining of Social Capital and institutions that had for centuries sustained the societal balance of intergenerational equity and welfare

Economic and Social Basis of Inequity and Deprivation of the Aged

Every society has a built-in system of age stratification that defines the role and the status of the aged. Kingsley Davis writes that 'all societies recognize age as a basis of status, but some of them emphasise it more than others'. Age stratification in societies, assign differing social roles and social status according to broad age groups. Age stratification theory proposes that age is a basis of social differentiation analogous to stratification by social class (Foner 1975). Stratification implies inequalities whereby society distributes resources unequally by age. Resources include, economic goods, social approval, acceptance and respect. Foner notes that 'as the individual ages, he too moves within a social hierarchy. He goes from one set of age-related social roles to another and at each level receives greater or lesser rewards than before'. Social mobility in the age hierarchy is 'inevitable, universal and unidirectional in that the individual can never grow younger'. The number of age strata and the prestige and power associated with each age strata is determined by social needs and the characteristics of people at each age. Europe had in the past had three age strata- infancy, adulthood and old age (Aries 1962), and power was concentrated in the hands of the older people. In contemporary societies at least seven strata are seen, infancy, childhood, adolescence, young adulthood, middle age, young old, and old old, with power typically concentrated in the hands of the middle-aged. However, social change occurs to the extent that successive cohorts do something other than merely repeat the pattern of behaviour of their predecessors (Norman Rider 1964). Modernization and rapid change in health and economic technologies, urbanization and education are leading to intergenerational competition, social distance, residential segregation and the inversion of states (Donald Cowgill 1979). Health technologies increase longevity and create intergenerational competition for limited jobs leading to the retirement of the aged, lower income and lower status. In pre-modern societies, the young aspired to move up to the status of their parents. In the modern context the urban jobs and occupations with the required skills, mobility and higher incomes favour the young and thus the relegation of the status of the elderly, because of changes in economic technologies. In the rapidly urbanizing world, parents have become peripheral in the lives of the young, creating segregation of residence, intergenerational social and physical distance depressing the status of the elderly. Rapid changes in educational technologies are creating intellectual and moral (Values) distances among the young and the old. Evidently, historical forces change the status of the elderly as well as the very character of the elderly. Tightly structured traditional, rural and agrarian societies are experiencing transition from the communitarian value system to that of the individualistic. The profound change in the foundational values of family structures are leading to socio-economic transformations that have a bearing on the patterns and degrees of vulnerability of the elderly. The emerging issue therefore is, whether modern families are prepared or equipped to address the modern phenomenon of exploitation, deprivation and emotional voids that has begun to constitute the world of the aged.

The Rural Context: The Socioeconomic Status of the Village Elderly

The village of Tabungkhok lies on the outskirts of Imphal and as such it is a village that has absorbed much of the social as well as the moral urban cultures of the town. In some ways one can imagine the social and moral processes that are taking place in the village as the precursors of the likely changes in the status of the elderly that are to occur in the rural areas of the state. The village has a population of 2288 persons and the proportion of the elderly is 7.6 per cent. Amongst the male population, the elderly constitute 8.9 per cent and amongst the female population the elderly constitute 6.5 per cent of their respective populations. The educational profiles of the elderly in the village, shows a contrasting picture between the men and the women population. Amongst the males, 47 per cent are literate as against only 11 per cent amongst the females. Thus 89 per cent of the women in the village are illiterate. In fact 12 per cent of the elderly males were graduates and 2 per cent were post graduates. However there was one post graduate woman in the village. The high levels of literacy amongst the elderly males are reflected in their occupational patterns (Table 1). Among the elderly males, 28 per cent were retired pensioners and another 9 per cent were government employees (many in the state understate their age in their certificates and as such continue to work in the government way beyond 60 years of age). Another 14 per cent of the elders were agricultural labourers, reflecting that the young old in the village are largely economically active. This fact is bolstered by another fact that only 37 per cent of the elderly male population in the village are economically inactive, being too old or disabled. On the other hand, 80 per cent of the elderly women are economically inactive and only 4 per cent were either pensioners or government employees reflecting the low levels of education among the elderly women in the village.

The socio-economic characteristics of the aged in the village indicates that the village is an ageing village and that the male elders are far more economically secure and educated than their female counterparts. The majority of the male elders are economically active(63 per cent) and almost half of them are literate whereas among the female elders only 20 per cent are economically active and only 11 per cent are literate. These high levels of differences in the economic and literacy status between the male and the female elderly apparently has a high correlation with the way the elderly in the village live their lives, are treated by the family members and whether they are neglected, maltreated, exploited or abused, even though cultural factors do play an intervening role.

Village Life and the World of the Elderly

There are some 173 elders above the age of 60 years in the village. For getting a detailed insight into the life of the aged, a sample of 25 men and 25 women, with an appropriate stratification was surveyed. The survey result reveals that on the whole, rural society in Manipur is yet to experience significant levels of intergenerational competition that leads to the lowering of the status of the elderly with its consequent marginalization of the aged.

Family structure: Historically there has been a dichotomy of family structures in the rural and the urban area. The capital town of Imphal mostly had Joint Family structures whereby two and three generations lived in the same house and in the same piece of land which was much smaller than those of the rural areas. On the other hand, in the rural areas, the more prevalent family structure was that of the extended family type whereby as the son married, he would build his own house and earn his living from the agricultural land that his father gave as his share. His house was built in his share of the homestead land that his father gave him. The patriarch of the family will ultimately live in his house with the youngest son and his family. Thus the patriarch was the head of the extended family living in the same plot of land that he owned. Growth of population and the limited space no doubt brought changes in the family structures but the dominance of the extended family structure is still visible in the rural areas of the state. The survey of the elderly reveals that 58 per cent of the aged lived in extended families whereas 30 per cent lived in joint families. Only 12 per cent lived in the emerging nuclear families (Table 3). The social norms would therefore be still a strong enough force to restrain large scale marginalization of the elderly. But the rising proportions of the extended and the nuclear families are clear indications of the change in the family structures in the state. In terms of the residential types, 76 per cent of the elderly lived in their own house and only 24 per cent lived in the house that their sons built.

Economic status: The majority of the elders possessed land and other assets, 68 per cent had both agricultural and homestead land and 52 per cent had some stock of cash and gold (Table 12). All the elders had homestead land and 36 per cent did not have agricultural land of their own. In terms of economic activity, 42 per cent of the elders earned income from all sectors of the economy. The average annual income of the 60-70 years male group was Rs. 46500 as against only Rs. 15000 for the same group of females (Table 6). This high level of divergence in the income levels is also replicated in the high levels of divergence in the earner and non-earner status among the sexes. Thus while 64 per cent of the male elders are earners only 20 per cent of the females are earners (Table 6). Among the females, only the younger old in the age group of 60-70 years earned some income whereas among the males only the age group of 80+ did not earn some income, 75 per cent of the earners among the males was in the age group of 60-70 years. Obviously this lower economic status of the female elderly has had a large bearing on their overall status as well as their welfare in the rural setting. This is visible in the relative decision making powers of the elderly within the family(Tables, 7,8,9). Overall, the elders of the village have 'much' say(44 %) and 'some' say(44%) in the decisions within the family and only 12 per cent of the elders had no say in family matters. However among the males, 60 per cent had 'much' say as compared to only 28 per cent among the females.

Neglect, deprivation and abuse: Inspite of the fact that the majority of the elders earn, have stocks of cash and assets, live in their own homes and have a say in the affairs of the households, they suffer from varying degrees of neglect and deprivations. On nutrition and diets, 88 per cent of the elders thought that they received sufficient amounts but only 80 per cent believed that the quality was not sufficient (Table 10). There is a significant feeling among the elders that they are deprived of clothes, health care and physical attention (Table16). A significant 40 per cent felt that they were deprives of cloths and 36 per cent felt that they were deprived of proper health care. However, only 4 per cent felt that they suffered from food deprivation. What is more significant is that the female is far more deprived in clothing, health and physical care than their male counterparts. Thus while 24 per cent of males felt deprived of cloths, 56 per cent of females felt they were deprived. Health deprivation was 16 per cent among the males as against 60 per cent among the females. Physical deprivation was 28 per cent among the males as against 44 per cent among the females. The majority of the elders (58 per cent) felt that they were not neglected but 36 per cent felt that they were somewhat neglected while only 4 per cent felt that they were absolutely neglected(Table 11). The females felt more neglected than their male counterparts. On the issues of labour, monetary and property exploitation, the degree was rather low at 12 per cent, 4 per cent and 6 per cent respectively (Table15).

Physical care and attitude towards death: The majority (56 per cent) of the elders perceived that death was God's wish. However 30 per cent feared death while14 per cent had no fear of death. Interestingly 44 per cent of the males feared death while only 16 per cent of the females feared death. Interestingly 80 per cent of the women perceived that death was a matter of God's wish (Table 16). The elders of the village spent most of their time with the children (36 per cent) and all the family members (32 per cent). The females spent more time with their daughters and the children than the males.

In the rural areas of Manipur, the traditional family structures are largely prevalent but the significant emergence of the nuclear families in the rural agrarian setting are definite signs of the beginning of the breaking up of the traditional structures. There are no homeless elders in the surveyed village as all had their own homestead land and 36 per cent of them lived in houses built by themselves. Living arrangements are therefore largely a matter of the elders choice. Most of the elders worked up to the age of eighty. There are however glaring gaps in the economic status of the male and female elders and as such the males had a greater say in social decisions. Because of the strong economic base of most of the elders, absolute neglect, exploitations and deprivation of nutrition are yet small. However there seems to be large deprivation in the matter of cloths and health care, especially among the women. On the whole, strong social norms and family structures are keeping exploitative or depriving norms from raising their heads strongly.

The Tip of the Iceberg: Old Age Homes and the World of the Elderly

The apparent social balance of status, intergenerational respect, lesser levels of exploitation and deprivation of the elderly and the social ecology of comparative justice and equity that one observes in rural Manipur, are tragically shattered in the world of the elderly who have chosen to inhabit the Old Age Homes of the state. Manipuri women throughout history have been the backbone of internal trade as well as part providers of the family, in a martial and constantly warring nation, where the man even did not have sufficient time to fully develop a trans-border trading culture. The tales of exploitation of the resilient labour of the mother, and the abuse of the innate cultural heritage of the Manipuri women, narrated by the inmates of the Old Age Homes, are facets of the unobserved reality of the contemporary world of the elderly in the state, as well as the pointers to the futures of the elderly.

The state has thirteen old age homes spread over the nine districts, according to the official records of the state Department of Social Welfare. These Homes are funded by the central government and there are no Homes funded by the state government. Imphal East district has three homes, Imphal West, the most populous district has only one, Thoubal district, six, Bisenpur, Senapati, and Tamenglong districts have one home each. There are no Old Homes in the tribal districts of Ukhrul, Churachandpur and Chandel. The majority of the Homes are reportedly not functioning though they receive central funds. Of the functioning ones we visited, the number of inmates varied from three to nine inmates. We were told that though the sanctioned capacity of the homes were twenty five and above, the actual intake swung widely through the year. Three homes that we visited were non-functional and the functionary of one, who was the General Secretary of the association of NGOs of the state, did not allow us to visit his Home on one pretext or the other for over fifteen days and we finally gave up. His Home was located in uneasy territory and he insisted that one of his men accompany us to the home. Definitely he seemed to have something to hide! The shady business of many NGOs in India are apparently also present here in the state. In the district of Thoubal, which the central government has also marked as having an inordinate number of NGOs, we were told of how come inspection time and one would see the shady ones make emergency arrangements to rent the requisite number of beds as well as inmates! One old lady had made a reputation of running her Home with exemplary dedication and devotion but we could not visit her home. We could not visit any home in the hill region also, though we intend to do so in the near future to complete the picture of the world of the Old Age Homes in the state. It is in this mixed world of the Old Age Homes that we entered to discover the very social dynamics of the elderly in Manipur that gave rise to the Old Age Homes themselves. The data provided here represent the findings from the survey of four 'Aged Home Centres', in the three valley districts of Imphal West, Imphal East and Thoubal.

Aged Home Centres in the state are almost an all women's affair according to our sample, where 90 per cent of the in mates were women and only 10 per cent were men. Seventy per cent of the inmates were in the semi active and inactive age group of 70 to 80 and 80+ age group, the rest thirty per cent were in the active age group of 60-70 years(Table 18).

All inmates of the Homes had earned a living and contributed to the incomes of their families before they came or during their active lives. Of the inmates, 50 per cent had worked in the tertiary sector and 20 per cent in the primary sector(Table 19). Thirty per cent had worked both in the primary as well as in the tertiary sectors. The range of occupations included shop keeping, various kinds of trading in primary as well as secondary sector goods, vending, firewood gathering from the hills, weaving, agriculture labour, etc.

Literacy levels among the elderly are extremely low, only 15 per cent of the inmates are literate. Literacy among the women reached only 10 per cent. The younger old are more educated and among the age group of 60-70 years, the literacy rate is 66 per cent and 33 per cent among the 70-80 years group (Table 21). All the inmates have no living spouse (Table 20). Twenty per cent of the inmates had no surviving relatives and as such had no one to call theirs'. Single daughter or single son inmates accounted for 20 per cent each of the inmates. Twenty five per cent of the inmates had only daughters and no sons (Table 25). The health conditions of the inmates are on the better side in that only 35 per cent had chronic ailments and the rest 65 per cent were comparatively healthy. The chronic ailments were Tuberculosis, coronary problems, paralysis, ophthalmic, psychiatric and renal (Table 25).

The decision to stay in the Aged Home was overwhelmingly voluntary. About 60 per cent of the inmates came to the homes after hearing about the facility, without anyone's intervention. Though the rest 40 per cent came on the suggestions of relatives or acquaintances, the decisions were voluntary. However the reasons for coming to the Homes varied, 60 per cent came for reasons of emotional insecurity, 35 per cent for homelessness and 25 per cent for physical insecurity (Table 23). Thirty five per cent of the inmates had no fears of dying and 25 per cent thought that dying was a matter of God's will. Fifteen per cent wanted to die (Table 7).

From the socio- economic data cited above, one can construct many of the social and moral issues that is coming up in the world of the elderly in the state, their angst, emotional traumas, psychological degradation, physical and economic exploitation, and the many hidden inequities and injustice that are structured in the social and economic system of the state. A distinct feature of the inmates of the Homes was that except one inmate, all the other women inmates were hardy women who had substantially contributed to the income of the family in their pre-home and younger days. Circumstances like, brutal and economically dependent husbands or sons exploiting her income and labour or selling off the family land and homestead, sonless widows being harassed, deprived of their property and other rights, having to live with their daughters, daughter-in-laws creating unbearable emotional stress, or being homeless, were but some of the reasons driving the elderly women to the desperate world of the Aged Homes. These factors acted either independently or in various combinations, to tilt the decision scale towards the Homes.

The case study of 'Thagoi', an eighty years old inmate of an Aged Home, provides a vivid example of the struggles that some issueless women with irresponsible husbands have to go through for sheer survival. Thagoi married young and gave birth to a son. Her infant son died at six months and she did not give birth to any other siblings. The truant husband married others, living in the women's homes and died. Her husband's family sympathised with her initially but as time passed and more so after her husband died, her stay in her husband's house became a bone of contention for everybody in the joint family. Her inheriting the husband's property in the absence of any sibling was untenable in the thinking of the other members. She was a trader of vegetables, sometimes gathering wood from the hills and trading them also, she also worked as agriculture labour, thereby being economically self-sufficient. The clear intent to physically disinherit her combined with the hostile emotional and moral environment in the family, ultimately drove her to her brother's house where she stayed for some time. In time her brother's sons enacted the same drama that she had suffered at her husband's home and she moved out once again. Being economically independent, she chose to take the extreme step of clearing a small space on the bank of the river and settled there in a small hutment. She could not stay there long, the rain God's chose to even deprive her of her home. A severe flood washed off her home one summer day and then began her saga for the hunt of a place to stay. Getting older, she was able to find a place to stay in many of the middle class homes of the capital town of Imphal. As nuclear families are mushrooming in this town, as more and more couples are working, the demand for house maids, specially the child maid, has grown tremendously in the recent years. In fact 'Human Capital' firms have sprung up to supply the much sought after maid. Women beyond menopause and who are either homeless or destitute, are much sought after to stay in the master's house and look after varied physical needs of the busy families. Thagoi stayed in many of these houses but when her utility was diminishing, as when a new bride arrives in the family, or the masters are retired, she had to leave again. This is how she landed in the Aged Home, forlorn, semi dependent and virtually abandoned. She is now above eighty years of age, dose not fear death and thinks that death is only a matter of God's wish. She finds good company among her peers and has still not lost the zeal to live, her spirit is yet to break.

Women with multiple issues are however not entirely immune from the many deprivations, exploitations and abuse that the mothers and widows suffer from, after the demise of their husband. 'Momon' a widow', has two sons and two daughters, she is sixty years old. During and after her husband's death, she provided for the family by selling vegetables. She is suffering from Tuberculosis and has not treated herself (she had not been treated by the Home also, we were rather surprised that the Homes that we visited and the women inmates were not aware that the T.B. centre of the state provided free treatment of T.B. patients). Her sons are married but she was constantly bothered by monetary demands. The daughter-in-laws also constantly bothered her inspite of her dwindling earnings. She had an accident and had her ribs fractured. Still not fully recovered, she continued plying her trade. Inpite of her deteriorating health, the demands of the family did not cease, though nobody ever bothered about her health. Unable to bear the emotional and the physical insecurity in the family, she finally decided to come to the Home. Non of her sons visit her and she preferred to die rather than live in her present state of physical as well as emotional insecurity.

Many widows without sons but having a single daughter, seem to have the common problem of physical and emotional violence in their homes, especially if she is earning. 'Ibeton' was a known weaver in Imphal and she was comparatively well off. But her crime was that she had no male issue. After her husband's death, property disputes and the physical violence by her nephews, pushed her to her daughter's home, where she stayed for quite some time. But emotional insecurity ultimately drove her to the Aged Home where she has been staying for the last seven years. She has high blood pressure and her only daughter visits her regularly providing some solace and emotional support. She is 80 years of age but she makes Agarbatties (Incense sticks) at the Home, earns about Rs. 50 per month and supplements the Rs. 150 that the Home gives her per month to maintain herself.

The old age homes of the state give us a peek into world of the independent minded hard working mothers of the state who have not been able to bear the psychological, emotional and physical stresses in the family that are largely outcomes of poverty, breaking down of traditional social norms, especially amongst the younger generations, and the changing economic structure of the state which has tremendously increased rural and urban unemployment. In the absence of industrialization and stagnating agriculture, the movement towards massive tertiarization of occupations is building up a commercial culture in the state that does not have much moorings in hard toils, sweat and labour, upon which was built many of the traditional institutions and the social capital that provided the safety nets and the social balance of intergenerational equity and welfare. The ethos of rural Manipur is getting fast absorbed into the vortex of urban cultures even though the productive base has remained agrarian.

Aged Population and Welfare Measures in the State

The population of the state has grown from 2.8 lakhs in 1901 to 22.9 lakhs in 2001. The proportion of the aged was 4.2 per cent in 1911 and has consistently risen. It reached 6.1 per cent in 1951 and stands at 6.9 per cent in 2001. The aged population in the state is higher than the Northeastern States' average of 5.52 per cent, but lower than the national average of 7.45. Only Tripura has a higher proportion of 7.27 per cent. The total aged population in the state is 145,471 persons, which is evenly distributed between the sexes.

There are three welfare schemes in the state that caters to the elderly. Under the Manipur Old Age Pension Scheme, 26,909 persons and under the Indira Gandhi National Old Age Pension Scheme, 72,514 persons, are being presently benefited in the state. The state plan scheme pension is worth Rs 100 per month and the National Plan Scheme is worth Rs 200 for each beneficiary. The total coverage is 99423 out of the 145471 aged in the state which represents a 68.35 per cent of the aged population. Over and above the pension schemes, the Annapurna Scheme distributes 10 Kgs of rice a month to 8590 beneficiaries who are not recipients of the pension benefits. The Social Welfare Department could not provide us with any ground level official reports from the districts on the actual working of the schemes, non seemed to exist. There are 13 old age homes on the records of the Department but here again there are no existing assessment report on the subject. The interest of the department in these homes are little, as the funds of the homes are directly going to the homes and the department is only a recommending authority, we were informed. There is therefore an urgent need for an assessment of the functioning of the welfare schemes of the aged in the state as the elderly in the villages simply refuse to believe that about 70 per cent of them are receiving old age pensions or 10 Kgs of rice a month!

Cultures, Traditional Institutions Social Networks and the Aged

The states of the North-East are poor communities that are going to depend on the doles of the centre for quite some decades. In the meantime the proportions of the aged are going to grow by leaps and bounds. The states will never have, at least in the coming few decades, the capacity or the capability to handle situations of the future, only on the basis of the hands of the state. How is the region going to cope with the impending crisis?

The cultural institutions in Manipur provide the elders with many safety nets and cultural practices that insure that they have vital ritual roles and responsibilities that secures their non-material status. Rituals relating to births, marriage and mortuary rites, are the domains of the elderly of any locality and their presence, views and decisions have the force of the community on the individual families. This has its origins in the ancestor worshipping pre–Vaishnavite and pre-

Christian cultures and traditions of the tribal and Hindu communities of the state. Festivities and religious ceremonies are also the domains of the elderly. In the highly ritualised, ceremonial and celebrative social practices around the year, the physical and ethically based circulation of the elderly provides them the social basis of their existence as well as emotional and the psychological substance that fill up many of the voids that are created within the family. This is perhaps the reason why the elders are still holding out in the villages of the state, inspite of the onslaught of the commercial and modern moral norms that are not only threatening their social status but also their economic status. The conditions of the abandoned or the forced out mothers in the Old Age Homes, are but the tip of the ice burg that fore tales the future fate of the elderly in a rapidly urbanizing state. There was a substantial and educated male pensioner in one of the Aged Homes who was living in the home as his son had pawned off even his pension book, his only income source. The shifting sands of age stratification and moral norms of society needs to be controlled for the North-East to prepare for a painless transition into the world of a welfare state that equitably balances intergenerational competitions justly and morally. Identifying the social institutions that are living, cultural norms and practices that are dovetailed to emerging modern norms and morality, and structuring welfare measures into them, is what the region has to plan for to address the needs of the aged, for nobody gets old without being young.

Table 1
Education level of the Aged of Taobungkhok village

	Male	*Female*
Illiterate	21	62
Literate	47	8
Matriculate	15	-
Secondary	4	1
Graduate	12	-
Post-graduate	2	1
PhD	-	-
Total	101	72

Source: Census survey by Silvia Lisam, Research Scholar, Dept. of Economics, M.U.

Table 2
Occupation of the aged of Taobungkhok village

	Male	*Female*
Government employee	9	1
Agricultural labour	14	2
Shopkeeper	0	1
Government teacher	1	0
Tailor	1	0
Vegetable seller	0	2
Fish seller	0	1
Private sector employee	5	0
Carpentry	3	0
Pensioner	28	2
Housewife	0	5
Brick field labour	1	0
Quake	1	0
Mat making	1	0
Old and disabled	37	58
Total	101	72

Source: Census survey by Silvia Lisam, Research Scholar, Dept. of Economics, M.U.

Table 3
Distribution of family types of aged in Taobungkhok Village

Age	*Joint Family*	*Nuclear Family*	*Extended Family*	*Total*
60-70	10	5	11	26
70-80	4	1	13	18
80+	1	0	5	6
Total	15(30%)	6(12%)	29(58%)	50(100%)

Source: sample survey

Table 4
P.C. distribution of income earner and non-income earner of Aged in Taobungkhok Village

Age	*Earner*	*Non-Earner*
60-7070-8080+	1740	9146
Total	21(42%)	29(58%)

Source: sample survey

Table 5
P.C. distribution of income earner and non-income earner of the aged in Taobungkhok Village

Age	*Male Earner*	*Non-Earner*	*Total*	*Female Earner*	*Non-Earner*	*Total*
60-70	12 (92.3%)	1 (7.7%)	13 (100%)	5 (38.5%)	8 (61.5%)	13 (100%)
70-80	4 (44.4%)	5 (55.6%)	9 (100%)	0	9 (100%)	9 (100%)
80+	0	3 (100%)	3 (100%)	0	3 (100%)	3 (100%)
Totals	16 (64%)	9 (36%)	25 (100%)	5 (20%)	20 (80%)	25 (100%)

Source: sample survey

Table 6
Distribution of average annual income of earners of the aged in Taobungkhok Village

Age	*Male*	*Female*	*Total*
60-70	46500	15000	61500 (67.2%)
70-80	300000	0	30000 (32.8%)
80+	0	0	0

Source: sample survey

Table 7
P.C. distribution of say in family matters of aged in Taobungkhok Village

Age	*NON*	*Much*	*Some*	*Total*
60-7070-8080+	222	1462	10102	26186
Total	6(12%)	22(44%)	22(44%)	50(100%)

Source: sample survey

Table 8
P.C. distribution of say in family matters (male) of aged in Taobungkhok Village

Age	*NON*	*Much*	*Some*	*Total*
60-7070-8080+	102	951	340	1392
Total	3(12%)	15(60%)	7(28%)	25(100%)

Source: sample survey

Table 9
P.C. distribution of say in family matters (female) of aged in Taobungkhok Village

Age	*NON*	*Much*	*Some*	*Total*
60-7070-8080+	120	511	762	1393
Total	3(12%)	7(28%)	15(60%)	25(100%)

Source: sample survey

Table 10
Distribution of nutrition/diets of the aged in terms of quantity and quality in Taobungkhok Village

Age	*Quantity Sufficient*	*Not Sufficient*	*total*	*Quality Sufficient*	*Not Sufficient*	*Total*
60-70	26	0	26	24	2	26
70-80	144	4	18	13	5	18
80+	4	2	6	3	3	6
Total	44 (88%)	6 (12%)	50 (100%)	40 (80%)	10 (20%)	50 (100%)

Source: sample survey

Table 11
P.C. distribution of deprivation of elders of aged in Taobungkhok Village

Age	*Food*			*Clothes*			*Health*			*Physical*		
	Yes	*No*	*total*	*Yes*	*No*	*total*	*Yes*	*No*	*total*	*Yes*	*No*	*total*
60-70	25	1	26	10	16	26	6	20	26	10	16	26
70-80	18	0	18	5	13	18	6	12	18	5	13	18
80+	5	1	6	5	1	6	2	4	6	3	3	5
Total	48	2	50	20	30	50	14	36	50	18	32	50
%	96 %	4 %	100 %	40 %	60 %	100 %	28 %	72 %	100 %	36 %	64 %	100 %

Source: sample survey

Table 12
Distribution of landholding according to type of land and ownership of assets of the aged in Taobungkhok Village

Age		*Land*			*Asset*					*Total*
	Home-stead Land	*Agricu-ltural Land*	*Both*	*total*	*cash*	*Gold*	*Econ-omic Asset*	*Cash and gold*	*ALL*	*nil*	
60-70	12	0	14	26	11	1	0	3	0	11	26
70-80	2	0	16	18	6	2	0	3	1	6	18
80+	2	0	4	6	0	0	0	0	0	6	6
Total	16	0	34	50	17	3	0	6	1	23	50
%	32%		68 %	100 %	34 %	6 %	0 %	12 %	2 %	46 %	100 %

Source: Sample Survey

Table 13
P.C. distribution of physical needs taken care of aged in Taobungkhok Village

Age	*Spouse*	*Son*	*Daughter*	*Daughter In-law*	*Others*	*Family*	*Mixed*	*Total*
60-70	4	0	4	14	1	0	3	26
70-80	0	0	3	7	0	0	8	18
80+	0	0	1	4	1	0	0	6
Total	4	0	8	25	2	0	11	50
%	8.00	0	16.00	50.00	4.00	0	22.00	100

Source: sample survey

Table 14
P.C. distribution of neglect of aged in Taobungkhok Village

Age	*Yes*	*No*	*Some*	*Total*
60-70	1	17	8	26
70-80	1	10	7	18
80-90	1	2	3	6
Total	3	29	18	50
%	6.00	58.00	36.00	100

Source: sample survey

Table 15
P.C. distribution of exploitation of elders of aged in Taobungkhok Village

Age	*Labour*			*Monetary*			*Property*		*Total*
	Yes	*No*		*Yes*	*No*		*Yes*	*No*	
60-70	5	21	26	1	25	26	1	25	26
70-80	1	17	18	1	17	18	1	17	18
80+	0	6	6	0	6	6	1	5	6
Total	6	44	50	2	48	50	3	47	50
%	12.00	88.00		4.00	96.00		6.00	94.00	

Source: sample survey

Table 16
P.C. distribution of attitude towards death of aged in Taobungkhok Village

Age	*Fear*	*No Fear*	*God's Wish*	*Total*
60-70	10	2	14	26
70-80	5	4	9	18
80+	0	1	5	6
Total	15	7	28	50
%	30.00	14.00	56.00	100

Source: sample survey

Table 17
P.C. distribution of most time spent of aged in Taobungkhok Village

Age	*Wife*	*SN*	*DT*	*CLD*	*FM*	*FR*	*Mixed*	*Total*
60-70	2		1	8	8	4	4	26
70-80			4	8	5	1		18
80+			1	2	3			6
Total	2		6	18	16	5	4	50
%	4.00		12.00	36.00	32.00	10.00	8.00	100.00

Source: sample survey

Table 18
P.C. age & sex distribution of inmates of Old Age Homes, Manipur

Age	*Female %*	*Male %*	*Total %*
60-70	30.00	0	30.00
70-80	40.00	10.00	50.00
80+	20.00	0	20.00
Total	90.00	10.00	100.00

Table 19
Percentage distribution of occupation (pre-home) of inmates of Old Age Homes

Age	*Primary %*	*Tertiary %*	*Both %*	*Total %*
60-70	10.00	15.00	5.00	30.00
70-80	10.00	30.00	10.00	50.00
80+	0	5.00	15.00	20.00
Total	20.00	50.00	30.00	100.00

Table 20
Percentage distribution of marital status of inmates of Old Age Homes

Age	*Widow %*	*Widower %*	*Total %*
60-70	33.33		33.33
70-80	44.44	10.00	54.44
80+	22.22		22.22
Total	90.00	10.00	100.00

Table 21
Percentage distribution of literates of inmates of Old Age Homes Manipur

Age	*Illiterate %*	*Literate %*	*Total %*
60-70	20.00	10.00	30.00
70-80	45.00	5.00	50.00
80+	20.00		20.00
Total	85.00	15.00	100.00

Table 22
Percentage distribution of decision to stay at inmates of Old Age Homes

Age	*Others %*	*Voluntary%*	*Total %*
60-70	20.00	10.00	30.00
70-80	15.00	35.00	50.00
80+	5.00	15.00	20.00
Total	40.00	60.00	100.00

Table 23
Percentage distribution of reason to stay at inmates of Old Age Homes

Age	*Emotional Insecurity %*	*Homeless %*	*Physical Insecurity %*	*Total %*
60-70	20.00	10.00	0	30.00
70-80	25.00	20.00	5.00	50.00
80+	5.00	5.00	10.00	20.00
Total	50.00	35.00	15.00	100.00

Table 24
Percentage distribution of contact with relatives of inmates of Old Age Homes

Age	*Non %*	*Monthly %*	*Occasional %*	*Weekly %*	*Total %*
60-70	20.00	5.00	5.00	0	30.00
70-80	40.00		10.00	0	50.00
80+	15.00			5.00	20.00
Total	75.00	5.00	15.00	5.00	100.00

Table 25
Percentage distribution of chronic ailments of inmates of Old Age Homes

Age	*No %*	*Yes %*	*Total %*
60-70	15	15	30
70-80	40	10	50
80+	10	10	20
Total	65.00	35.00	100

17

Aging in Meghalaya

C J Thomas & F T Diengdoh

Aging is a natural process which involves every individual and affects every society. Aging or becoming old is associated with the gradual deterioration of the organs of the human body leading to physical and psychological problems. The Aging population was initially thought to be a cause of concern only of the developed nations because of the growth in the population of this particular section of the population. However, the past decade or so, surveys and census data show there is a rise in the elderly population even in the developing countries as well.

There are enormous amount of literature worldwide indicating an upward trend of the elderly population globally. According to the United Nations (1988), the most dominant trend from the mid-Eighties to the middle of the 21st century is likely to be the aging of the population in the developed as well as the developing world. The number of the elderly may increase to one billion by the year 2030 and about 50 per cent of these would be from Asia, with major contributions from India and China (Thakur: 2002).

The increase in the population of the elderly is a major boost reflecting the advancement of science and technology like better health facilities, better nourishment and improved standards of living resulting in the decrease in birth rate and reduced death rate especially of the elderly. However, the rise in population in among the elderly also poses as a challenge to the concerned authorities to cater to the welfare and specific needs of this vulnerable group of people which affects the economy of a country.

Recognizing the importance of this particular age group, in 1990, the UN General Assembly designated October 1 as the *International Day of Older Persons* for celebrating and acknowledging the contribution of older people to society. The United Nations Principles for Older Persons, adopted in 1991, are best summed up in the logo: *To add life to the years that have been added to life.*

As has been reflected earlier, India being a developing country with a large population, one of the many challenges facing the country is the growth of elderly population, which is growing much faster than the overall global population. The United Nations too declared that India would become an ageing society where the aged would account for more than seven per cent of the total population in the world.

This trend is also seen emerging in the North-Eastern part of the country whereby there seems to be an increase in the population of the elderly and hence some problems associated with it have been observed. The available literature on this issue in this particular region is scanty as it was not a cause of concern for the elderly, family or society then. However, similar trend experience elsewhere indicating the growth of this section of the population and simultaneously the problems associated with it therein, have very recently raised questions on the welfare of the elderly persons.

Meghalaya too is not lagging behind in the increase of the elderly population. The recent project report sponsored by the Department of Social Welfare, Government of

Meghalaya undertaken by our Centre (ICSSR-NERC) on the *Magnitude of the Magnitude of the Problem of Elderly Persons in Meghalaya* during the year 2005, clearly indicate an upward trend in the growth of the elderly population and the many issues related with it. The objective of this sample survey was to assess the general profile of the elderly in the State, their socio-economic status as well as health and age-related issues.

Data for the survey was obtained mainly through a broad questionnaire that was circulated among 231 randomly selected elderly respondents, covering seven district headquarters of Meghalaya. This was supplemented by observations, interviews and informal discussions with the respondents as well as selected Key Informants, comprising headmen, social/community workers, NGOs and State officials concerned. The report, is not an exhaustive study on Ageing and the elderly population, but it clearly outlines the basic profiles of the elderly population in Meghalaya and some of its main concerns and how these may be addressed by the various stakeholders. Through this exercise, it is hoped, the department of Social Welfare will be able to formulate appropriate policy for the elderly in Meghalaya.

It is generally viewed that being a matrilineal society, in which traditional customs and values are deeply entrenched, the elderly are well looked after in Meghalaya, and so until recently, there has been little focus on the quality of life of the elderly population in Meghalaya. This sample survey, even if it has been done on a small scale, indicates that with changing time certain problems are affecting the elderly population in Meghalaya, too, which deserve attention and mitigation.

In 1991, Meghalaya had a population of 1,774,778 with 51.14 per cent male and 48.58 per cent female. The elderly constituted 4.5 per cent of the total population. Their absolute number was 78,742. Of the total elderly, 55.1 per cent were males and 44.9 per cent were females. While in the rural areas, proportion of the elderly males was higher than the females, in the urban areas their proportion was almost the same.

In 2001, while the population of Meghalaya went up to 2,318,822, with 50.72 per cent male and 49.28 per cent female. The total number of elderly was 1,05,726. Of the total elderly, 51.09 per cent were males and 48.91 per cent were females. A comparison between the 1991 and 2001 population census reveals that while the decadal growth rate of population in Meghalaya has been 30.65 per cent, the same for the elderly population stands at 34.27 per cent. This clearly indicates that elderly population in Meghalaya is growing at a faster rate than the decadal growth rate of the overall population. Thus, as far as the change in age-composition of population is concerned, Meghalaya exhibits a similar trend as has been observed elsewhere. Therefore, public authorities in Meghalaya have reasons to be concerned about the problems of the elderly. This trend calls for appropriate public interventions in order to ensure the welfare of the elderly in the State.

Key Findings

Trends in growth of elderly population

- Elderly population in Meghalaya is growing at a faster rate than the overall growth of population.
- While the decadal growth rate of population has been 30.65 per cent during 1991-2001, the same for the elderly population stands at 34.97 per cent.
- Growth of the elderly population is not evenly distributed across the state.
- Growth of the elderly population is concentrated in

three districts, viz., Jaintia Hills, West Khasi Hills and East Garo Hills.

- Rural Meghalaya bears much of the burden of the elderly population than its urban counterparts.

Trends in Old Age Financial Security

- About 56 per cent of the respondents have reported that they are facing financial problem.
- Elderly people face more financial problem during the early years of their retirement from active life. It is perhaps because a time lag is needed to adjust their consumption and spending habits with their reduced financial status. Financial problem is less pronounced among the people of very old age (above 75 years of age).
- In Meghalaya, the elderly males face relatively more financial problem than the females. Matrilineal social formation may be the reason for this inter-sex disparity.
- The problem of old age financial security is acute among the Garos, moderate among the Khasis and less among the Jaintias.
- It has been found that the problem of old age financial security bears some inverse relationship with the educational qualifications of the respondents. The lesser the educational qualification, the higher is the magnitude of the problem of old age security and vice versa. It is evident that education instills skills in individual. The higher the level of education, the better is the prospect of formal jobs which fetch higher income. With formal sector jobs come old age security provisions. Moreover, higher income enables individuals to save more for the old age and thereby reduces financial dependency.

- It has been observed that about 80 per cent of the elderly associated with agricultural activities suffers from financial dependency. Only 39 per cent of the elderly associated with non-agricultural activities has reported financial dependency.
- Education, occupation, income and old age financial security are all related. Better education enables an individual to find better jobs and earn higher income. The higher the level of income, the better is the financial position of an individual at old age. It has been noted that less number of respondents having higher income reported to have financial problem.
- It has, thus, been observed that the illiterates, self-employed, low-income groups are more vulnerable to old age financial insecurity than the literate and formal sector employees group of people. Old age security measures have to be focused on this vulnerable section of the elderly.
- As age progresses, more and more old adults retire from active life. This is obvious as ageing incapacitates individuals from doing physical work. Surprisingly, about 72 per cent of the elderly in the age group of 60-65 is still active. About 51 per cent of the elderly in the age group of 65-70 also remains active.

Trends in Status of Health of the Elderly

- About 50 per cent of the respondents reported to have health problems. It has been observed that with age health problem increases. While 44 per cent of the elderly of the age group of 60-65 have reported health problems, this per centage rises with the age and about 85 per cent of the elderly of the age group of 80 plus reported to have health problems. Thus, problem of health bears a positive relation with age. This is a general trend and Meghalaya sample shows no exception.

- Contrary to the general believe that male elderly suffer from more health problems than the female elderly maybe due to greater exposure of the former towards stress related activities and unhealthy habits like drinking, smoking, etc., higher per centage of female elderly in Meghalaya reported to have health problems than their male counterparts. While 57 per cent of male elderly reported to have health problems, 65 per cent of the female elderly have reported the same. This contradictory finding calls for deeper investigation of the phenomenon.
- However, this trend is also consistent with facts that majority of the Jaintia elderly (51.35 per cent) reported to have health problems. Next to the Jaintias, 50 per cent of the elderly of Garo origin reported to have health problems. Least number of the Khasi elderly (38.46 per cent) reported to have health problems.
- Contrary to conventional wisdom, sample data exhibits a negative relationship between educational level and income on the one hand and health condition of the respondents on the other. It has been observed that the higher the educational and income level, the more is the health problems. One probable explanation may be that higher level of education is associated with higher level of income and higher level of income is, in turn, associated with greater profligacy. Extravagance leads to health hazards. A further study is needed to look into this apparent contradiction.
- it has been observed that about 91 per cent of them suffer from age-related diseases. The old adults associated with agricultural activities suffer less than those peers associated with non-agricultural activities.

Moreover, old female adults suffer less from age-related diseases than their male counterparts.

- Age-related diseases like heart problems, blood pressure, blood sugar, asthma, rheumatism, etc., are most common among the elderly. Public health policy needs to be thoroughly informed of this trend so that public health care services can focus on the health problems of the elderly. Adequate infrastructure in terms of both men and materials need to be created in public health centers in order to cater to the needs of the elderly.
- About 40 per cent of the elderly suffering from health problems has complaints about the quality of health care services provided by public health care providers.
- It has been observed that the elderly of high income group prefer health care services from the private health care providers, whereas elderly of low income group access the same from the public health care providers. As majority of the elderly in our sample belongs to low income group, deterioration of public health care services directly impinge upon their welfare.

Trends in Psychological Status of the Elderly

- It has been found that more number of elderly suffer from psychological adjustment problems particularly during the early years of their retirement from active life. This primarily happens due to the role erosion, as the elderly, immediately after their retirement, are stripped of the various roles and duties, both at home and workplace. It is difficult for an individual to reconcile with this change in his roles. As time passes, he gradually adjusts himself/herself with the facts of life and hence experiences lesser psychological problems. It has been found that these problems decline with the age of the elderly.

- It has been observed that the old male adults suffer more from psychological adjustment problems than their female counterparts. Probably, for the women, the role erosion is much less at old age.
- As educated and well off people can better plan and manage their old age, they face less psychological adjustment problems than those are illiterate and poor. The per centage of people facing psychological adjustment problems declines with higher educational achievements. People with formal sector employment also exhibit less psychological adjustment problems at old age than people with informal occupations.

Trends in Informal Care giving to the Elderly

- In matrilineal social system in Meghalaya, the responsibility of care giving to the elderly vests with the daughter in a family. Due to this, daughters play a crucial role in providing informal care to the elderly. About 56 per cent of the elderly in our sample fully depends on their daughter for financial support. Another 26 per cent depends on their daughters partially.
- Informal care givers are the prime source of support for the elderly.About 97 per cent of the elderly respondents said they stay with their family members and relatives. Thus, elderly in Meghalaya do not suffer much from familial and social isolation.
- *It has been noted that the average family size in Meghalaya is large. On an average, an elderly is having more than five children. We find hardly any relation between the informal care giving and the number of children a person is having. That is, having

more children does not guarantee higher level of informal care. Moreover, we do not find any discrimination in informal care giving to the elderly across the sex of the children – male or female.

- *It has been observed that instead of number of children, the income level of children is positively correlated with the level of informal care giving to the elderly. The level of informal care giving is interpreted in terms of the attitude of the children towards the elderly. If the needs of the elderly are attended to, it is interpreted as sympathetic attitude. It has been observed that the higher the level of income of the children, more sympathetically the elderly is treated and vice versa.

Recommendations and Suggestions

Old Age Security

1. It is difficult for any government to provide adequate and full proof old age security in view of the enormous cost involved in supporting a growing population of the elderly. However, the Government can provide a bare minimum financial support. It can create market and non-market instruments, and through these, encourage people to plan and save more for the old age. Government may explore various options, which will encourage people to save more during their active and working life.
2. Eligibility conditions for the old age pension need revision. Amount of pension should be considered keeping inflation and purchasing power in mind. The base amount needs upward revision.
3. The transaction cost of pension needs to be reduced.
4. Old age pension amount should be decided based on the basic need principle.

5. The delivery mechanism needs to be simplified and accessibility of the elderly needs to be improved.
6. Awareness campaign needs to be strengthened so that elderly in remote areas can avail the assistance.
7. Whatever limited old age assistance programmes are available, their distribution should focus on the self-employed, illiterate and rural elderly who are most vulnerable to old age insecurity.

Health Care Services

8. Health care services offered by both public and private health care providers need to be improved. Not that all elderly depend on public health facilities. For example, many elderly in the Jaintia Hills face less financial problem and often access private health care services. The government should encourage the private health care providers to cater medical services to the elderly at subsidized rates as part of a social commitment of the corporate entity.
9. Public health care providers need to be sensitized and made more accountable to the needs of the elderly.
10. Public health care services need to be strengthened and improved for the elderly with special units in hospitals and assured supply of medicine. It is also important to examine various models of health care so that the system can be improved.
11. Health centers exclusively for the elderly can also be considered. Health check ups and other related services need to be provided at the doorsteps to those who are immobile. Mobile medical services can go a long way in this regard.
12. Primary health centers need to be revitalized.

13. Health awareness programmes need to be organized and NGOs need to be vigorously involved in this effort.

14. Public health care institutions need to be provided with adequate infrastructure – in terms of professionals, equipments and medicines – so the elderly are better looked after.

Psychological Support

15. Informal care givers provide the psychological support to the elderly. Society needs to be sensitized about the problems of the elderly. This may be done through both formal system of education and informal socialization process. Government may launch public awareness campaigns about the need for better care of the elderly through school curriculum and also encourage community organizations and NGOs to disseminate the same.

16. Government may take initiative to introduce social service as part of school curriculum and encourage the younger generation to help and serve the elderly in surrounding areas of a school.

17. Government may declare a day for the elderly population and encourage various social institutions and civil society organizations to observe the same. Popular community leaders, officials, intellectuals and local celebrities may be involved to sensitize people on that day about care, respect and support that the elderly need.

18. On the other hand, the community too may encourage the elderly to participate in various social and community works as they are the store house of experience and knowledge. This will give them a purpose and help reduce the shocks of role erosion

from which they suffer during the post-retirement life.

19. Involvement of the local community like the *Durbar Shnongs* to organize regular check up programmes may be of immense benefit.
20. As the educated elderly can better manage the retired life and suffer less from psychological adjustment problems, government may vigorously campaign for adult literacy.

Institutional and Policy Support

21. In order to achieve transparency and full implementation of the old-age pension and other schemes for the elderly, the State government may consider the following: a) create a data base of the elderly population (village wise), identify the BPL families and enlist those elderly who are entitled to the existing two schemes, old-age pension and one-time medical grant. A village-wise household list has already been computerized by the C&RD, which is available online; b) the identified BPL elderly in each village may form an SHGs, which will ensure that the money reaches the identified beneficiaries and records/books are maintained properly; c) Another option may be the use of tiny cards, a no-frill account scheme aimed at facilitating micro-credit to poor farmers, which is being promoted by the SBI to fulfill its mandate of financial inclusion. The tiny card, just like the ATM/debit card, contains the biometric information, a digital picture of the account holder and his/her thumb impression, which authenticates the identity of the individual account holder. The same kind of no-frill accounts can be made available to the identified elderly. The government may just transfer the old-pension amount to their account, which the

elderly can access through the tiny cards at their convenience. A method may be worked out to update the list of surviving elderly NOAP beneficiaries once in a year or half-yearly basis.

22. Besides, a reliable database on the health status, morbidity and disability in terms of sex, locality and socio-economic status needs to be developed.
23. An in-depth review of the existing pattern of care for the elderly at the state, community and family levels should be initiated.
24. Institutional care like Old Age Homes and Nursing Homes for the elderly need to be promoted and strengthened.
25. As income, and not the number of children, is positively correlated with the level of elderly care, society needs to be sensitized to restrict the family size so that parents can invest more on their children. More investment on children will make them better educated. Better education will enable them to get better jobs and higher income. This will enhance the family capacity to better look after their old adults.
26. Finally, but not the least, media can play an important role in sensitizing the society about the problems of elderly and need for elderly care

REFERENCES

Atal, Yogesh. (2001). 'The United Nations and Ageing' in: Sharma K L. Indian Journal of Gerontology, *Quarterly Journal Devoted to Research on Ageing,* 15(1-2). Rawat Publications, New Delhi.

Census of India. (2001). *Primary Census Abstract*-Tripura, Meghalaya, Assam & Sikkim.

Sinha, A.C. (1992). *Senior Citizens of Meghalaya: A Study of the Problems of the Aged and Need for Social Intervention.* North Eastern Hill University, Shillong. (Mimiographed Report on a project sponsored by Ministry of Welfare Government of India, New Delhi).

Thakur, M K. (2002). 'Genetic Determinants of Aging: Prospects in the New Millenium'. *Indian Journal of Gerontology,* 16(1-2).

18

Aging in Mizoram: Challenges for Society

Lianzela & Vanlalchhawna

Introduction

Elderly population occupies a crucial position in society though the importances attached to them culturally vary from society to society. The status enjoyed by older persons in many societies has changed with time and place. Mizo society which has witnessed tremendous social transformation over the last century also saw rapid changes in the status given to older persons. In the past, older persons commanded respect and were accorded high status in society as they controlled power, wealth, land etc. Under jhum economy, older persons look after the household including the children since the young and middle aged persons had to work in the jhumfield everyday. However, with the coming of modern education and development, there has been drastic change in the way of life of the Mizo which automatically changed the way older persons are treated and taken care of. Power centres in the family and the community shifted to younger generations; administrative, churches and the community-based organisations played increasingly a dominant role in society undermining the traditional authority exercised by the aged in the community. The changing lifestyle has led to decrease in the role played by the older persons which becomes less and less as they grow older and older. They thus, gradually become more and more withdrawn within their own family and the community in which they lived.

Demographic Profile of Elderly Persons in Mizoram

People 60 years and over have increasingly a larger share in the total population of the state of Mizoram. From 4.42 per cent in 1981, the share of old age population has increased to 5.52 per cent in 2001. The elderly population (aged 60 and above) grew much faster than the total population over the last three decades. Between 1981 and 2001, the total population grew by 80 per cent from 493,757 persons in 1981 to 888,573 persons in 2001 while the elderly population increased from 21832 persons to 49023 persons, showing an increase of 124 per cent. During 1981-1991, the population 60 years and over increased by 52 per cent, from 21832 persons to 33185 persons. In contrast, the total population increased by about 40 per cent from 493,757 persons to 689,756 persons. In 2001, 60 years of age and over numbered 49,023 in Mizoram, showing a decadal growth rate of 48 per cent during 1991-2001. The total population has shown a growth rate of only 29 per cent during the same period. (Table1).

The share of elderly male and female population in the total population has been rising. Between 1981-2001, the number of elderly male increased from 11,270 to 24,800 persons. In 1981, the elderly males accounted for 4.38 per cent of the total male population and the share rose to 5.40 per cent in 2001. The elderly female grew from 10,562 to 24,223 persons, showing an increase in their share from 4.47 per cent to 5.64 during the same period. The share of elderly population in rural and urban areas is also increasing steadily.

In rural areas, the share increased from 4.60 per cent to 5.74 per cent. The share of elderly population recorded an increase from 3.89 per cent in 1981 to 5.29 per cent in 2001

Table 1

Growth of old age population (persons 60 years and above) and total population (all ages), Mizoram, India, 1981-2001

Year	*Total Population*	*Old Age Population*		*Decadal Growth Rate (%)*	
		Total	*Per cent*	*All Age*	*60 years and over*
1981	**493,757**	21832	4.42	-	-
1991	**689,756**	33185	4.81	39.70	52.01
2001	**888,573**	49023	5.52	28.80	42.70

Sources:

1. *Census of India 1991. Ageing Population of India - An Analysis of the 1991 Census Data, Registrar General, India, New Delhi.*
2. *Census of India, 2001, Mizoram Primary Census Abstract Directorate of Census Operation, Mizoram.*

The population 60 to 69 ages showed the highest growth rate during 1981-1991. The growth rate was nearly 70 per cent as against the growth rate of 52 per cent recorded for 60 years and over population and another 40 per cent for total population (all ages). The number of persons in the age group 70-79 grew by 28 per cent and 80 years and over population by 30 per cent during the same period. In contrast, those ages 70 to 79 showed the highest growth rate among the older population between 1991 and 2001. While the number of persons in the age group 60-69 increased by only 36.36 per cent, the age group 70-79 increased by nearly 80 per cent. For persons aged 80 years and over, the growth rate was 42.11 per cent. For the elderly males as well as the females, the age group 60-69 showed the highest growth rate

Table 2

Persons aged 60 + and their percentage share in total population by sex and residence, Mizoram

Year	*Total*			*Rural*			*Urban*		
	Total	*Male*	*Female*	*Total*	*Male*	*Female*	*Total*	*Male*	*Female*
1981	21832	11270	10562	17091	9072	8019	4741	2198	2543
1991	33186	17013	16173	18948	9876	9072	14238	7134	7101
2001	49023	24800	24223	25683	13322	12361	23340	11478	11862
Percentage share in total (all ages) population									
1981	4.42	4.38	4.47	4.60	4.70	4.48	3.89	3.41	4.43
1991	4.81	4.74	4.89	5.10	5.08	5.11	4.48	4.34	4.63
2001	5.52	5.40	5.64	5.74	5.72	5.75	5.29	5.07	5.53

Sources:

1. Census of India 1991. *Ageing Population of India - An Analysis of the 1991 Census Data,* Registrar General, India, New Delhi.
2. Census of India, 2001, *Mizoram Primary Census Abstract,* Directorate of Census Operation, Mizoram.

during 1981-1991. However, both elderly men and women in the age group of 70-79, recorded the highest growth rate during 1991-2001 (Table-3).

Table 3
Percentage decadal growth rate of population aged 60+ and total population (all ages) by age and sex, Mizoram 1981-2001

Age group	*Period*	*Per centage decadal growth rate*		
		Total	*Male*	*Female*
60-69	1981-91	69.56	59.36	82.38
	1991-01	36.36	33.69	51.22
70-79	1981-91	27.82	39.66	17.44
	1991-01	79.59	79.02	80.14
80 +	1981-91	29.82	31.94	28.09
	1991-01	42.11	42.42	41.91
60+	1981-91	52.01	50.96	53.12
	1991-01	47.72	45.77	49.77
All ages	1981-91	39.70	39.55	39.85
	1991-01	28.80	27.88	29.84

Sources:

1. Census of India 1991. *Ageing Population of India - An Analysis of the 1991 Census Data,* Registrar General, India, New Delhi.
2. Census of India, 2001, *Mizoram Primary Census,* Abstract Directorate of Census Operation, Mizoram.

The number of elderly persons declines with increase in the age. In 1981, about 57 per cent belonged to 60 to 69 years, nearly 30 per cent in 70 to 79 years and 13 per cent in 80 years and over. In 1991, the proportion of the population 60 to 69 years has increased, constituting 74 per cent of the elderly persons. The share of 70 to 79 years and 80 years and over in contrast declined to 25 per cent and 13 per cent respectively. In 2001 Census, there were 28932 persons (59 per cent) in the age group 60-69, 14783 persons (30 per cent) in the age group 70-79. Population 80 years or over numbered 5308 persons (11 per cent) (Table 4)

Table 4
Persons aged 60 years and above and their per centage share by age 1981-2001, Mizoram

Age/Year	*1981*		*1991*		*2001*	
	Total	*Per cent*	*Total*	*Per cent*	*Total*	*Per cent*
60 to 69 years	12513	57.31	21217	63.93	28932	59.02
Males	6969	61.84	11106	65.28	14851	59.88
Females	5544	52.49	10111	65.52	14081	58.13
70 to 79 years	6442	29.51	8234	24.81	14783	30.15
Males	3008	26.69	4201	24.69	7519	30.32
Females	3434	32.51	4033	24.94	7264	30.00
80 years and over	2877	13.18	3735	11.25	5308	10.82
Males	1293	11.47	1706	10.03	2430	9.80
Females	1584	6.54	2029	12.54	2819	11.64
Total	21832	100.00	33186	100.00	49023	100.00

Sources:

1. Census of India 1991. *Ageing Population of India - An Analysis of the 1991 Census Data,* Registrar General, India, New Delhi.
2. Census of India, 2001, *Mizoram Primary Census,* Abstract Directorate of Census Operation, Mizoram.

The sex ratio (the number of females times 1000 divided by the number of males) has increased over the years. In 1981, there were 11270 men and 10562 women aged 60 and over, yielding a female-male ratio of 937. In 1991, the ratio increased to 950 and in 2001, it had further grown to 976. The elderly sex ratio i.e., the number of elderly female per elderly male increases steadily increases with age group. In 2000, there were 14851 men and 14081 women in the age group 60-69, giving a sex ratio of 948. In the 70-to-79 age group, the female-male ratio was 966 and in the 80 years and over group, the ratio was 1160. The sex ratio in each age group did not show any consistent growth pattern. In 1981, the sex ratio in the age group 60-69 was 795; this rose to 1074 in 1991. In 2001, the ratio slides back to 948. In the 70-to-79 age group, the sex ratio fell from 1142 in 1981 to 960 in 1991 and then increased again to 966. In the 80 years and over, the ratio hand fell down steadily (Table 5).

Table 5
Number of females per 1000 males by age, for the 60 years and over population 1981, 1991, & 2001

Age	*1981*	*1991*	*2001*
60 years and over	937	950	976
60 to 69 years	795	1074	948
70 to 79 years	1142	960	966
80 years and over	1225	1189	1160

Sources:

1. Census of India 1991. *Ageing Population of India - An Analysis of the 1991 Census Data,* Registrar General, India, New Delhi.
2. Census of India, 2001, *Mizoram Primary Census Abstract Directorate of Census Operation,* Mizoram.

The number of centenarians increased during 1981-1991. There were 67 centenarians in 1981 Census consisting of 29 males and 38 females. The number had increased to 215 persons in 1991 Census with 162 males and 53 females. The number of centenarians increased by 283 per cent over the decade 1981-1991 while male centenarians showing an increase of 459 per cent grew faster than female centenarians which were increasing approximately at 39 per cent.

Access to Health Care Services by Elderly Persons

While the numbers of elderly population are increasing phenomenally over the years, the current health care delivery system, however, have not duly addressed their health care needs. An ICMR study done for rural areas has highlighted the following health problems among elderly persons over the age of 60 years:

Table 6
Health problems among the elderly persons (60 years over)

Sl. No	*Ailment*	*Reported %*
1.	Visual impairment	88.0
2.	Locomotive disorders, joints, muscles	40.0
3.	Neurological complaints	18.7
4.	Cardiovascular diseases	17.4
5.	Respiratory diseases	16.1
6.	Skin conditions	13.3
7.	Gastro intestinal disorders	9.0
8.	Psychiatric problems	8.5
9.	Hearing loss	8.2
10.	Genitourinary disorders	3.5

The state of geriatric health care services in Mizoram is still inadequate though various attempts have been made to provide special health care / package to elderly persons. The state government of Mizoram implemented a Centrally Sponsored Scheme called National Programme for Control of Blindness, which cater for the health of the elderly citizens under which sight is restored through cataract operations. One of the initiatives undertaken is implementation of a World

Health Organisation programme "Community Based Health Care for the Elderly in Mizoram" with effect from first November 2005. The objectives of this programme are: (i) providing health care for identified diseases like hypertension, diabetes, and special sensory impairments; (ii) providing simple physiotherapy and fitness exercises for affected persons; (iii) developing a medium for social interaction; (iv) increasing health awareness among the elderly. The programme runs its weekly clinic at the Headquarters of Mizoram Senior Citizens Association which is centrally located and easily accessible. This has enabled large numbers of patients to attend the clinic. The programme also runs monthly Clinics at Agapia Social Centre, in one of the localities of Aizawl city. The pattern of cases attended in the clinic Headquarters of Mizoram Senior Citizens Association during 10 months duration may be summarised as follows:

Table 7

Patterns of cases attended in the clinic at the headquarters of Mizoram Senior Citizens Association, Aizawl

Sl. No	*Complaints*	*No. of cases*
1.	Endocrinology system	181
2.	Sensory organs & peripheral nervous system	131
3.	Digestive system	125
4.	Respiratory system	99
5.	Cardio vascular system	89
6.	Bone & Joint Disease	49
7.	Excretory System	24
8.	Skin	21
9.	Central Nervous System	14
10.	Dental Disease	3
11.	Gynaecological Disease	2
12.	Others	90
	TOTAL	828

Source : Dr. Jane R. Ralte (2007)

A study of the health care requirements of the elderly persons in Mizoram was also undertaken covering both government and private hospitals in the capital city by Dr Jane R.Ralte (2007). Profile of patients attending the Out Patient Department (OPD) of Civil Hospital, Aizawl and Narareth Medi-Tech Hospital was studied retrospectively for a period of 4 and 12 months respectively. The age group considered in this study is over the age group of 50 years to match the figures considered as members by Mizoram Senior Citizens Association. The total number of patients examined constitutes 25,264 patients in which patients aged above 50 years were 2,619 (10.36%). The study from the OPD attendance in selected departments of Medicine, Surgery, Gynaecology, Orthopaedic, ENT, Eye etc for 4 months revealed the following information:

Table 8
Findings at Civil Hospital, Aizawl- Patients ages above 50 years

I. Diagnosis-Sex distributions:-

Sl No	*Diagnosis*	*Male*	*Female*	*Total*	*%*
1.	Visual impairments	292	360	652	24.89
2.	ENT disease	234	305	539	20.58
3.	Gastroenterology	140	112	252	9.62
4.	Locomotors, joint & muscle disease	134	107	241	9.20
5.	Respiratory disease	120	93	213	8.13
6.	Gynaecological disease	-	185	185	7.06
7.	Genito-urinary disorder	81	48	129	4.92
8.	Cardiovascular disease	45	35	80	3.05
9.	Diabetes mellitus	42	29	71	2.71
10.	Cholelithiasis	21	40	61	2.32
11.	Neurological disorder	28	25	53	2.02
12.	Infection	30	13	43	1.64
13.	Skin disease	21	16	37	1.41
14.	Ano-rectal disorder	17	8	25	0.95
15.	Appendicitis	9	5	14	0.53
16.	Malignancy	6	2	8	0.30
17.	Goitre	1	3	4	0.15
18.	Others	9	3	12	0.45
	Total	1230	1389	2619	100%

II. Diagnosis-Age group distribution:-

Sl. No.	*Diagnosis*	*50-59*	*60-69*	*70-79*	*>80*	*Total*
1	Visual impairments	329	165	128	30	652
2	ENT disease	270	159	80	30	539
3	Gastroenterology	141	68	33	10	252
4	Locomotors, joint & muscle disease	119	74	37	11	241
5	Respiratory disease	105	57	40	11	213
6	Gynaecological disease	139	35	11	-	185
7	Genito-urinary disorder	50	42	30	7	129
8	Cardiovascular disorder	37	28	14	1	80
9	Diabetes mellitus	31	22	9	9	71
10	Cholelithiasis	32	24	4	1	61
11	Neurological disorder	21	23	6	3	53
12	Infection	15	25	1	2	43
13	Skin disease	15	15	7	-	37
14	Ano-rectal disorder	8	7	9	1	25
15	Appendicitis	6	8	-	-	14
16	Malignancy	4	3	-	1	8
17	Goiter	4	-	-	-	4
18	Others	-	12	-	-	12
Total	1326	767	409	117	2619	

Source: Dr. Jane R. Ralte (2007)

The findings at Nazareth Medi-Tech Hospital, Aizawl also revealed interesting results. Here, the profile of the total OPD attendance was studied in detail for a period of 12 months. Total number of patients was 903 and patients ages above 50 years comprise 176 (19.49%).

Table 9
Findings at Nazareth Medi-Tech Hospital, Aizawl

I. Diagnosis-Sex distribution:-

Sl No	*Diagnosis*	*Male*	*Female*	*Total*	*%*
1.	Malignancy	30	23	53	30.11
2.	Infection	26	17	43	24.43
3.	Gastroenterology	20	18	38	21.59
4.	Diabetes mellitus	6	6	12	06.81
5.	Cardiovascular disease	7	4	11	06.25
6.	Respiratory disease	5	5	10	05.68
7.	Psychiatric problem	2	2	4	02.27
8.	Locomotor disorder, joint & muscle	2	-	2	01.13
9.	Neurological disorder	1	1	2	01.13
10.	Genito-urinary disorder	1	-	1	00.56
	TOTAL	100	76	176	100.00

II. Diagnosis-Age group distribution:-

Sl No	*Diagnosis*	*50-59*	*60-69*	*70-79*	*>80*	*Total*
1.	Malignancy	31	6	13	3	53
2.	Infection	19	13	10	1	43
3.	Gastroenterology	26	9	2	1	38
4.	Diabetes mellitus	7	3	1	1	12
5.	Cardiovascular disease	5	6	-	-	11
6.	Respiratory disease	1	3	3	3	10
7.	Psychiatric problem	4	-	-	-	4
8.	Locomotor disorder, joint & muscle	2	-	-	-	2
9.	Neurological disorder	2	-	-	-	2
10.	Genito-urinary disorder	-	-	1	-	1
	Total	97	40	30	9	176

Source: Dr. Jane R. Ralte (2007)

The elderly persons constitute 10.36% of total attendance in Civil Hospital, a government institution, with more number of female elderly patients (53%). The attendance of elderly patients is almost double (19.49%) in the private hospital surveyed, which may be due to the availability of easily accessible services. The number of male elderly patients is higher at 76% in the private hospital. A common trend observed is that the per centage of attendance progressively decreases with the increase in age in both hospitals. Attendance was found to be 50-55% between the age group of 50-59 years, 22-29% between the age group of 60-69, 15-17% between70-79 and 4-5% above 80 years. The most common disease conditions in the elderly are visual impairments, hearing impairments, malignancy/cancer, problems of the gastro-intestinal tract etc.

As per the statistics available from the on-going WHO sponsored geriatric programme (November 2005-August 2006, a period of ten months), the maximum number of clients attending these clinics are aged between 71-80 years. Diabetes mellitus accounts for 21% of all cases, hypertension accounts for 10%, followed by lung diseases 7%, cataract 5% and osteoarthritis 4%. The existing health care services in the state and the on-going programmes are not adequate to meet all the health care needs of the elderly. The health care institutions in both public and private sectors of Mizoram are also not particularly geared up for the elderly citizens. There is deficiency in the infrastructure and physical facilities which adversely affects the delivery of health care to this group of population. There is also deficiency in the knowledge level, attitude and orientation of the health staff towards geriatric care. In other words, the whole system is not very conducive towards providing comprehensive health care for the elderly citizens. Some attempts have been made by the Department of Health and Family Welfare in this area. However, there is still much left to be done.

The goal of health services to the elderly would have to be based on the general principle of providing affordable services of adequate and acceptable quality as near the beneficiary as possible. It is recommended that special rates of user charges be levied for the elderly so as to lessen the burden on the household and to induce them to seek medical attention for the elderly with no hesitation It is in this context that schemes for health insurance become important. Health care services for the elderly persons will have to be delivered at three different levels, namely primary, secondary and tertiary levels. The primary health care system would have to be the main provider of such services to the elderly, because of its reach. It would have to be strengthened and oriented for this purpose because the health and medical problems of the elderly would often be accompanied with disability, loss of some faculties and psychological problems. These problems are not always manageable at home or would require special training or orientation in those who cater to the needs of such elderly persons. Geriatric care facilities would have to be provided at the secondary and tertiary care levels. The private health institutions should be encouraged to provide such facilities, and Government could provide incentives for any initiatives undertaken by private players. This would reduce the immediate investment that would, otherwise, have to be made to provide such facilities in all public health institutions. The management of both public and private institutions would need to be sensitized to the special needs of the elderly. Certain measures can be undertaken to improve services for the geriatric patients like provision of single point counters to avoid multiple trips to various counters, barrier free passage ways, elimination of long waits etc.

The issues relating to the elderly are complex since they include social welfare and cultural parameters. These issues need to be dealt with in a comprehensive manner so as to ensure that the elderly lead comfortable lives with assured minimum health care, sustenance and shelter, preferably within the family system. The role of the "care-givers" who are an important component in ensuring the health of the elderly in their own families needs to be recognized and built upon. Orientation of care givers so that they can recognize presentations of the common ailments of this age group and who will be able to provide basic treatment at home is essential. This will take care of the "pre-hospital" component of care. An important aspect that needs to be recognized is that elderly women are more disadvantaged than men.

The process of aging is something which no one can ignore or escape from. However, steps can be taken to make it less traumatic while giving more dignity to this process and at the same time imposing less financial burden on the elderly themselves or their relatives. Many factors which contribute to the disease burdens associated with aging are potentially responsive to preventive interventions. For example, if tobacco consumption is stopped it can lead to a healthier life style and prevent many diseases in later years. It is therefore essential to design and implement preventive strategies which are appropriate and socially acceptable for the specific community so as to reduce various risks and also maintain functional independence. Disease prevention strategy in the elderly has great potential to improve their quality of life and increase life span.

Social and Economic Security Programme for Elderly Persons

The State Government, recognising the importance of the older persons and their contribution to the society as a whole has taken various steps for their welfare. The important ones provided by the state are old age pensions, old age home and in recent years the formulation State Policy for Older Persons and various supports given to NGOs who provide help to the elderly.

Old Age Pension: In Mizoram Old Age Pension was introduced soon after it achieved the status of Union Territory, and as many as 150 people were selected to receive Old Age Pension. In the beginning Rs 30/- was given monthly, totalling Rs 360/- annually. As the years passed and with rising inflation, Rs 30/- of monthly pension was considered meagre and was increased to Rs 60/- a month in 1981-82 and in 1993-94 it was again increased to Rs 100/- a month. On 15thAugust 1995, the 50th anniversary of India's Independence, the Prime Minister of India announced a new programme called 'National Social Assistance Programme'. The main purpose of this programme is to help the poor and the needy. In Mizoram this programme was implemented through the Social Welfare Department.

One of the schemes under NSAP is the 'National Old Age Pension Scheme.' The assistance for older persons is provided by this scheme in the form of Old Age Pension. According to the guidelines approved by the State Government those who are eligible to receive Old Age Pension are : (i) He / she has attained the age of 65 (sixty five) and is a resident of Mizoram, provided that in case of physically and mentally handicapped person, the minimum age limit shall be 55 (fifty five); (ii)He/ She is a person living under the poverty line. (iii) He/She has no relation who can maintain him/her and (iv) He/She has been a resident of Mizoram for not less than 10 years on the date of making application.

All the applicants are screened by the recommending body at the village level comprising such as Village Council, Young Mizo Association, Mizoram Upa Pawl (Mizoram Senior Citizens Association) and Mizoram Hmeichhia Insuihkhawm Pawl (Mizoram Women Organisation) under the supervision of the CDPO concerned by strictly following the criteria laid down. As per Government of India Guidelines, all benefit payments should be made through the Bank Account of the beneficiary in the Post Office Savings Banks or in a commercial Bank or through Postal Money Order. However, due to non- availability of Bank/ Postal Services in many remote areas of Mizoram, payment through such agencies are considered not feasible in some interior villages for timely release of assistance. Mode of payment, therefore, has been modified in order to suit the local needs. The CDPOs make door to door benefit payment to all the beneficiaries under NOAPS in cash through pay books issued by Social Welfare Department. In this task, the CDPOs utilize the services of Circle Officers and Anganwadi Workers so that the pension money is delivered to the rightful beneficiary.

Since the State Government is perpetually facing a fiscal crisis, the people receiving Old Age Pension under the State Government have all been transferred to NOAPS. The total number of people receiving Old Age Pension comes up to 10525. The Central Govt. grants only Rs 75/- a month per person and the State Government has to bear for Rs 25/- in order to bring the monthly disbursement per individual to Rs 100/-. Therefore, the annual expenditure of State Government for this sponsorship amounts to Rupees thirty-one lakhs fifty seven thousand and five hundred (Rs 3,157,500/-) a year. For both the Central and State Government combined the amount spent for the 10525 old age pensioners in a year totals to Rs 12,630,000/- (Rupees one hundred and twenty six lakhs thirty thousand) a year.

Old Age Home: The first Old Age Home was started on 1st March 1989 by Social Welfare Department. This is the only Home for the Aged (60+) in Mizoram. The aims and objectives are to provide care and protection, both physical and mental, to the aged (60+) both men and women, having no relatives / supporters to look after him / her. The applicant must be a permanent resident of Mizoram. Applicants having communicable diseases may be denied admission to the Home. Admission is done only after spot verification and interview by Departmental Officer. The Home is having a capacity of

10 (ten) seats. All the basic needs (shelter, food, clothing, recreation) and services (washing, cooking, bathing etc.) are freely provided to the inmates. Balanced and nutritious diet, as per approved diet scale & rate for various Homes under Social Welfare Department are provided to the inmates. Special diet is provided on National Days & Festivals.

Recreational facilities such as Television (cable connection), Tape Recorder, Radio, Carrom Board, Books etc. are provided. They are also allowed to keep kitchen garden near the Home for their recreation / enjoyment. Inmates are allowed to attend the Local Church Meeting. As most inmates are physically weak, devotion programmes are conducted in the home regularly.

The physical healths of the inmates are regularly checked by Medical Officer working in Social Welfare Department. All prescribed medicines are provided freely. If necessary, the inmates are also taken/admitted to the Hospitals. All necessary expenditures for their treatments/Hospital bills are borne by the Department. Inmates who are not able to take bath himself/herself are helped by the staff. The inmates are not allowed to go outside the locality of Govt. Complex, Luangmual without the permission of Care Taker / Warden. When the inmates died in the Home, they are buried in the cemetery of the local area where the Home is located, with the help of the local people and church if there is no claimant of the dead bodies. All necessary funeral expenses are borne by the Department.

The Government of Mizoram also assist and aid the Mizoram Upa Pawl, an organisation working for the welfare of older persons in the state, in many areas. Besides Mizoram Upa Pawl, there are also other NGOs working for older persons, some of them are running Day Care Centres for Older Persons and the State Government gives its full support to the various NGOs working for the older persons.

The State's Social Welfare Department under the sponsorship of the Ministry of Social Justice and Empowerment, Government of India, has already formulated the State Policy for Older Persons (See Annexure).

Role and Activities of Mizoram Upa Pawl (Mizoram Senior Citizens' Association)

The Mizoram Upa Pawl (The Mizoram Senior Citizens' Association) was founded as a non-government organisation in 1957 to address problems and issues facing older persons in Mizo society. However, the constitution was formally adopted in 1961. It was registered under Societies Registration Act XXI of 1860 in 1977. The motto of the association is "To be a blessing to many others". The aims and objectives of the Society may be summed up as follows: (a) To make the senior citizens to be able to meet their special biological, social and emotional needs so that they could continue to enjoy healthy and happy life. (b) To advise and assist public leaders. (c) As far as practicable to maintain and uphold the Mizo customary laws, cultures, traditions and practices from ancient time and if necessary to help in amending or improving those which on careful examination are found no longer suit the present ways of life. (d) To offer opinions to the concerned authorities in matters concerning economic development. (e) To be very watchful of the political, social and economic life of the Mizo and to help guide the people from wrongful and undesirable trend towards more beneficial and honourable targets. (f) To offer advice wherever the association feels it to do so to the state Govt. for the efficient management of any of its machineries. (g) To be ready, when situation demands to work together with other voluntary organisations for a common good cause.

Total membership was 50400 as on 31 August, 2008, comprising 25000 males and 25400 females. The MUP at present has more than 548 units, 67 areas and 6 Sub-

Headquarters all over the state. It has its own 4-storeyed building and also run Old Age Home with 7 inmates. The budget of the headquarters amounted to more than 20 lakhs during 2007-2008. Their main activities include publishing of monthly bulletin (5100 copies), running library, announcing the year as Anti corruption year, instituting Charity Fund for the benefit of the needy, assisting the Govt of Mizoram in its venture for Environment Protection, holding General Assembly annually, conducting excursion/short trip (pleasant tour) for members, some units maintained Centres used for recreation for members, condolense meeting conducted in honour of the deceased member, visiting and helping sick members, making calender and selling at a nominal price -each year they made 25,000 copies

Members of the Mizoram Upa Pawl (MUP) in every unit and area are engaged in finding out destitute among their fellow members in particular and the poor and needy in general within their local limit and give them financial assistance from their own contribution and sometimes by rendering physical work. To make their life more enjoyable and occupied, they always organize meeting in which recreational items of different descriptions including cultural items, games and dancing which every member could enjoy were chalked out and included in the programme. Sometimes lectures on various subjects like health education, sanitation, care of the aged and how to rear successful family are given by qualified resource persons which include doctors, professionals and others. The MUP has instituted awarding of MIZO MEDAL to those who exhibit extra ordinary bravery, scholarship, high quality of social works. In political and economic fields, the organization gives awareness to the general public of the need of having good and clean administration where the rule of law could reign and where economic self-sufficiency could be achieved. The organisation declared 2006 as "Year of Anti-Corruption". Delegates of the organization used to have special interactions with Ministers and high officials of the state giving them constructive advice on issues concerning public interest.

The organisation has never been involved in party politics. Any Indian citizen who has crossed over 50 years of age residing in Mizoram could become a member. There is no discrimination on the basis of community, creed, rich and poor. The Executive Committee, one of the most important decision making bodies used to meet at least 4 times a year and the biggest one is the annual assembly of the association.

The executive committee has recently resolved to constitute CHARITY FUND amounting to at least Rs. 50 lakhs to assist the needy members of the association. In this way the association has been trying its level best to be a blessing for others. The state government by itself and through the Central Government schemes has been implementing various schemes for the benefits of the elderly people. However, the schemes and projects of the government are still far from satisfactory. For example, the old age pension given to the deserving older persons in Mizoram since 1974 is still very small and payment irregular in comparison with the amount given by other states. Mizoram government has given, at irregular interval, only a sum of Rs. 100 per month, not at their doorstep but at Aizawl, the state capital. The total recipients in Mizoram come to 10,525 elderly persons.

The MUP very much welcomes the new national policy on older persons of India (NPOP) announced by the Government of India in 1999. The Central Government has already instructed all the states and U.Ts. to prepare State Action Plans for older persons to implement the policy. The MUP members were happy to learn that the long awaited State Action Plans are now prepared by the Government of Mizoram. However, in connection with this State Action Plan, the MUP suggested another 20- point new scheme to be included in the State Action Plan. Of the said suggestions, only a few may be mentioned here below: (a) Setting up of State Council for Older Persons. (b) Introduction of income generating schemes for senior citizens. (c) Inclusion of representatives of MUP in State Loan Boards and other state-level committee. (d) To help solve the health problems of the elderly a Geriatric Department/Wards in District Civil Hospitals of the state.

The state government, recognizing the vast experiences and wisdom of elderly people, appointed MUP members in 36 standing developmental committees under different state government departments. In addition, the state government quite often sponsor local workshops and seminars for the aged. The State Government also run and looked after Old Age Homes since 1989 where the aged people who have no relatives to look after them, are taken care of, providing them with amenities and medical facilities. Other facilities provided by state government, churches and private organisation include organizing occasional free medical check up for them by the Health Department, Government of Mizoram, granting of Old Age Pension to eligible members, concession of bus fare to those who are above 60 years by private bus owners association, observance of Old Age Day and distributing gifts to older people including Christmas gifts by the churches etc. Every year first October is observed as Old Age Day in Mizoram. The organization is pressing hard the state government to implement National Policy for Older Persons/ State Policy for Older Persons and provision of government fund for construction of Old Age Home in their own plot of land at Zemabawk, in one of the localities of Aizawl. For this purpose, the Ministry of Social Justice and Empowerment (GOI) has been approached but till now, no positive response had been received from the Ministry.

REFERENCES

Census of India, (2001): *Census of India-Aged Data in in 2001 Census,* Mizoram Directorate of Census Operation, Aizawl, Mizoram.

Census of India, (1991): *Ageing Population of India-An Analysis of the 1991 Census Data*, Registrar General, India, New Delhi.

Census of India, (2001): Mizoram Primary Census Abstract, Directorate of Census Operation, Mizoram

Lalbiakkimi (2007): "Social and Economic Security Programme for Elderly Persons in Mizoram: Role of State Government" in Lianzela & Vanlalchhawna (Eds) in *Ageing in North East India-Magnitude of the Problem of Elderly Persons in Mizoram,* Volume 1 (ICSSR-NERC), Akansha Publishing House, New Delhi.

Lianzela & Vanlalchhawna (Eds) (2007): *Ageing in North East India-Magnitude of the Problem of Elderly Persons in Mizoram,* Volume 1 (ICSSR-NERC), Akansha Publishing House, New Delhi.

Ralte, Dr, Jane R., "Health Conditions and Access to Health Care Services by Elderly Persons in Mizoram" in Lianzela & Vanlalchhawna (Eds) in *Ageing in North East India-Magnitude of the Problem of Elderly Persons in Mizoram,* Volume 1 (ICSSR-NERC), Akansha Publishing House, New Delhi.

Thangchungnunga (2007): "Social and Economic Status of Elderly Persons in Mizoram" in Lianzela & Vanlalchhawna (Eds) in *Ageing in North East India-Magnitude of the Problem of Elderly Persons in Mizoram,* Volume 1 (ICSSR-NERC), Akansha Publishing House, New Delhi.

Thanseia (2007): "Aging Gracefully: Role and Activities of Mizoram Upa Pawl" in Lianzela & Vanlalchhawna (Eds) in *Ageing in North East India-Magnitude of the Problem of Elderly Persons in Mizoram,* Volume 1 (ICSSR-NERC), Akansha Publishing House, New Delhi.

Vanlalchhawna (2007): "Magnitude and Growth of Elderly Population in Mizoram" in Lianzela & Vanlalchhawna (Eds) in *Ageing in North East India-Magnitude of the Problem of Elderly Persons in Mizoram,* Volume 1 (ICSSR-NERC), Akansha Publishing House, New Delhi.

State Policy for Older Persons

(Formulated by Social Welfare Department,
Government of Mizoram)

With a wealth of ideas and suggestions contributed in the state level workshop held on 9th & 10th October, 2003 at I & PR Auditorium by the Social Welfare Department under the sponsorship of the Ministry of Social Justice and Empowerment, Government of India, the State Policy for Older Persons (SPOP) has been prepared.

I. **State Council for Older Persons (SCOP):** Instituting the State Council for Older Persons with the Chief Minister as the Chairperson of the Council assumes the first important policy.

II. **The State Policy for Older Persons (SPOP)** have been formulated thus:-

III. **Psycho-Social**

(a) The Social Defence Branch of the Social Welfare Department is entrusted and specially assigned to deal with matters concerning the needs and welfare of older persons.

(b) Making uniform age of 60 for extending concessions.

(c) To enumerate the aged of 60 years old and above from the electoral list and to acknowledge the EPIC cards as confide proof for senior citizens identification.

(d) Taking every possible step for the security of older persons by government and especially the community based organisations.

(e) To teach the younger generation to acknowledge and celebrate the value of old age.

(f) To propagate and encourage the family as the primary caregivers for the aged.

(g) Suitable projects should be formulated for older persons where by they would be in a position to utilize their knowledge, wisdom and talent and to encourage them to work where they can.

(h) To set up old age home and recreational complexes in every district from available resources of the state and central government.

(i) A scheme for excursion for senior citizens to be formulated to enable them to see places of importance within the state and the country.

(j) To allow for concessional rates in Mizoram Houses and Government Accommodations for older persons.

(k) To encourage and assist the elders- especially of the age group of 60-70 years to organize their pool of human resources-discipline – wise, with a view of utilize their knowledge and experience for the advancement and benefit of the younger generation (example: Tutorial Institutions by the education discipline resources groups would go a long way in up-gradation of merit of students with potential for meritorious performance especially for the poorer sections of the society).

(l) To introduce a subject in the college and university curriculum regarding "Ageing" with a view to understand the perspective of aging academically and built up a wealth of data and studies which would serve to be a valuable resource for the planning process of the state government.

IV. Health Sector

- Transit Accommodation for the older persons who come to Aizawl and Lunglei for medical treatment.
- Setting up a hospice for terminally ill and cancer patients. This is to be taken up by the nodal department on a project mode.
- Organize free mobile clinic for the elderly in every district of Mizoram.

- Geriatric Ward to be opened in Civil Hospitals.
- Seminar and awareness programs should be organized to acquaint the elderly of the common ailments and diseases that befall them and are prone to.
- Concessions to be extended to older persons in respect of medical consultation fees. This should however be determined by their income bracket.

V. **Economic Empowerment**

1. The state government to take initiative for full coverage of old age pension in the state and raising the amount of old age pension from the existing rate.
2. Introduction of income generating schemes for senior citizens sourced from both state and central funding.
3. To impress upon the nationalized Banks to offer assistance in fostering savings with a special focus on the welfare of the senior citizens as well as for the citizen at large with a view to inculcate the need to save for their evening of their lives.
4. Steps to be taken with the active participation of the Financial Institutions and Bank not only to encourage savings but to educate the elders on the scope of availing loans.
5. To seek the active participation of the various Insurance Companies to educate the elders on the merits of availing suitable policies for the aged.
6. Special dispensation for the deprived aged in availing of Housing Loans and Residential House site allotment by the government.
7. The nodal department should facilitate the convergence of various state and centrally funded schemes for the benefit of the elder citizens. Special reservation should be made with proportionate percentage reservation of the budget against various

developmental schemes, e.g SGRY, Housing, Welfare, other development department, etc. for the elderly.

VI. Transportation(Mobility)

- Concessions to be made for the older persons in MST Bus, City Bus and Town Bus.
- To utilize the voter ID card for concessions in MST Buses, Town bus and City Buses.

VII. Legal Provisions

The foundation of legal protection for older person is inherent in the Fundamental Rights of the Constitution. With special reference to the older persons there are a number of statutory provisions that affirm the protection of their rights. For instance, there is the Code of Criminal Procedures, 1973 Section 125 which inter alia, guarantees the safeguard for the older persons whereby if the children are not willing to take care of their aged parents through this law they can be taken to court.

- The state government should set up special cells to cater to the legal needs and advise of the elderly especially in upholding their rights – e.g. property matters, inheritance issues, and other financial related issues and disputes, legal education on writing of Will and other documentation.

VIII. Other Self – Actualisation Measures

Media exposures and special programs: Special forums e.g. discussions in TV programs, and topical talks on various categories of events and issues which may be cultural, social, political, historical etc. These may be facilitated in AIR, DD and other local channels and media.

IX. Multi Sectoral Intervention

- All departments must be impressed to be prompt in settling the terminal claims of their retiring functionaries.

- All Departments to be advised to set aside a special welfare fund from out of their budget for the aged. The rationale behind this being that the welfare of the aged is a multi-sectoral responsibility and that each department should contribute in the welfare activity of the elderly persons in society.
- Non-developmental departments also have equally important part to play in the welfare of the elderly. For instance, the Accounts & Treasury Department may organize Pension(Adalats) Court as is practiced in some larger states of the country. These adalats are highly laudable intervention, which are basically meant to be a fast track re-dressal camp/programme for pensioners.

Action Arising Out of the Spop

The state government through the nodal department i.e. Social Welfare Department shall draw up a comprehensive State Action Plan. The Action Plan which will emerge from the above stated policy for older pensions will set out clear goals both long and short term. The affirmative centres, which will unequivocally spell out the various roles assigned to the various wings and departments of the state government and also to the banks, insurance agencies, other financial institutions, NGOs and community based organisations etc., as well.

(LALRAMTHANGA TOCHHAWNG)
Secretary
Social Welfare Department
Government of Mizoram

19

The Trend of Aging in Nagaland: A Sociological Perspective

A. Lanunungsang & Visielie

[This paper is based on empirical study conducted in 2008 covering major urban and rural areas in the state of Nagaland. It investigates dynamic changes of aging that are taking place in Naga society as a result of rapid urbanization, socio-politico changes, identity formations and growing individualism amongst the tribal population- a great challenge for researchers and planners. It deals with the problems of old aged, and how societies understand them and response to their problems. Basing on facts and figures, it gives a clear projection on the trend of ageing in Naga society from a sociological perspective that can form a part study of the trend of aging in North-East India. After examining various inter-related issues, it suggests remedial measures addressed not only to the government but the NGOs, churches, civil societies and every individual, a challenge to recognize the importance of old aged persons].

Introduction

For decades, sociologists have observed that increasing

age brings about changes in roles, rights, expectations, opportunities, behaviors and responsibilities (C. Richard Crandall.1980). Martha Baum and Rainer C. Baum (1980) stated that unlike in other societies, Knowledge and skills wear out fast in modernity, and older people are consigned to premature obsolescence. Gerben, J. Westerhof and Emmanuel, Tulle (2007) pointed out that increasing dependency and decreasing productivity, are constructed as inherent aspects of old age posing social problems that have to be solved. Acharya and Das (1989) in their study on 'Aged Tribals of Phulbani, Orissa, pointed out that the trends of materialism and individualism are growing rapidly among the modern youths. Upala Barua (1996) pointed out that changing socio-cultural ethos initiated and sustained by increasing urbanization and industrialization and growing individualism at the cost of kinship ties pose problems for the aged in future. Narendra Kumar and Pushpa Saxena (1989) in their study on Gonds tribal of Madhya Pradesh stated that even in the rural and tribal set up the family ties and social values have been undergoing changes which are not favorable to the aged. P.Venkata Rao (1999) in his study on the Chenchu tribe observed that urbanization, industrialization, occupational mobility and migration are affecting the living conditions of the aged. K. Mahadevan and M.Sumangala (1992) declared that changes in the institution of the family, marriage, and property ownership also diminished the leadership of parents in the family. To quote Saraswati Mishra (1987) 'In addition to the rise in percentage of old people, the more important factor is the roles and status of the old people are declining in the present society.

Aging is a process of biological development and a universal phenomenon to be faced by every individual gradually. Getting old is a result of the interplay of biological, social, psychological etc - the last stage of life cycle that needs to be understood from different perspectives. This stage is one of the most critical periods of life that faces various problems such as, food and shelter, clothing, nutrition, psychological problems, loneliness, family separation, negligence by society and family, Government, non-availability of opportunities such as hospital, health-care, doctors and nurses, medicines etc. All these problems need special attention with due recognition not only by family circles and dear ones but also by the government, societies and institutions.

Naga society is a casteless society and there is no joint family system. According to national census report, state of Nagaland has recorded the highest growth of population in India (64.41%) during the last two decades (1991-2001). A high degree of migration from rural to urban is noticed since recent years though rural population is still much higher than the urban area (82.25%). As a result, its population is now concentrating in urban areas mostly in Dimapur, the commercial hub and Kohima, the state capital and other growing district headquarters like Mon, Mokokchung, Wokha etc. This is one of the reasons affecting various dimensions of ageing in contemporary Naga society coupled with many other issues.

Basing on facts and figures, it gives a clear projection on the trend of ageing in Naga society from a sociological perspective that can form a part study of the trend of aging in North East India. After examining various inter-related issue, it suggests remedial measures addressed not only to the government but the NGOs, Churches, civil societies and every individual.

Method

This is a case study covering both rural and urban areas of Nagaland state. Out of 1317 villages in the state, we have purposefully identified ten major villages in the first place i.e. five each from Kohima and Mokokchung districts that represents rural areas in the state and in the second place, 100 (50 males and 50 females) elderly persons of 60 years and above have been randomly selected as our samples from rural areas. The basic data furnished in this paper represent only rural areas from 10 villages as case study. However, some preliminary information collected from three major towns namely Kohima, the state capital, Dimapur, commercial center in the state and Mokokchung, the district headquarters of Mokokchung district have also been incorporated in this analysis. Thus, the materials used in this study are absolutely of ours collected from the fields in the month of June to August 2008 by employing research assistants. Questionnaire scheduled was used in the process of data collection followed by personal discussion and observation methods. The aged of 60 and above have been categorized into five groups as indicated in Table 1. As a case study it has its own limitations. The study was conducted in a tribal and Christian dominated egalitarian society in the state of Nagaland that may not necessarily represent the universe of study.

Results and Discussion

In order to understand the trend of ageing in Nagaland from a sociological perspective, we have attempted to examine various inter-related issues in this exercise. The age structure, living condition, educational qualification, economic conditions, recreational facilities, medical treatment, ailment, family and societal concerns have been dealt in brief in this exercise. Those issues have been discussed item by item in order to discover the reality of aged in Naga society. The discussions of every item selected for this purpose are furnished below with the help of simple tables reflecting the result of our discussion. The present study found that marital status has a great impact on the life style of the aged. Losing the spouse in old age brings extreme hardship in the passage of ones life and the living partner has to face all the problems of old age as the graveyard awaits them. In this situation, many aged prays to God that they should be allowed to depart from this world early but nobody knows when they will experience the last breath.

Table 1 shows a detailed account of the aged respondents in rural areas. The number of married men and women is 63 (41 males and 22 females). The data also shows that the age group of 60-65 has the highest number of married with 20 respondents' (11 males and 19 females). 27 (9 widowers and 18 widows). 9 divorced respondents has also found in the study of which 4 are males and 5 females. Visielie in his Study of 'Ageing in Nagaland: A Sociological Study' pointed out that the most obvious factors of the predominance of widows over widowers is greater longevity of the women than men, in addition, women tend to marry men older than themselves, and wider age gap of difference in marriage which compound the likelihood of women outliving their husbands (*Visielie. 2007. p 46*). Further, there is a wider social acceptance of remarriage among widowers than widows. One unmarried respondents, a spinster of the age group of 60-65 is also found in the study. After 80 plus, there is high degree of decline.

Living Arrangement of the Aged

Table 2 indicates clear picture of status of living arrangement of our respondents. Out of 100, 16 respondents (3 males and 13 females) are living alone. 20 respondents (12 males and 8 females) are living with their spouse. Furthermore, 45 respondents consisting of majority of the respondents (27 males and 18 females) are living with their spouse and unmarried children. Of the 45 respondents 27 (23 males and 5 females) are chief bread earners, 10 respondents comprises of (3 males and 9 females) as part-time earners and 3 respondents consist of (1 male and 4 females) are wholly dependent to their children. 10 (4 males and 6 females) respondents are living with their married sons.

Table 1
Age-Sex composition and marital status

Age Groups	*Unmarried*		*Married*		*Widowers/Widows*		*Divorced*		*Total*
	Males	*Females*	*Males*	*Females*			*Males*	*Females*	
60-65	-	1	11	19	1	3	3	3	41
66-70	-	-	10	2	2	5	1	1	21
70-75	-	-	8	4	-	3	-	1	16
76-80	-	-	6	1	4	3	-	-	14
80 and Above	-	-	2	-	2	4			8
Total	1	1	41	22	9	18	4	5	100

4 respondents (3 males and 1 female) are living with their married daughters and 5 respondents (1 male and 4 females) are living with their grand children.

Table 2
Living Arrangement of the Aged

Living Arrangement	*Males*	*Females*	*Total*
Living Alone	3	13	16
Living with Spouse	12	8	20
Living with Spouse & Unmarried Children	27	18	45
Living with Married Sons	4	6	10
Living with Married Daughters	3	1	4
Living with Grand Children	1	4	5
Total	50	50	100

Educational Levels of the Respondents

The introduction of formal education is not an old phenomenon in Naga society. This is because Nagas has just crossed around 50-60 years of urbanization. In this study, (table 3) out of 100 aged a little more than 50%, 54 of the respondents (21 males and 33 females) are illiterates. 46 of the respondents (29 males and 17 females) are literates of which 32 respondents (20 males and 12 females) have studied under matric. 8 respondents (4 males and 4 females) have studied up to pre-university. 4 respondents (3 males and 1 female) have passed degree and 2 respondents both are male have done their post- graduation.

From the glance of the table it clearly shows that being a patriarchal society female were less educated among in Naga society. Out of 50 male respondents more than 50% of the aged 29 males are literates, where as out of 50 females' respondents 17 females less than 40% are literate. In the past, more preference was given to son for education rather than the daughter. This is the reason as to why female literacy rate is still lower than the male today. The overall literacy rate in the state was recorded 67.11% of which males 71.77% and females literacy rate was recorded 61.92% as per 2001 census.

Table 3
Educational Levels of the Respondents

Educational Level	*Males*	*Females*	*Total*
Illiterate	21	33	54
Undermatric	20	12	32
Pre-University	4	4	8
Degree	3	1	4
Post- Graduate	2	-	2
Technical Education	-	-	-
Total	50	50	100

The well-being of the elderly is intimately linked to their education. Longevity also has a strong association with education as literacy levels and life expectancy at birth is highly correlated. Education, apart from providing economic stability, also enables smoother adaptability towards the socio-economic tradition in the society.

Though the current literacy level among the elderly is not high, the future elderly are expected to be more literate and will be demanding more from the government for social security and other benefits.

Earners and Non- Earners

Table 4 presents the picture of capability of earnings at old age. 48 (37 males and 11 females) are the chief bread winner of the family. 31 (8 males and 23 females) are part-time earners and 21 (5 males and 16 females are totally dependent. Even in at old age, majority of them are still found as main bread earners.

Table 4
Earners and non-earners

Status of the Respondents	*Males*	*Females*	*Total*
Chief Bread Earners	37	11	48
Part Time Earners	11	35	31
Totally Dependent	2	4	21
Total	50	50	100

Sources of Monthly Income

Our respondents are found enjoying seven sources of income as indicated in table 5. The study reveal that 32 (11 males and 21 females) are getting income from farming. 17 (14 males and 3 females) are getting pension from the Government. 12 (7 males and 5 females) from business. Another equal numbers 12 (8 males and 4 females) getting income from rent. 10 (3 males and 7 females) from old age pension. 4 (2 males and 2 females) are getting salary as their source of monthly income. In the analyses of 4 respondents who are getting salary. 2 males 1 is working as Church Chowkidar and the other is a plumber in P.H.E Dept on fixed pay basis. Of the 2 female respondents 1 is working as a primary teacher in a private school and the other is a sweeper in one private company. 6 respondents (2 males and 4 females) are without any sources of income and all are dependent to their children and grand children respectively. Interestingly there is no respondent found begging as their source of income in the study.

Monthly Income of the Respondents

Their monthly income sources are projected in table 6 which are categorized starting from Rs. 2000 below to 20000 above. In the income level of below 2000, we there are 48 respondents (17 males and 32 females) females outnumber the males, while in the remaining income groups' males outnumber females. It shows that there is a greater degree of dependence of female respondents than that of males.

Table 5
Sources of monthly income

Sl. No	*Sources*	*Males*	*Females*	*Total*
1.	Salary	2	2	4
2.	House Rent	8	4	12
3.	Profit from Interest	3	4	7
4.	Business	7	5	12
5.	Govt. Pension	14	3	17
	Old Age Pension	3	7	10
6.	Farming	11	21	32
7.	Any others	2	4	6
	Total	50	50	100

Table 6
Monthly incomes of the respondents

Sl. No	*Monthly Income*	*Males*	*Females*	*Total*
1.	Below 2,000	17	31	48
2.	2,001-5,000	11	10	21
3.	5,001-10,000	7	4	11
4.	10,0001- 15,000	6	3	9
5.	15,0001-20,000	6	2	8
6.	20,000 and Above	3	-	3
	Total	50	50	100

The aged those who are not getting any sources of income had to depend on their children in meeting their needs. As an elderly man and woman in the society they have an obligation to perform like attending marriages or funeral rites etc. In such a situation they are obligated to give in terms of cash or kind as a gift or token of love. For meeting all these needs, they face economic and psychological tensions. Without any source of income, the aged finds it difficult to meet these social obligations and they feel uncomfortable to ask from their children and on the other hand feel guilty if they could not do as it is obligated.

58 respondents (42 males and 16 females) are having assets like land, forest and buildings. 22 (15 males and 7 females) are having saving in the banks. 6 (3 males and 3 females) are having cash at hand. 14 (6 males and 8 females) expect contribution from their children and grand children for their livelihood as they solely depend on them.

Interestingly, 82 (44 males and 38 females) are living in their own constructed houses. Whereas 16 (6 males and 12 females) are living with their children or grand children. Surprisingly no one is living in rented house. This is because by tradition Nagas have a very high regards for aged, widowers and widows as an asset in society so in the case of the death of spouse or children or issueless man or woman. The family members, clan or the community come to the rescue and are always ready to donate a piece of land in helping the aged and the needy people in constructing house and also even helping them in their fields and other activities.

Furthermore, 71 (42 males and 29 females) are self dependent and 28 (7 males and 21 females) are dependent to their children and grand children. 1 female depends on her relative due to death of her spouse and children. It is also found that 76 (43 males and 33 females) are taking care of their needs where as 24 (7 males and 17 females) depend on their children.

In our attempt to study the pattern of utilization and free time of the aged (table 7) 17 (12 males and 5 females) spend their leisure time by going for a stroll. 14 (5 males and

9 females) visits friends during leisure time. 27 (10 males and 17 females) spend time in baby sitting and playing with grand children. 12 (9 males and 3 females) spend time in watching TV. 6 (5 males and 1 females) spend time in listening to radio. 8 (2 males and 6 females entertained friends at home. 2 males by reading newspapers and Bible and 14 (5 males and 9 females) by visiting church.

Table 7
Leisure and recreation

Sl. No	*Leisure*	*Males*	*Females*	*Total*
1.	Going for a Stroll	12	5	17
2.	Visiting Friends	5	9	14
3.	Playing with Grandchildren	10	17	27
4.	Watching TV	9	3	12
5.	Listening to Radio	5	1	6
6	Entertaining Friends at Home	2	6	8
7.	Reading Newspapers	2	-	2
8.	Visiting Church	5	9	14
	Total	50	50	100

When quarried what kind of social problems they are facing, 7 (2 males and 5 females) are facing housing problems, another 14 (8 males and 4 females) commented the threat by the youth, 13 (6 males and 7 females) replied negligence by the family circle, 25 (11 males and 14 females) stated disregard by the society, 43 (23 males and 20 females) replied facing none of the above.

Status of Medical Treatment

On the basis of data collected through interview schedules on status of medical treatment, (table 8) 50% (25 males and 25 females) have reported getting treatment from the professional doctors. Furthermore, a little more than 40%, 43 (21 males and 22 females) gets treatment from the indigenous medical practitioners. Most of these aged respondents who avail indigenous medical practitioners are happened to be the farmers and part- time bread earners. In addition, it was found that 7 (4 males and 3 females) respondents do not go for any kind of treatment. The reasons for not undergoing any kind of medical treatment was due poverty 2 (1 males and 1 females) and 3 respondents (2 males and 1 females) considered as natural ailment of elderly people and 2 (1 male and 1 female) are found frustrated as they lost interest in life.

Table 8
Systems of medical treatment

Sl. No	*Type of Medical Treatment*	*Males*	*Females*	*Total*
1.	Private Allopathic Doctors	8	11	19
2.	Govt.Clinics/Hospitals	17	14	31
3.	Indigenous Medical Practitioners	21	22	43
4.	Any Others	4	3	7
		50	50	100

Physical Ailments of Aged

The present study reported 9 types of physical ailments by the aged, but it has also to be to mention that no physical impairment or disabilities like blind, crippled, paralytic or deaf and dumb was found among the samples. The above statement is clearly supported by table 9 that 18 respondents (7 males and 11 females) are having gastrointestinal and are recorded as the highest number of ailment in the study. Most of these aged who are having gastrointestinal problem stated in the later stage of life this problem is prompt to the aged because of their diet and food habit. 8 respondents (3 males and 5 females) having toothache. 4 (3 males and 1 female) suffering from asthma problem. 11 (5 males and 6 females) complained of indigestion problem. 12 (4 males and 8 females are having arthritis problem. 9 (4 males and 5 females) giddiness problem. 11 (5 males and 6 females) complaint backache problem. 7 (4 males and 3 females) suffering from diabetes. 8 (6 males and 2 females) are having liverish of which 3 males are alcoholic and 1 had stop after developing this problem and the other 5 (3 males and 2 females) are not into drinking habit. 12 respondents (9 males and 3 females) have no health complaint of which 7 males and 2 females are in the age group of 60-65 and 1 male and 1 female in the age group of 65-70. 1 male in the age group of 75-80 a retired under secy.

Table 9
Physical ailments of aged

Sl. No	*Ailments*	*Males*	*Females*	*Total*
1..	Gastrointestinal	7	11	18
2.	Toothache	3	5	8
3.	Asthma	3	1	4
4.	Indigestion	5	6	11
5.	Arthritis	4	8	12
6.	Giddiness	4	5	9
7.	Backache	5	6	11
8.	Diabetes	4	3	7
9.	Liverish	6	2	8
10.	Others	9	3	12

Feeling of Love and Care from Children and Grand-children

Table 10 shows to understand the level of love and care

from the children and grand children to the aged. 55 respondents (27 males and 28 females) are contented with their children and grand children. 23 (13 males and 10 females) complaint that they were loved but don't care well. 17 of which 9 males and 8 females' complaint that they have no concerned. 5 (1 male and 4 females) have no comments. From the present Table it show that out of 100 respondents 40% of the aged are not contended with the love of children and grand children. Therefore, we can arrive to a conclusion that the love and care of the elderly people is deteriorating which was never a problem in the in the history of the Naga society since time immemorial.

Table 10
Feeling of love and care from children and grand-children

Sl. No	*Love and Care*	*Males*	*Females*	*Total*
1.	Very Much	27	28	55
2.	They love me but don't care me well	13	10	23
3.	They have no concern for me	9	8	17
4.	Cannot say	1	4	5
	Total	50	50	100

Frequency of children visit to their aged parents

To know the level of proximity and sharing of affection the respondents were asked the frequency of visits by their children. 45 (20 males and 25 females) says children pay a regular visits everyday. Out of, 22 respondent, (12 males and 10 females) visit weekly, 20 (14 males and 6 females) once in a month. 17 (9 males and 8 females) visit once in a year and 1 female once in two years.

Frequency of aged visit to their children

Out of 100 respondents 28 (12 males and 16 females)

visits their children daily. 30 (14 males and 16 females) visits weekly. 22 (12 males and 10 females) visits once in a month. 17 (9 males and 8 females) visits once in a year. And 3 males once in two year.

To have a deeper understanding of the aged and their grievances, the aged respondents were asked their expectation from the family members on three variables. From the analyses of the above table 11 it clearly shows that 73 (42 males and 31 females) expect love and care from their family members. 20 (8 males and 12 females) expect health care from their family members. 7 all of which are females expect shelter from their family.

Table 11
Expect from family members

Sl. No	*Expect from the Family*	*Males*	*Females*	*Total*
1.	Health Care	8	12	20
2.	Shelter	-	7	7
3.	Love and Care	42	31	73
	Total	50	50	100

When they were asked about feeling of loneliness 86 (47 males and 39 females) replied no feeling of loneliness. Whereas 14 (3 males and 11 females) replied having a feeling of loneliness. In the analyses of these 14 respondents, 7 (1 male and 6 widows) answered it is because of death of spouse and children expired before the parents etc. 5 of which 1 male and 4 females complaint because of drinking habits of their children and irresponsible at works. And 2 respondents (1 male and 1 females) complaints negligence in studies by their children.

Respect from the Society

The data in Table 12 shows that 23 respondents (8 males

and 15 females) feels that aged are highly respected by the society which is supposed to be the highest as per the cultural aspect. 31 (16 males and 15 females) explained that aged are respected by the society. 38 (21 males and 17 females) feels that the aged are fairly respected by the society. And 8 (5 males and 3 females) have no comment on it.

Listen to advice of the Aged

In regard to listening to the advice of the aged the table 13 shows that 34 (13 males and 21 females) agreed that society listen to the advice of the aged in accept to do. 53 (28 males and 25 females) answers that they listen carefully but rejected the opinion. 13 (9 males and 4 females) explained that the society totally rejected the opinion of the aged.

With regard to getting respect and listen to the advice of the aged by the society table 12 and 13 clearly explained that the attitude of the younger generation is changing very fast. The table indicates a crisis of generation gap in the Naga society. The table pointed out that the level of respect and advice of the aged has ignored and taken a U turn in the present Naga society. This is because the data shows that level of respect and regard which is supposed to be very high from the cultural point of view seems to be waning in the Naga society. The arguments can be clearly supported by the Tables 12 and 13.

Table 12
Respects from the society

Sl. No	*Judgement*	*Males*	*Females*	*Total*
1.	Highly Respected	8	15	23
2.	Respected	16	15	31
3.	Fairly Respected	21	17	38
4.	Cannot Say	5	3	8
	Total	50	50	100

Table 13
Listen to advice of the aged

Sl. No	*Listen to Advice*	*Males*	*Females*	*Total*
1.	Accept in to do	13	21	34
2.	Listen carefully but rejected the Opinion	28	25	53
3.	Totally Rejected	9	4	13
	Total	50	50	100

Decision-making on the Family Matters

Table 14 gives a clear picture of decision on the family matters by our respondents. 49 respondents (32 males and 17 females) take part in decision making of their children's in marriage. 27 (9 males and 18 females) by the respondents' children. 18 (7 males and 11 females) take collective decision. 6 respondents (2 males and 4 females) children are unmarried.

In property matters 70 (38 males and 32 females) take decision in property matters. 26 (11 males and 15 females) by the respondents' children. 4(1 male and 3 females) take collective decision.

In matters of children's education 43 (25 males and 18 females) take independent decisions and 34 (12 males and 22 females) respondents' children take decisions. And 23 (13 males and 10 females) takes a collective decision.

In employment matters 23 (11 males and 12 females) takes decision for children's employments. 60 (27 males and 33 females) respondents' children decides and 17 (12 males and 5 females) take collective decision.

Pertaining to vote casting during the last general election in 2007, 26 (23 males and 3 females) exercised their votes according to their own decision. 42 (16 males and 26 females)

Table 14
Decisions-making in the family matters

Decision-making	*Respondents*		*Respondents' Children*		*Collectively*		*Unmarried*		*Unemployed*		*Total*
	Males	*Females*	*Males*	*Females*	*Males*	*Females*	*Males*	*Females*	*Males*	*Females*	
Marriage of Children	32	17	9	18	7	11	2	4			100
Property Matters	38	32	11	15	1	3	-		-	-	100
Children's Education	25	18	12	22	13	10	-	-	-	-	100
Children's Employment	11	12	27	33	12	5	-	-	-	-	100
Vote casting during election	23	3	16	26	11	21	-	-	-	-	100

exercised their votes according to decision of their and 32 (11 males and 21 females) took collective decision.

General Observations

Mobility of aged from rural to urban- As a normal practice, Naga parents are living in the villages where as their children are working in different towns. In this situation, most children use to pull out their parents from the villages and keep with them in order to avail better medical check up and health care while living with them. As a result, there is a high degree of mobility of aged from rural to urban in Naga society. However, in most cases, this is only a temporary shiftment because elderly people cannot stay longer period away from their home in the village whatever facilities they are given in the towns.

Increase in longevity of life- Study shows that longevity of life in modern society has increased a lot due to better medical facilities, higher degree of health consciousness, education and economic factors. They take better balance diet, avail better timely medical check up that keep them healthy and strong. In rural areas, 70-80 years old are found working in the field, earning their livelihood. They are accustomed to do hard works daily that keep them physically strong even in old age. In addition, the climate, food habit and the environment where they live promote healthy living and longevity of life. There are many aged over 100 plus in Naga society. For instance, one Mr. Watiangshi a retired teacher, 102 years old and Mrs. Medemakla in her 109 from Mongchen village are still very active who can read bible and news paper without spectacle today. Mr.Watiangshi in 102 resides in middle *khel* use to go to lower and upper *khel* every day walking without any support who can walk miles after mile a day. There are many aged persons like him in many Naga villages today.

Male-female ratio—The study shows that among the aged, female respondents prolong more than the males in most cases. As a result, there are more number of females aged than the males in every village and towns.

Health problems—Study shows that most aged suffer from gastrointestinal (18%) followed by arthritis 12%. In one of the recent studies conducted in Mokokchung town, it was found that most aged suffers from joint pain/ache 89% followed by cataract 42% (*A. L.Ao 2007*) In addition, study shows that loneliness, mis-adjustment and depression are the major problems faced by aged. Study shows that aged in Nagaland are still strong and healthy as compared to many other places and they have less problem of shelter and clothing.

Regard and respect—Formation of senior citizens' forum in different towns and villages and conduct of regular programs for elderly persons by churches and NGOs are found to be very effective, a new trend in Naga society. Elderly people are duly respected by the people in Naga society. During any given crisis, hardly any decision is taken without consulting them because they are the guardian of society who acts as advisors and consultants on many issues of critical in nature including political decision. Once an aged shakes his head that indicates his opinion on the mater in Naga society.

Social roles—Aged people are looked after by the family members. Neglect of an aged is considered as social shame and a prestige issue in Naga society. In absence of children or hirer, they are looked after by clan members and in absence of clan members they are looked after by the villagers and community people. Fire wood, water and warm clothing are given by *khel* members and churches. Youngsters and *khel* members will keep watching the aged persons helping them in times of needs. A matured tree standing nearby the village gate is reserved for aged persons for firewood. The women folk will provide head load of fire wood from time to time as a routine. This practice is not found in many places. Today, there is a high degree of realization of societal roles about the care of aged in Naga society.

Role of aged—Younger people normally refrain from speaking in presence of elderly people. They first listen carefully to them and share their opinions with permission from elderly persons and final decisions are normally uttered by elder ones in society. After listening from the crowd carefully, certain selected elderly people will speak which becomes final decision of the house. In absence of written customary laws, aged are the sources of information that have been transmitting from generation to generation. Unfortunately, many valuable oral traditions, folklores and songs etc are vanishing gradually along with the death of aged. As a result there is a decline in preserving customary laws, and culture and traditions.

Dead and funeral of aged—According to Naga customary practice, the dead body of an aged should be buried only in their own common village graveyard. This is their belief that once the dead body of an elderly person is buried away from their village graveyard, there will be no blessings in the village in future and their male clans members will not be progressive. For this reason, it is restricted not to burry the dead body of aged in other place. They carry the dead bodies to their native village and burry there with great honor and respect. There are instances where dead body buried in other place was dug out and the skeleton was re-buried in their own graveyard where their parents were buried.

Recommendations

Basing on the empirical data in our hand and our practical involvement in the issue, the following suggestions are made that are addressed not only to the government and, society but to every concerned individual.

1. Setting up *Old Age Home* in every town creating all possible facilities making regular and suitable programs for the aged. This will be highly essential.

2. Functioning of traditional *social institution* (*Semtu/ Salang*) system found in traditional society in different *khel* of every Naga village needs to be revived creating more opportunities for aged such as recreational facilities like T.V, rural telephone network, play games, traditional crafts making, and free medical check up from time to time. Youngsters can learn folklores, songs and customary practices from aged if such institution could be activated. This approach will be very effective in rural areas where as establishment of Old *Age Home* in district headquarters will be essentially required.

3. Provision of *Old Age Certificate*-Issuance of old age certificate be made available to all the deserving persons by competent authority, and by producing this certificate they should be given subsidized rates on essential commodities, concession in taxi/bus fare, railway, air tickets etc.

4. Provision of *Old Age Pension Schemes*—Creation of awareness education is a must specially in rural areas because many elderly people are not aware of it as a result, they are deprived of old age pension both state and national pension schemes. There is a need to enhance the old age pension amount at least from 200/-at present up to Rs.500/- for State pension and from Rs. 75/-to Rs. 200/-for National Old Age Pension. The qualifying age to get state pension is 60 years and above and 65 years and above for National Old Age Pension. In one of the recently conducted survey

in Mokokchung district, only 1800 aged get state pension and 3900 National Old Age Pension, which is too found to be very low as compared to the number of aged persons in the district.(*A.L.Ao.2007*).

5. The state government should consider for opening a separate *Pension Directorate Cell* specially to deal with Pensioners and Family Pensioners in every state.
6. *Free medical checkup* should be arranged in every village/town as a regular program under communitization programs and to provide subsidized health care in town for aged with separate geriatric units in every hospital with free or highly *subsidized medicines*
7. *Due recognition* of elderly people be given by inviting them to participate in public meetings, and at time honoring them with citation and gifts,
8. The State government/civic bodies should provide *financial assistance for self entrepreneurship* or re-employment to those who are capable to do so.
9. There is need to *set up counseling/training centers* creating for self help groups on different subjects having a well defined object and course syllabi. Regular seminar programs, debate and sharing of ideas in informal level will be of great relief for the aged in every locality. We must create awareness among them about the various welfare schemes and its timely implementation; invite them for discussion, dialogue and seminar on various themes.
10. In tune with working of *Senior Citizens' Forum* in Mokokchung, Kohima and Dimapur, there is a need to set up senior citizens forum in the state level. Every district and village should have such forums that could be financed by state government.

11. State department, NGOs and educational instructions should *conduct surveys* related to socio-economic and health conditions of the older people particularly in remote rural areas to identify their problems for possible policy implementation.
12. Above all, the tradition of *'family bondage'* should be strengthened to solve problems of the aged by introducing family value education in educational institutions and religious organizations.

It is expected that by translating these suggestions into action by concerned authorities at different levels, much of the problems of aged could be solved. This is the need of the hour.

Conclusion

Study of aging is becoming one of the challenging areas in contemporary society from different perspectives. Industrialization and modernization are the main responsible for population explosion affecting the entire socio-cultural aspect including the conditions of aged people. Medical science has brought tremendous change in the over all aspects health and human longevity in modern world. On the other hand, family value system, morality, socio-cultural value system, customary practices, gender biasness, traditional value system, occupational structures etc are under threat due to modernization and westernization coupled with information technology revolution where this natural world is turning into a highly sophisticated and mechanical world. In this crazy world there is every possibility of neglecting aged in every society who needs extreme care and recognition. As trend of aging enters into a new dimension, society must pave the ways for aged making them comfortable and a satisfactory ending of life. They need maximum care, protection, love, affection, company, regard and respect in every society. These are missing in many families and societies without realizing the value of aged. Many children and grandchildren feel that caring of their parents or grandparents is a burdensome and of no use. As a result, they use to neglect them who are nearing to the graveyard. Giving a helping hand to aged and living more closely with them is the responsibility of family, society and government. It is the responsibility of younger generation to understand the problems and the needs of aged.

REFERENCES

Acharya and P.K Das. (1989). '*Socioeconomic Status and Health Condition of the Aged Tribals of Phulbani, Orissa*', in R.N Pati and B.Jena (eds). *Aged in India*, New Delhi: Ashish Publishing House.

Baum and Baum. (1980). *Growing Old: A Societal perspective*. New Jersey: Prentice- Hall, Inc.

Barua, Upala.(1996). *Some Aspect of the Problems of Elderly Persons: Communities of North East India. An Anthropological Perspective:* in Das, Ahmed. Farida and Barua (ed). New Delhi: Mittal Publications. pp-188-196.

Brubaker, Timothy.H. (1897). *Ageing, Health,and Family: Long-Term Care* (ed). Londond: Sage Publication.

Chowdhry,D.Paul. (1992). *Ageing and the Age*. New Delhi: Inter-India Publications.

Crandall,C. Richard. (1980). Gerontology. A Behaviuoral Science Approach. U.S.A: Adison-Wesley Publishing Company.

Mahadevan. K and Sumangala, M. (1992). *Approaches to the Study of Elderly Population*, (ed) in Mahadevan.K and Sumangala. M. Delhi: B.R.Publishing Corporation.

Mishra, Saraswati. (1987). *Social Adjustment in Old Age*. Delhi: B.R Publishing Corporation.

Kumar,N. and P. Saxena. (1989). '*Aged among the Tribals of Madhya Pradesh*', in R.N Pati and B. Jena (ed). *Aged in India*, New Delhi: Ashish Publishing House.

Rao, P.Venkata. (1999). '*Aging in the Tribal Context: A Study of Chenchu*' in Deepak Kumar Behera and George Preffer (eds). *Contemporary Society: Tribal Studies*. Volume Four, Social Realities. New Delhi: Concept Publishing Company.

Soodan, K. Singh. (1975). *Ageing in India.* Calcutta: Minerva Associates (Publication) Pvt.Ltd.

Visielie. 2007. '*Ageing in Nagaland: A Sociological Study*', Ao. A. Lanunungsang (ed). Ageing in North East India: Nagaland Perspective,. New Delhi: Akansha Publishing House.

Ao. A. Lanunungsang (ed) (2007). Ageing in North East India: Nagaland Perspective,. New Delhi: Akansha Publishing House.

Westerhof,Gerben.J and Tulle, Emmanuel. (2007). '*Meaning of Ageing and Old Age: Discursive Contexts, Social Attitudes and Personal Identities*', John and et.al (ed). *Ageing in Societies. European Perspective on Gerontology.* London: Sage Publications.

20

Aging Among Tribes in Tripura

Manoshi Das

Introduction

As a white candle in a holy place,
So is the beauty of an aged face.

-Joseph Campbell

Aging is a natural and irreversible process of human life. According to P. Gorman, "The aging is of course a biological reality which has its own dynamic, largely beyond human control". *Oxford Dictionary* defines old age as the later part of the normal age. Elderly or old age cannot be defined exactly because it does not have the same meaning in all societies or countries. It differs from society to society and is linked with the life expectancy of the society's population. In many parts of the world, people are considered elderly or old because of certain changes in their activities or social roles. In some societies, people may be considered old when they become grand parents or they began to less or different work.

But in Indian ancient scriptures which is Manu scripts, where we can found the definition of old age. Manu divided the whole span of into four stages these were Brahmacharya or celibacy, then Grihastha or householder next Vanaprastha which entailed giving up worldly pursuits in order to follow spiritual growth by leaving home for the forest and the final stage was Sanyasa or renunciation and asceticism. Among these four stages Vanaprastha indicated old age which winding down social obligations from the life.

In traditional Indian society, older people enjoyed a sense of honour and authority, had the responsibility of decision-making in the family, with its extended structure, and was a stable unit due to low migration rates and the imperatives of the family mode of work required in agriculture and trade. The transition to a modern society since has dealt a body-blow to social institutions of yore like the joint family; parallel to this is the loss of the traditional authority of older people in most areas of decision making and their growing dependence on the younger generation.

In tribal societies, older adults commonly function as a storehouse of knowledge about such things as family lineage, religious rituals, lore and myth that explain tribal origins and identity as well as in-depth knowledge about the environment and how to exploit it for survival. Among many African tribal peoples, older adults are the gatekeepers for the ritual management of life, from the naming of children to the planting songs chanted by West African village women to assure the younger female farmers that the harvest will be good.

Despite the respect that relative age often generates in tribal societies, many anthropologists find that chronological age itself is seldom the basis for respect or authority. Pamela Amoss and Steven Harrell have proposed that there are two key factors that determine how older adults fare in their particular cultural settings. The first is the relative balance between the contributions older persons make and the costs to society that they represent; the second is the control older persons have over resources that are important to younger members of the community. Amoss and Harrell sum this up succinctly by predicting that "the position of the aged in a given society can be expressed in terms of how much old people contribute to the resources of the group, balanced by the cost they exact, and compounded by the degree of control they have over valuable resources" (1981, p. 6). A series of global statistical studies have corroborated in many respects the association of status and deference with the control of informational and administrative roles, as well as with valued activities and extended family integration (Silverman). This research shows that, in terms of resource and information control, only certain types of control, particularly administration and consultation, correlate with beneficent treatment of the elderly. Some forms of supernatural information control, especially transformational powers are, in fact, a potential threat to the elderly. This fact is highly relevant to some historically known situations of massive societal change, such as in Europe during the thirteenth through the sixteenth centuries, where the majority of persons burned at the stake for their transformational knowledge (witchcraft) were middle-aged and older females (Bever).

The construct of a stage of elderhood or of later adulthood appears to exist in all tribal societies and is largely based on combining social and functional definitions of one's place in the life cycle. Often there is a distinction between elderhood as a marker of social maturity in relation to others in the community contrasted to boundaries of old age that can take some of the criteria of elderhood and combine them with how a person's physical being and behavior reflects the biological aging process. Elderhood on the one hand is a relative status marker, accomplished by passing through ritual transitions, and is not necessarily tied to extended chronological years.

Persons who do not pass these ritual markers will not be considered elders no matter what their age. Among Australian aboriginal tribes as well as in Africa, persons could enter the beginning ranks of elderhood in their early thirties and proceed over time and through ritual passage into different elder statuses.

Older adulthood on the other hand links changes in the persons physical being (reduction of work capacity, beginning of menopause) with social changes (such as the birth of grandchildren) to create a culturally defined sense of oldness, which like elderhood, can have various gradations that can even extend beyond the point of death. Steve Albert and Maria Cattell make a helpful distinction between old age, ancients, and ancestors. The first notion of *old age* typically begins in tribal societies between the fourth and fifth decades of life, with a change in social/economic role being the most common beginning marker (Glascock and Feinman).

Factors such as invalid status and senility are quite rare as primary indicators of a general designation of old, since tribal culture begins using such labels before such changes are likely. However, many tribal societies also recognize those truly ancient adults who show sharp declines in functional skills as a different category of old, which may lead to a dramatic loss of status and even neglect and actions that hasten a person's death (Glascock).

Despite the strong male dominance in many tribal societies, some authors have begun to document a pattern of positive changes of role, power, and status by women as they pass into the middle and later adult years. These occur when women enter their postreproductive phase, and culminate when mastery of the domestic sphere is complete—as marked by control of the daughter-in-law and other adult female kin, influence over married sons and their children, greater authority over life-cycle ritual, and the gradual withdrawal of a woman's older spouse out of his public domain and into her hearth-centered life. As the women become older they often assume more authority, become more assertive, tender their advice more frequently and interfere where the activities of any of their kindred are likely to run contrary to the tribal law.

In some tribal societies where age is used as the most powerful organizing principle, different spans along the life cycle are sharply set apart by highly managed images involving spectacular ritual, distinct dress, specialized tasks, modes of speech, comportment, and deferential gestures. Persons move through the life cycle collectively and form tightly bound groups, or age-sets, performing specific tasks. Societies where age plays such a powerful role in ordering social life have been found in Africa, among certain Native American groups and Australian aborigines, and in Papua, New Guinea (Bernardi).

Some worldwide statistical studies have dealt with the darker side of aging, including various types of nonsupportive, and even harsh, treatment directed toward the elderly. This work makes it clear that being old in a small-scale, traditional, face-to-face community does not necessarily prevent cultural variants of death hastening from occurring. Anthony Glascock found that killing of the aged was found in about one-fifth of his global sample, and that 84 percent of the societies exhibited various forms of nonsupportive treatment. However, few societies enforce a single treatment of their elderly, and it was commonly found that both supportive behavior and death-hastening behavior coexisted in the same social setting. Glascock's study demonstrates that cultural distinctions drawn between intact, fully functioning older adults and decrepit individuals who find it difficult to carry out even the most basic tasks are critical. It is persons placed in this latter category toward which geronticide or death hastening is most frequently applied.(Jay Sokolovsky, 1997)

In Tripura among the tribal society like Tripuri, Reang, the elderly are considered as an asset since time immemorial. Inspite of the marked changes brought about by urbanization, modernization and globalization somewhat the status and situation of the elderly people in these tribal societies of Tripura have not undergone any significant changes. Tribal society of Tripura is to a large extend joint family and the elderly people are cared by the family members. Their role in the household is very important and indispensable. They follow a traditional system named *Muikwthar* in which they kept untouched curry aside for the elderly person in case the other members of the family wants to have meal earlier than the elderly or old age person.

The status of elderly persons among the tribal society is different in economically, socially and culturally in allover India and the world. But still now they are holding higher status than the other societies. In this paper an attempt has been taken to draw a picture about the different socio-economic, cultural and health status of the tribal population of Tripura. This paper is divided into three parts. In part-1, an introduction on old-age and the status of tribal elderly persons was discussed. The demographic aspects of aged tribal population in Tripura in compare to India and other north esatern states were illustrated in part-2. An emperical look towards various socio-economic and cultural dimesion and health conditions of the aged person in the Tripuri community and the challenges faced by them were highlighted and also guided some suggessetions to change the status of the olders in part-3.

Aging in India

According to UN General Assembly President, Han Seangsoo (2002), "Older persons must be seen as an asset, not a burden". The number of older persons rises dramatically along with the proportion of the population.A million men and womenturn sixty every month, 75% of them in the developing world. The situation of aging in India has reached alarming proportions. From 25.6 millions in 1961, the number those over 60 years is expected to touch 340 millions in 2061. Between 1961 and 2061 while the total population would climb five times; the number of the elderly population would soar 13 times. The majority of older people resides in rural India and is denied the specialized health and social services that may be available to their urban counterparts. The rush of migration of the young from rural to urban areas in search of new opportunities has left the old to fend for themselves. Their prolems are compounded by the fact that as they age, their physical and mental strength are affected. Their inability to fulfil or perform certain roles and types of work decreases their earning capacity.

The present situation of the elderly population was was clearly presented in Table-1.

Table-1
Elderly persons in India, 2001

Number of elderly persons in India	77 million
Elderly persons living in rural areas	75% of the total population
No. of women elderly persons	48.2% of the total population
No. of widow elderly women	55% of the total population
No. of elderly persons who are illiterate and dependent on physical labour	73% of the total population
No. of elderly persons living below proverty line	One third of the total population
No. of elderly persons living just above proverty line	66% of older persons
No. of elderly persons working in unorganized sector	90% of the total population

Source: http://www.helpageindia.com/

Table-2
Total old age population of India by residence and sex (2001)

	Number of old age population (60+)		
	Persons	Male	Female
Total	76,622,321	37,768,327	38,853,994
Rural	57,444,714	28,359,605	29,085,109
Urban	19,177,607	9,408,722	9,768,885

Source: Census of India, 2001

From thes table it clearly noticed that the greying population is higher in rural area than urban area and the greying population among female is also higher both in rural and urban ares.

Table-3
Changing pattern of 60+ Age-Group in India from 1960-2050

Year	*60+ Age-Group*	
	Male	*Female*
1960	5.5	5.8
1970	5.9	6.0
1980	6.4	6.6
1990	6.5	7.2
2000	7.1	8.2
2020	10.4	11.9
2040	16.4	18.4
2050	20.0	22.3

Source: UN World Population Prospects and Projections, 1998

This table brings out the over time changes in composition of 60+ male and female. These details were provided to show the increasing of persons in higher ages with an edge by the female over their male counterparts. The most significant growth may however be noted for population above 60 from 5.5% to 20% among male and 5.8% to 22.3% among female during the period under reference. It looks even more striking in absolute numbers- i.e., a jump from 70 million in 1999 to 324 million 2050.

Tribal Aging in Tripura

In the North-East corner of India, Tripura is a tiny and hilly state. According to the former president of India Mr. R. Venkatraman, Tripura is the gem of brilliant necklace of India. Its population is heterogeneous. Diverse ethnic elements can be traced in it. Thus, Tripura is a fertile field to study Anthropology and Sociology for its colorful tribes like Tripuri, Riang, Chakma, Jamatia, Noatia, Mog, Halam, Uchai, Kuki etc. The greying population in Tripura among the tribal is highest than other North Eastern States. The data from the following tables showed the numerical strength of elderly population in Tripura.

Table-4

Percentage distribution of 60+ population among the general, the scheduled caste and the scheduled tribe- India and North-East Region-2001

India/State	*General*	*Scheduled Caste*	*Scheduled Tribe*
India	7.7	6.9	6.1
Sikkim	5.2	4.5	6.2
Arunachal Pradesh	2.8	2.1	5.5
Nagaland	2.6	No SC population	4.8
Manipur	7.1	7.3	6.0
Mizoram	2.0	0.4	5.7
Tripura	7.9	7.1	6.3
Meghalaya	4.6	4.8	4.6

The table showed that the percentage of 60+aged population among general and scheduled tribe was highest in Tripura than other seven North Eastern States and all India.

Table-5
Dependency ratio for the 60+ population among the general, the scheduled caste and the scheduled tribe- India and North-East Region-2001

India/State	*General*	*Scheduled Caste*	*Scheduled Tribe*
India	134	125	112
Sikkim	Neg	Neg	108
Arunachal Pradesh	Neg	Neg	106
Nagaland	Neg	No SC population	Neg
Manipur	116	119	101
Mizoram	Neg	Neg	Neg
Tripura	128	120	116
Meghalaya	Neg	Neg	Neg
Assam	104	114	92

Source: Census of India, 2001

The dependency ratio of tribal aged persons was highest in Tripura among the other North-Eastern States. It was also higher than all India.

Table-6
Total old age population (60+) of North-East Region by residence and sex

State	*Total/Rural/ Urban*	*Number of old age population*		
		Persons	*Male*	*Female*
Sikkim	Total	29,040	16,391	12,649
	Rural	26,699	15,117	11,582
	Urban	2,341	1,274	1,067
Arunachal Pradesh	Total	49,916	26,417	23,499
	Rural	45,973	24,263	21,710
	Urban	3,943	2,154	1,789
Nagaland	Total	90,323	50,736	39,587
	Rural	81,294	45,300	35,994
	Urban	9,029	5,436	3,593
Manipur	Total	145,470	73,233	72,237
	Rural	102,047	52,272	49,775
	Urban	43,423	20,961	22,462
Mizoram	Total	77,955	24,800	24,223
	Rural	25,683	13,322	12,361
	Urban	23,340	11,478	11,862
Tripura	Total	232,549	112,206	119,893
	Rural	190,501	93,023	97,478
	Urban	42,048	19,633	22,415
Meghalaya	Total	105,726	54,016	51,710
	Rural	85,718	44,633	41,085
	Urban	20,008	9,383	10,625
Assam	Total	1,560,366	800,585	759,781
	Rural	1,361,247	696,202	665,045
	Urban	199,119	104,383	94,736

Source: Census of India, 2001

From this table it was revealed that in Tripura the number of elderly women higher than the male elderly persons in both rural and urban areas. But in other States the number of male aged persons was higher than female aged. It was also noticed that the number of greying population was higher in rural areas than that of urban areas.

Table-7
Total old age population (60+) among Scheduled Tribe of India and North-East Region by residence and sex (2001)

State	*Total/Rural/ Urban*	*Number of old age population*		
		Persons	*Male*	*Female*
India	Total	5,128,500	2,433,168	2,695,332
	Rural	4,806,063	2,283,103	2,522,960
	Urban	322,437	150,065	172,372
Sikkim	Total	6,915	3,795	3,120
	Rural	6,398	3,537	2,861
	Urban	517	258	259
Arunachal Pradesh	Total	38,866	19,713	19,153
	Rural	37,432	19,083	18,349
	Urban	1434	630	804
Nagaland	Total	84,652	47,118	37,534
	Rural	78,719	43,629	35,090
	Urban	5,933	3,489	2,444
Manipur	Total	44,729	23,539	21,190
	Rural	42,847	22,599	20,248
	Urban	1,882	940	942
Mizoram	Total	48,035	24,164	23,871
	Rural	25,367	13,092	12,275
	Urban	22,668	11,072	11,596
Tripura	Total	62,581	32,405	30,176
	Rural	61,534	31,907	29,627
	Urban	1,047	498	549
Meghalaya	Total	90,712	45,868	44,744
	Rural	77,962	40,480	37,482
	Urban	12,750	5,488	7,262
Assam	Total	1,73,758	90,447	83,311
	Rural	168,870	87,824	81,046
	Urban	4,888	2,623	2,265

Source: Census of India, 2001

The total number of aged tribal population was noticed higher in rural areas in all North-Eastern States and all India in this table. In all India the female aged population was higher than male aged. In Tripura the number of elderly women was slightly lower than the elderly men in rural areas but in urban it was higher among female aged.

The data from the Table 8 showed the present picture of household with aged persons in Tripura.

Table-8
Elderly households in Tripura 2001

Total number of household	663662
Number of households with no aged person	472607
Household with one aged person	145284
Number of single member household	7656
Aged male members in single member household	2053
Aged female members in single member household	5603
Sex ratio of single member aged households	2729
Percentage of single member aged households tohousehold with one aged person	5.3

Source: http://www.helpageindia.com/

An Empirical Study among Tripuri Tribe of Tripura

There are 19 tribes belonging in Tripura. Among them Tripuri is the largest tribe. The total tribal population is 31.13% of the total population of Tripura and majority of them is Tripuri tribe (17.04%). For this reason, the Tripuri tribe was selected.

Objective of the study

The broad objectives of the study were:

- To investigate various socio-economic and cultural dimesion of the aged person among the Tripuri community
- To find out the challenges faced by the aged persons.
- To suggest some recommendation for betterment the status of the olders.

Material and Methods

The study was conducted among the Tripuri tribes of two tribal villages under Bishalgarh subdivision of West Tripura district. The study areas were selected in purposive sampling method. From these two villages 76 old age persons (33 male and 43 female) were selected randomly from the household with old age persons. A pretested scheduled were used to collect data from the elderly persons through direct interview method. The numerical data were analysed in computer.

Major findings

i) ***Socio-economic Status of the Old-age persons:*** The socio-economic status was revealed from the table-9. The showed that-

- Among the total elderly persons majority of them are females (56.58%).
- Majority elderly persons are married. Among them male married persons (72.73%) were higher than the females (27.27%).
- The economic level of the maximum elderly persons families were above proverty line (65.79%).
- Among three family types, the elderly persons were living in the joint families (59.21%) than the nuclear (35.53%) and extended (5.26%) families.
- The majority of the elderly persons (96.05%) of these two villages haven't changed their religion from hindu to other religion. Only few (3.95%) were converted into christianity.
- The percentage of the own house land was higher (88.15%) than the Govt. Khas land (11.85%).
- The literacy rate was higher among the male elderly persons (32.89%) than that of their counterparts (11.85%).

- The membership in village administration was only 21.05%. Among them majorities were the male (36.36%) and very few (9.3%) were female.

Table-9

Socio-economic status of the old-age persons

Sl.No.	*Category*	*Old-Age Persons*	
		No.	*%*
1.	Total No. of Elderly Persons	76	100.00
2.	Male	33	43.42
3.	Female	43	56.58
4.	Marital status		
	Married	40	52.63
	Widowed	36	47.37
5.	APL	50	65.79
6.	BPL	26	34.21
7.	Family Type		
	Nuclear	27	35.53
	Joint	45	59.21
	Extended	4	5.26
8.	Religion		
	Hindu	73	96.05
	Christian	3	3.95
9.	Ownership of house land		
	Owner of land	67	88.15
	Govt. Khas land	9	11.85
10.	Education		
	Illiterate Male	8	10.52
	Illiterate Female	34	44.74
	Literate Male	25	32.89
	Literate Female	9	11.85
11.	Membership in village Administration		
	Yes	16	21.05
	No	60	78.95

ii) ***Occupational Status of the Aged Persons***

- The previous occupations among the male aged persons maximum were the agricultural labour (66.67%) and very few were in services and other activities. The majorities of the female aged persons were housewives (30.23%) and agricultural labour (27.91%). But the cultivators were higher among the female (13.95%) than the male aged persons (6.06%).
- At present 54.2% male aged persons and 4.63% female aged persons are agricultural labour. Majority of the female aged are housewives (62.79%). Some females are doing small business (16.28%) which higher than the male aged (4.2%).

iii) ***Economic Conditions of the Families and the Elderly Persons***

- The main earning member of the maximum families were the sons (63.15%) and 25% were the elderly persons. Among them 42.4% were the male and 11.63% were the female aged persons.
- Monthly contribution in the family more than 2000 rupees by the 30.3% male and 6.98% female aged persons.
- Total monthly income of the family above 3500 in the maximum families (43.42%). Only one family having income less than 500 rupees and others varing between 500 to 3500 rupees.
- All the male aged persons (43.10%) except one and only 25% female aged have the assets like ponds, tila, robber garden and others .
- Among the male 25% having savings account in Bank and only 3.94% have in Post Office. !5.79%

females have account in Bank and 2.63% saving money in Post Office.

iv) ***Family Activities and Social Activites of the Elderly persons***

- The elderly people never sit idle. Most of the elderly male making baskets and others things from bamboo or fencing with bamboo.
- The elderly women were helping in the kitchen for cooking, brewing rice beer or looking after their grandchildren or great-grandchildren, clearing house, getting firewoods etc.
- Only few male and female aged persons were engaged with social activies, maximum were busy in family activities.
- Majority of the elderly persons both male (72.73%) and female (74.42%) have the decision making power in the family.

v) ***Arrangement of Living of Aged Persons***

- The maximum elderly men (81.82%) and women (83.72%) were living inside the main house and very few were living outside the main house.
- In theses two villages the elderly men (42.4%) and women (32.55%) have their own house. 42.4% male and 51.16% female aged were living in their sons house. Among male only 9.1% and female 2.33% living alone. Very few were living with their daughters.

vi) ***Health Status of the Elderly Persons***

- The elderly persons of the study areas have cronic diseases like Stomackache, Asthama, Eye problem, Blood presser, Gastric problem, Paralysis, diabetes etc. Cronic diseases were noticed higher among the elderly women than the male aged persons. But majority of them both male (51.51%) and female (25.59%) haven't any cronic diseases.

- The maximum aged persons getting treatment support and care from the family members.
- More than half portions of the elderly persons both male (51.52%) and female (55.81%) were dependent upon quack doctor and others were going to hospitals and primary health centres.
- Monthly expenditure for health purpose nearly 200 rupees among 30.3% male and 34.88% female aged persons. Some elderly persons in both male (15.2%) and female (6.98%) have to spend money above 500 rupees.
- In this community both male and female aged persons were addicted by bidi, hukka, hand made wine etc. Among them elderly women (55.32%) were more addicted by bidi than male(50.00%) and male aged (27.78%)were addicted by hand made wine than women (14.89%).
- Physically only 15.2% male and 2.33% female aged persons were dependent on family members.
- Maximum elderly persons both men (39.4%) and women (44.19%) were not facing any difficulties in movement and daily activities. Some of them who were very aged and having paralysis, Asthama, High blood presser wee facing difficulties in movement and other activities.

vii) ***Spending of Leisure Time of the Elderly Persons***

- Generally the male elderly persons were spending

liesure time gossiping with same aged persons and female elderly persons were spening these time with the family members.

- In the evening most of the elderly people both men and women will be telling stories or folk tales to their grandchildren or great grandchildren.
- Very few of them were watching TV or listening radio.

viii) ***Traditional Indigenous Knowledge***

- The traditional knowledge like folk knowledge, traditional wisdom or science, knowledge in medicinal plants, religious beliefes and thoughts are passed from generation to generation by the words of mouth and cultural rituals.
- These oral cultures and knowledge are controlled by the community and the elderly people both men and women.

ix) ***Perception on Aging***

Percption on ageing is more or less same among the Tripuri elderly men and women. They thought that when they will not be able to do family work or any type of physical work, they become old. Some of them thought that advanced age, physical and mental weakness make people aged. Cronic diseases and excess hard work also help to increase age. They also feel them as aged persons when they became grandmothers or grandfathers. Very few them thought that when a man or woman need stick or any support for walking he or she became old.

x) ***Govt. Support for the Elderly People***

Under National Old Age Pension Scheme

(NOAPS) 42.42% male and 13.95% female aged persons getting benefits in tese study areas.

- Only 3.03% men and 2.32% women were under Arnapurna Scheme and 12.12% male and 6.97% female wee getting support from Antordaya.
- Many of them both men (42.42%) and women (72.09%) were not getting any support from Govt. schemes.

Recommendations

For betterment of the status of the old age persons following steps can be followed:

i) The PHC should have minimum requirement for health care of aged or geriatric care because maximum number of aged persons are dependent on PHC, quack doctor or ojha in the tribal villages.

ii) The elderly women have more cronic diseases than elderly men, because they donot think about their health care. The family members and volunary organigation should aware them.

iii) The elderly persons who are living alone should be cared by Govt. and other Non Government Organizations. They need proper care and support.

iv) To improve the health status of the elderly persons, there is a need of indepth research studies in different tribal areas to identify various factors related to health problems.

v) To develop proggrammes for the elderly persons , it is important to carry out more investigations to gather information about the actual proportions of the elderly population who are alone or disable and psychologically distress.

vi) There are many national policies and schemes for older persons. But all the aged persons residing in rural areas specially in tribal villages are not aware about the schemes and not getting benefits from the schemes properly.

vii) Government support should be given to all ederly persons equally without any political favours.

Conclusion

"The aged and elderly are not afraid of death, but are afraid of life". It is the fact of every aged person's life. In modern time family members treat them as burden. But still now in tribal societies the elder persons respected lot than other societies and it was also noticed in this emperical study among the Tripuri tribes of Tripura though their economic conditions were not very well. The tribal cultural ethos gives a special respect to the elderly persons as wise and counselors of the community. The younger generation should more aware about the elderly population because the experience and wisdom of old age is the treasure for any community. In evolving any policy on aging care both geriatric support and social empowering should be given to improve the competence of the aged people and to ensure their active participation in society. Like other global issues such as enviroment or poverty eradication, ageing should be given much attention. Government must emphasize the mainstreaming of ageing into national policy and implement it carefully and must strive to achieve the empowerment of older persons and their full participation in all aspects of society. Every body should respect and take care the aged persons, because no one can escape the fact old age.

21

Pattern of Population Aging in Tripura

Paramita Saha

I

Population ageing refers to a situation when number of elderly people increases much more rapidly than the rest of the population, leading to the increase in the proportion of older persons in total population. While population ageing is not a new phenomenon, the rapid pace at which the number and proportion of the elderly are growing particularly in developing countries, has led to widespread concern. Ageing of population is basically the result of a two-dimensional demographic transformation: on one hand the decline in overall mortality results in longer life- expectancy; and on the other, decline in fertility results in decreasing the proportion of children and young adults in the population. The relative strength of these two forces acts together to determine the proportion of elderly in the population.

Tripura a small northeastern state of India had an elderly population higher in proportion (7.01 per cent) than the national figure (6.55 per cent) in 1991. Tripura may be considered a state with population classified as 'old' following

United Nation's classification of populations with more than 7 per cent aged above sixty years as old. In 2001 this figure has increased to 7.27 per cent.

The present paper aims to highlight the regional dimension of population ageing, which is not reflected in the aggregate national figures, on the basis of census data from 1961 to 2001. Thus the paper documents and analyses the dynamics of population ageing in Tripura and also brings out the distinctive pattern of the ageing process in urban and rural areas in the state.

The paper is divided into six sections. After a brief introduction in section I, section II traces the growth rate of elderly population in Tripura. The situation in the neighbouring northeastern states (except Sikkim) are provided in section III. Section IV analyses the various dimensions of population ageing in Tripura. The importance of evolving an appropriate measure of population ageing is discussed in Section V and policy challenges are discussed in the concluding Section VI.

II

As population grows over time the age structure also undergoes changes, raising the absolute number of the elderly, (defined as person of age sixty years and above) as well as their proportion in the population (Table 1). In the year 1991 the proportion of elderly persons in total population showed a marginal decline but it has remained above seven per cent since 1981. At this point it is worthwhile to look into the pattern of changes in total population and the elderly population in order to understand their interrelation and possible future implications.

Changes in the proportion of population in a given age group between different dates depend on the relative rates of growth of the age group in question and of the total population (Shryock and Siegel, 1976). It has been shown that each unit increase in the rate of growth of stable population is associated with a corresponding drop in the proportion of elderly people (Keyfitz, 1975). In Tripura annual average growth rate of total population has declined from 3.62 per cent in 1961-71 to 1.60 per cent in 1991-01 (Table 2). However, during 1981-91 the population growth rate increased to 3.42 per cent per year from the 3.19 per cent per year experienced during the previous decade 1971-81. Consequently the proportion of elderly population recorded a decline from 7.05 in 1981 to 7.01 in 1991 (Table 1) i.e. by 0.55 per cent. *In all other years when population growth rate declined, proportion of elderly population recorded an increase. The increase in the proportion of elderly population* in the forty years from 1961 to 2001 *has been 34.13 per cent taking 1961 as the base year.* If the previous census year is taken as the base year, in each decade the change in proportion of the elderly persons has been 21.5 per cent in 1971, 7.07 per cent in 1981, -0.55 in 1991 and 3.68 in 2001.Thus, till 1981 the proportion of elderly persons increased at a decreasing rate; it declined in 1991 and picked up again during 1991-2001 by 3.68 percent If the population growth rate continues to decline, proportion of elderly persons will increase. However, for the purpose of policy formulation and public action, not only the proportion but also the growth rate of absolute number of the elderly is equally important as is the age distribution of the elderly population.

Generally it has been found that increase in the growth rate of elderly population is accompanied by a decline in the growth rate of general population (Rajan et al 1999). *In Tripura, however, average annual growth rate of both elderly population and the total population have recorded a decline over the years 1961 to 2001(Table 2).* Except for 1981-1991, the average annual growth rate of elderly population has remained above the average annual growth rate of general population (Table 2), which explains the increase in the proportion of the elderly population.

If the present trend continues, the number and proportion of elderly persons in future will depend on the size of the age cohort that is likely to enter the elderly age group, and their age-specific mortality rates.

III

The aging situation in Tripura is quite distinct from the other northeastern states. The elderly population (2,23,373) in the seven states together comprises of 5.82 per cent of the total population (3,83,16,918) of the region in the year 2001(Table 3). Assam has the highest number of elderly population among these states. 69.86 per cent of total elderly population in the region belonged to Assam in the year 2001.

Tripura, the smallest state *has 10.41 per cent of total elderly population of the northeast in 2001.* While Tripura has the second largest absolute number of elderly persons, *it has the highest proportion of elderly population (7.27 per cent) among the northeastern states and has recorded lowest growth rate of elderly population in 1991-2001(Table 4).* With the co-relation coefficient between growth rate of elderly population in 1991-2001 and proportion of elderly population in 2001 being negative (-0.6), it seems higher the proportion of elderly population lower is the growth rate of elderly population.

The figures thus reveal that the pattern and extent of population ageing is very diverse among the different states of the northeast. Similar diversity is also observed when population is grouped according to, locality of residence, gender and economic conditions. These are analysed in Section IV.

IV

When the elderly population is disaggregated with respect to their place of residence, age, gender and age groups several important aspects of the pattern of population ageing become apparent.

Though most of the elderly persons in the state live in the rural area it is observed that in Tripura the *proportion of elderly persons living in the urban area has been gradually increasing from 10 percent in 1981 to 18 percent in 2001* (Table 5). Percentage of elderly persons in urban population increased more (from 6.64 in 1981 to 7.7 in 2001) compared to percentage of elderly persons in rural population (from 7.1 in 1981 to 7.18 in 2001). While for the years 1981 and 1991 the percentage of elderly persons in rural population was higher than that in the urban population, *in 2001 the percentage of elderly persons in the urban population (7.7) exceeds the percentage in rural population (7.18).*

In the year 2001, both in the urban and rural areas number of elderly female exceed their male counterparts. *Elderly sex ratio in the rural area has increased to 1047 in 2001 and in the urban area the ratio is 1141.* The implication is that in both rural and urban areas, the life conditions for females have improved so as to result in increasing presence of women in the older age group.

If the different districts of Tripura are considered it is observed that proportion of elderly population is highest in the West Tripura District followed by South Tripura District (Table 8). *Elderly sex ratio is highest in South Tripura (1094), which is even higher than the figure for the state as a whole (1064).* It is lowest in the North District.

One prominent aspect of population ageing world over, is the ageing of the aged i.e. increase in the proportion of older elderly persons in elderly population. The structural change of the elderly population can be studied by dividing them into young-old (60-69 years), old-old (70-79 years) and very old (80 years and above) categories (Table 6).

Categorisation of the elderly population into various age groups helps in need assessment for policy-interventions for them. While persons in the young old category may still have a number of productive years ahead, policies to integrate them to economically productive and useful enterprises will be beneficial to the economy. For the old-old category the emphasis will be on healthy ageing, so that when they progress to the very old group they could remain functionally as fit as possible. Nevertheless at this stage various physical ailments and impairment creep in, and medical expenses and care become an important issue. Policies are needed to address these issues.

The annual average rate of growth during the period 1981 to 2001 of the old-old category is the highest at 3.81. The proportion of the young old and the very old, in the elderly population have declined from 1981 to 2001. It is the old-old category, which has increased, in proportional terms from 27.91per cent to 30.6 per cent in 2001 (Table 6).

Another feature of an aging population, experienced globally, is that, the female share increases over time and is termed as 'feminisation of the elderly' (Dhar Chakraborty, 2004). Disaggregating elderly population of Tripura in different census years according to gender shows that number of elderly female in total elderly population of Tripura has increased steadily over time and in 2001, female elderly has outnumbered their male counterpart (Table 1). The elderly sex ratio has improved continuously since 1961 and has remained above the overall sex ratio since 1981. It may be noted here that the *elderly sex ratio in Tripura is even higher than that of Kerala (1058) as per the 2001 Census figures (Table 7).* Also the growth rate of female elderly population has always remained above the elderly growth rate and growth rate of male elderly (Table 2). *Proportion of the elderly persons among female population of Tripura has been increasing steadily over the years (Table 7).* Presence of higher number of women in the older age group means that a large number of them will be widows probably with little economic resources to fall back upon and consequently will be in need of public support.

V

The median age is often used as a basis for describing population as young or old. Populations with median under 20 are described as 'young', populations with medians 30 or over as 'old' and those with medians 20 to 29 as of intermediate age. And when the median age of a population distribution rises it indicates aging of population. *The median age for Tripura increased from 21.1 in 1991 to 23.32 in 2001.* Though it means that *Tripura still is in the 'intermediate age' category it may be regarded as indicative of gradual ageing of population.*

The *'old age ratio' i.e. 'proportion of aged persons in total population'* is generally taken as a summary indicator of the extent of population ageing and shows a marginal increase in the proportion of elderly population from 7.01 per cent to 7.27 per cent during the period 1991to 2001 as discussed earlier.

However, in order to highlight the socio- economic impact of population ageing different dependency ratios are constructed. *Aged dependency ratio or Old age dependency ratio i.e. number of elderly persons per hundred population in the working age-group of 15 to 59 years* is intended to bring out the potential of the working population supporting the dependent elderly population. Particularly in a pay- as - you -go type of social security system where the ongoing pensions contribution from the labour force are used for current pension benefits the old age dependency ratio can be regarded as consumption – production ratio impact of population ageing. *From 1981 the aged dependency ratio has recorded a gradual decline, from 13.37 in 1971 to13.13 in 1981 to 12.86 in 1991 and to 12.32 in 2001* (Table 9).

Total dependency ratio (UN 1968) *is the number of population in the 0 to 14 years age group and in the elderly age group taken together per hundred population in the working age-group.* It represents the total potential burden on the working age population, of supporting the elderly and the children. *This has also recorded a decline from **93.39** in **1961** to **69.34** in 2001.*

The increasing share of working age population in the total population has caused the decline in the aged dependency ratio and total dependency ratio. The population in 15 to 59 years age group was 49.22 per cent of total population in 1971. It rose to 53.58 per cent in 1981, to 54.60 per cent in1991 and then to 59.05 per cent in 2001 (Table 12).

It is important to remember here that neither everyone in the 15 to 59 years age group is working, nor every elderly individual is dependent. *An index of real burden of old age dependency should therefore be based on the ratio of non-working elderly persons to working population of all ages.* Workers in different age groups are calculated by subtracting the non-workers from the population in that age group. These are then added to obtain the total number of workers. From 1991 to 2001 the newly defined burden also shows a decline even when the elderly workers are included and non-workers in the 15-59 years age group are excluded in calculating the total number of workers. *Burden of population ageing is calculated as number of elderly non-workers per hundred workers in the economy. This also shows a decline from **14.39** in **1991** to **12.31**in 2001*(Table 10). The underlying reason is the increase in the number and proportion of elderly and non-elderly workers in total population of elderly and working age population respectively. While the proportion of elderly workers in elderly population increased from 37 per cent to 39 per cent, that among the working age population increased from 51 per cent to 55 per cent. However, it needs to be mentioned here that this particular index also has its limitations. Firstly, workers of all the age categories as defined above include main as well as marginal workers. Secondly, it does not give any idea about the level and adequacy of income of the elderly persons who are working as either main or marginal workers. Moreover, in addition to income there are other needs typical of the elderly population, e.g. medical and daily care at an advanced age, which need to be taken care of. This aspect is not addressed by this index.

All the indices of population ageing discussed so far considers the elderly population as a homogenous group and do not account for the changing age composition of the elderly age group. It is observed that the conditions and need of the elderly person above 80 years of age will be very different than someone in the 60 to 65 years age group. Many have suggested a composite index that combines the number of the aged and also their extent of oldness (Basu and Basu, 1987;Chakravarty and Chakravarty, 1993). Thus the age difference index I (p), reflect the oldness of the elderly population. The P-index and the Q-index combines both the proportion and intensity of ageing. These are particularly useful in planning for geriatric health care.

The age difference index I (p) is an average of the extent of oldness of the old. Let Y_i be the age of individual i. Sixty years be the cut off age. Then $(Y_i - 60)$ is the age gap of the individual and $(Y_i - 60)/60$ is the extent of his or her oldness. Average of this extent of oldness is obtained by taking sum of the extent of oldness for all elderly individuals and dividing the sum by the total number of elderly persons q (p). Thus the age gap index is given as

$$I(p) = \frac{1}{q(p)} \frac{\Sigma(Y_i - 60)}{60}$$

If the proportion of elderly persons in the population is denoted by H(p) = q (p) / n (p), where n (p) is total population and q (p) is the number of elderly above the cut off age of 60, then the Q-index is the product of age gap index I (p) and H(p). It is further modified to derive the composite index P (p).

Thus, Q (p)= H (p) x I (p) and

$$P(p) = \frac{1}{n(p)} \quad \frac{\Sigma(Y_i - 60)^2}{60^2}$$

In case of Tripura, the age difference index I (p) show a little decline while there is an increase of 3.68 per cent in H (p) during 1991 to 2001 (Table 12). However, during the same period the Q (p) increased by 2.6 per cent and P (p) increased by 5.91 per cent. Though the age gap index has declined the proportion elderly population has increased. This has resulted in a comparatively steeper increase the P-index P (p). The modified P-index is more sensitive and records larger increase in the extent of population ageing compared to both H (p) and I (p).

Increasing proportion of population in the working age group has been the result of high population growth and high birth rate in the earlier years. This has caused larger cohorts to reach the potentially productive age group of working population. If birth rates and age-specific death rates in the later ages of life, remains constant or declines further, successively larger cohorts will enter the elderly age group and will raise the number and proportion of elderly even further.

Declining birth rates have already resulted in the lowering of the percentage of population in 0 to 14 years age group (Table 11). Therefore when the age cohorts of present 0 to 14 years enter the working age group, the number and proportion of population in the 15 to 59 years are likely to decline, if the birth rate remains constant or falls and large-scale in-migration does not take place. This will raise the relative share of older persons.

Increasing proportion of population in the working age group has been the result of high population growth and high birth rate in the earlier years. This has caused larger cohorts to reach the potentially productive age group of working population. If birth rates and age-specific death rates in the later ages of life, remains constant or declines further, successively larger cohorts will enter the elderly age group and will raise the number and proportion of elderly even further. Thus the old age dependency ratio may show an upward trend in future. With the proportion of elderly increasing, even if there is any fall in the age gap index, the P-index will increase, making it imperative to take appropriate policy measures.

VI

As discussed in the earlier sections population aging is the combined effect of falling fertility and mortality. Therefore, declining fertility and population ageing need not imply higher resource cost. The relative cost to the economy of a child and an elderly person need to be compared and the resources released by falling fertility rate need to be estimated to have a proper assessment of economic impact of population ageing.

The consequences of increasing proportion of elderly persons are felt at the micro level in the households with elderly members and also at macro level as it has implications for national productivity. It needs to be noted that while advances in medical technology has made major improvements in scope and quality of medical care it has also increased per capita healthcare costs. It is established that the aged have an above average demand for health services which largely remains unmet in countries like ours. The need for social security in the context of prevalent poverty, rising needs of pension in the organized sector, rising health care costs combine to create increasing strain on the ability of the working generation to finance pensions and health services for the elderly population.

At the policy level India has the provision of old age pension for elderly persons belonging to households below poverty line (NOAP), in each state, it only gives partial coverage. A large number of workers in the unorganized sectors face the prospect of an insecure old age. In the organized sector the pension scheme is under threat due to shrinking work-force and increasing number of retirees. The policy response to the rising cost of pensions has centered on measures replacing the publicly funded system based on Pay-As-You-Go (PAYG) pension scheme by private saving for retirement. There has also been strong support for the expansion of private health insurance and private provision of health services. These are presented as the only alternatives available without adequately discussing the fundamental issues concerning insurance market failure, transaction costs and social allocation of risk which, were the raison de tire for the existence of the publicly funded system.

Moreover, a key effect of switching from a PAYG to a funded pension system is to require the present working generation to pay twice- they must save for their own retirement while continuing to pay taxes that finance the pensions of the currently retired and other old age security schemes. All these issues require further research.

REFERENCES

Basu, A. and Basu,K.(1987) "The Greying of Population: Concepts and Measurement, *Demography India*, 16,79-89.

Chakravarty, S.R. and S. Chakravarty (1993) "A General Index of Aging", *Demography India,* Vol.22, No.1 89-96.

Keyfitz, N. (1975) "How do we Know the Facts of Demography?" in *Population and Development Review* 1(2).

Shryock, H.S. and J.S. Siegel (1976) *The Methods and materials of Demography*, New York .Academic Press.

United Nations (1968). *The Concept of Stable Population*, New York ST/SOA/SER.A/39.

Table 1
Elderly Population of Tripura (1961-2001)

Year	*Elderly Male*	*Elderly Female*	*Total Elderly*	*Total Male*	*Total Female*	*Total Population*
1961	33522	28365 (5.42)	61887	591237	550768	1142005
1971	55192	47276 (6.58)	102468	801126	755216	1556342
1981	75358	69372 (7.05)	144730	1054846	998212	2053058
1991	97939	95356 (7.01)	193295	1417930	1339275	2757205
2001	112656	119893 (7.27)	232549	1642225	1556978	3199203

Source: Census of India, Socio-Cultural Tables, 1961, 1971, 1981, 1991, Age - data 2001, RGCCI, New Delhi.

Note: Figures in the parentheses are percentages of elderly population in total population in respective years.

Table 2
Annual average growth rate of population in Tripura(1961-2001)

Year	*Total Population*	*Elderly population*	*Elderly Male*	*Elderly Female*
1961-71	3.62	6.55	6.46	6.66
1971-81	3.19	4.12	3.65	4.67
1981-91	3.42	3.35	2.99	3.74
1991-01	1.60	2.03	1.50	2.57

Source: Same as above

Table 3
Elderly persons in the North-Eastern States

	1981 Population		*1991 Population*		*2001 Population*	
States	*Elderly*	*Total*	*Elderly*	*Total*	*Elderly*	*Total*
Tripura	*144730* (7.05)	*2053058*	*193295* (7.01)	*2757205*	*232549* (7.27)	*3199203*
Meghalaya	59170 (4.42)	1335819	78742 (4.43)	1774778	105726 (4.55)	2318822
Manipur	83466 (5.87)	1420953	111105 (6.04)	1837149	145470 (6.70)	2166788
Mizoram	22806 (4.61)	493757	33186 (4.81)	689756	49023 (5.50)	888573
Arunachal	30093 (4.76)	631839	37560 (4.34)	864558	49916 (4.50)	1097968
Nagaland	46022 (5.93)	774930	63777 (5.27)	1209546	90323 (4.50)	1990036
Assam	NA	NA	1194460 (5.33)	22414322	1560366 (5.85)	26655528
Total	386287 (5.75)	6710356	1712125 (5.42)	31547314	2233373 (5.82)	38316918

Source: Same as above. Figures in the parenthesis denote proportion of elderly persons in total population of the respective states in each year.

Table 4
Annual average growth rate of elderly population in North-Eastern States

	1981 - 1991	*1991 – 2001*
Tripura	3.35	2.03
Meghalaya	3.30	3.42
Manipur	3.31	3.09
Mizoram	4.55	4.77
Ar. Pradesh	2.48	3.28
Nagaland	3.85	4.16
Assam	NA	3.06

Source: Same as in the previous Table 3.

Table 5
Number of elderly persons in rural and urban areas of Tripura

Elderly	*1981*		*1991*		*2001*	
	Rural	*Urban*	*Rural*	*Urban*	*Rural*	*Urban*
Male	68189	7169	84358	13581	93023	19633
Female	61566	7806	79651	15705	97478	22415
Total	129755 (90)	14975 (10)	164009 (85)	29286 (15)	190501 (82)	42048 (18)
Proportion*	7.1	6.64	7.02	6.94	7.18	7.7
Sex Ratio	902	1088	944	1156	1047	1141

Source: Same as above.

Note: Figures in the parentheses denote percentage of elderly persons residing in rural and urban areas.
*Proportion is the number of elderly persons per hundred populations in urban and rural areas.

Table 6
Age-composition of the elderly population

Years	Young old60-69 yrs.	Old-old 70-79 yrs.	Very-old80 +	Elderly Persons
1981	79548 (54.96)	40404 (27.91)	24778 (17.12)	144730
1991	103329 (53.45)	55795 (28.86)	34171 (17.67)	193295
2001	126101 (54.22)	71204 (30.6)	35244 (15.15)	232549
Growth rate*	2.92	3.81	2.11	3.03

Source: Same as above.

Note: Figures in the parentheses denote percentages among the elderly persons in each year.

* Refers to annual average growth rate during 1981- 2001.

Table 7
Greying of female population in Tripura

Year	Proportion of Elderly Female in elderly population (in percent)	Proportion of Elderly Female in female population (in percent)	Proportion of Elderly Male in male population (in percent)	Elderly Sex Ratio*	Overall Sex ratio *
1961	45.83	5.15	5.66	846	932
1971	46.13	6.25	6.88	856	943
1981	47.93	6.94	7.14	920	946
1991	49.33	7.12	6.90	973	945
2001	51.55	7.70	6.85	1064.	948

Source: Census of India, Socio-Cultural Tables, 1961, 1971, 1981, 1991, Age-data 2001, RGCCI, New Delhi.

Note: * Sex ratio denotes number of female per thousand male.

Table 8
Elderly population in different districts of Tripura, 2001

Districts	*West*	*South*	*North*	*Dhalai*
Elderly Male	54377	26746	21195	10338
Elderly Female	60012	29265	20556	10060
Total Elderly	114389 (7.46)	56011 (7.29)	41751 (7.06)	20398 (6.62)
Elderly Sex Ratio	1103	1094	969	973
Total Population	1532982	767440	590913	307876

Source: Age Data 2001.RGCCI
Note: Figures in the parentheses are proportion of the elderly in the population of the different districts.

Table 9
Indices of aging, Tripura (1961-1971)

Ageing Indices	*1961*	*1971*	*1981*	*1991*	*2001*
Old Age Ratio	5.41	6.58	7.05	7.01	7.27
Aged Child Ratio	12.64	14.90	17.90	18.30	21.62
Aged DependencyRatio	10.48	13.37	13.13	12.86	12.32
Total DependencyRatio	93.39	103.15	86.58	83.14	69.34

Source: Social and Cultural Tables, 1961-1991, Age Data 2001 RGCCI.

Table 10
Burden of population Aging

Year	*Elderly Non worker*	*Elderly Worker*	*Non worker 15-59*	*Worker 15-59*	*Total worker*	*Burden of population ageing*
1991	121093 (62.64)	72202 (37.35)	732953 (48.79)	769126 (51.20)	841328	14.39
2001	139913 (60.16)	92636 (39.83)	842857 (44.68)	1043440 (55.31)	1136076	12.31

Source: Economic Tables, Census of India, 1991, 2001.
Note: figures in the parentheses are percentages in population of the respective age group in each year.

Table 11
The changing population age structure of Tripura

Age-group	*1961*	*1971*	*1981*	*1991*	*2001*
0-14 yrs.	42.9	44.2	39.3	38.3	33.7
15-59 yrs.	51.7	49.2	53.6	54.6	59.1
60+ yrs.	5.4	6.6	7.1	7.0	7.3

Source: Social and Cultural Tables 1961-1991. Age Data 2001.
RGCCI, New Delhi

Table 12
Modified indices of aging

Years	*H (p)*	*I (p)*	*Q (p)*	*P (p)*
1991	0.0701	0.1645	0.01153	0.002771
2001	0.0726	0.1628	0.01183	0.002935

Source: Authors' calculations.

22

State's Response to Oldage Persons in Tripura: An Assessment

Jayanata Choudhury & Elizabeth Sangliana

The increase in population, both in the country and the state, is directly or indirectly a result of the improving conditions in health, economy, education, and increase in the welfare activities by both the Central and State Governments. With modernization, change in social structure and, value system in our society, the aged are being affected adversely.

The aged women owing to gender bias are suffering more and this is evident in their greater presence in terms of their numbers in the old age homes and day care centers for the elderly not only in the country, but also in our state of Tripura. The increase in the aged and infirm population over the years calls for the need for greater care of the aged which has now assumed greater importance.

The aged continue to be a neglected lot. The welfare needs of the aged are not properly met due to limited resources of the Government and the belief that the family needs to take care of the aged. Expenditure on social welfare is generally treated as non development expenditure. But, as their number is increasing and social changes in the elderly are taking place, they are increasingly attracting the attention of the State.

The Directive Principles of State Policy enjoins on the State the responsibility of public assistance to the older and Article 41 of the Indian Constitution, makes provisions for this purpose. The Hindu Adoption and Maintenance Act, 1956 imposes obligation on a person to maintain his or her aged or infirm parents. Section 125 of the Criminal Procedure Code (CrPC) 1973 makes it mandatory for a person (including daughter) with adequate means to maintain their parents.

The definition of the aged differs from society to society and is linked with the life expectancy of the society's population. In India, with the life expectancy increasing from 27 yrs, the retirement age has also gradually increased from 55 yrs to 58yrs and 60 yrs (in Central Govt.). Reaching retirement age under Government service means that a person above 58 yrs or 60 yrs is considered aged or elderly. The concept of age has a frame of reference such as chronological, social, psychological, temporal and cultural.

Tripura has a total population of 31,99,203 as per the 2001 census of which 85 % is adult population and 7 % of the total population is above 60 years of age. By 2010, the number of the elderly in Tripura is expected to rise to 9 %.There are 84,000 elderly persons covered under the social security scheme in Tripura. 2,500 families are covered under Annapurna Scheme where 10 Kgs. of rice is given free of cost per month to the BPL families who could no be covered under the old age pension scheme.

In Tripura, social welfare measures for the senior citizens have been going on since 1978 in the form of the Tripura Old Age Pension Rules, 1978 coming into effect. A pension of Rs.30/- was given every month to old persons who had attained the age of 80 and above unable to do any work. Only one member in a family (i.e. either husband or wife) was eligible to receive this pension. Old age pension was later modified to cover different categories like Old age pension including ex-military, Widow pension (Old age), Jhumia pension (Old age), Landless agriculture workers pension (Old age), Blind and physically handicapped including leprosy pension, Old Aged Rickshaw Pullers pension. All these pensions have now been amalgamated under the National Old Age Pension (NOAP) scheme.

Besides providing social security in the form of old age pension, the state government of Tripura, has felt the need to help the elderly through the different machinery of the Government by formulating a 'State Policy' on Older Persons on 28th November 2000 aiming at highlighting the different aspects of difficulties faced by the elderly especially the poorest of the poor, providing financial security, food security, extending health facilities and strengthening social and family ties.

The policy makes a conscious effort to give dignity and a sense of purpose of living for the elderly. It also encourages society to involve itself increasingly in caring for the older persons by roping in the family members of the old, NGOs, Panchayat etc and also through research and evaluation studies by academic institutions and bodies to improve the over all situation of the elderly especially, the elderly poor.

In order to carry out the state policy on older persons, a State Level Action Plan was formulated by the Social Welfare and Social Education Department, Government of Tripura in a meeting with the various Heads of Departments under the Chairmanship of the Chief Secretary of Tripura on 29.1.2004. The concerned departments have been asked to provide various services in making the life of the elderly more comfortable.

The Study

The objectives of the evaluation study are as follows:

1. To assess the performance of each type of programme and project currently being implemented in Tripura for older persons under the Social Welfare and Social Education Department.
2. To assess the participation by the concerned departments and village panchayats in implementing programmes for older persons in Tripura.
3. To identify the drawbacks and suggest ways and means for improvement in implementation of the present programmes for older persons.

Methodology of the Study

Except for old age pension, all other facilities extended to the better living and comfort of the senior citizens have been implemented since the enactment of Tripura State Policy on Older Persons on 28th November 2000 and an action plan for the implementation of the policy was drawn on 29.1.2004. The study therefore, confines itself to the implementers of the programme and verifying the practical implementation of the policy through interviews, spot verification and discussion with the old age pension beneficiaries and the local public.

The study will cover the whole state of Tripura which includes the four districts and forty blocks. In each block, four Gram Panchayats (GP) in non - ADC areas and Village Development Councils (VDC) in the ADC areas were randomly selected which covers 15% of the total GP / VDCs i.e.160 GPs / VDCs,

In each GP/VDC, three respondents have been interviewed who was either an old age pension beneficiary, an old person, Panchayat Secretary, GPIVDC members, member of NGO or a local public. But in some places more than three persons were interviewed making it a total of 678 respondents at the GPIVDC level. At the block level one person was interviewed who was the BDO, Panchayat Extension Officer or CDPO. At the Sub-divisional level also one person was interviewed who was either the SDM/ Addl. SDM or a member of the Panchayat Samity /Block Advisory Committee, At the District level the DM or ADM or a member of the District Grievance Redressal Cell for Older Persons was interviewed.

Regarding the implementing departments concerned with the implementation of the state policy for older persons, departmental officials at the various levels were interviewed. Spot or site visits were also conducted where ever possible like banks, gas distribution agencies, post offices, hospitals, transport ticket counters like bus stations, rail way ticket counters and airline ticket counters like the Indian Airlines City Office, electricity bill payment counters, LIC offices etc. Therefore, a total of 117 officials and members of NGOs were interviewed for the study. In all a total of 795 persons were interviewed and 158 site visits were carried out.

Findings of the Study

In Tripura, an *Action Plan* for implementing welfare programmes for older persons was prepared in a meeting by the Social Welfare and Social Education Department, Government of Tripura in a meeting with the various concerned heads of Departments under the Chairmanship of the Chief Secretary of Tripura on 29.1.2004. In the action plan, concerned departments have been asked to provide various services in making the life of the elderly more comfortable. A *Coordinating Committee* to coordinate the matters relating to implementation of the State Policy for Older Persons and to monitor its progress throughout the State was constituted.

i) ***Shelter***

Shelter being a basic human need, the Rural Development Department and Urban Development Department may be requested to earmark three percent houses for older persons from IAY, PMGY (Housing) schemes. But no such action has been taken up in informing the R.D. Department about earmarking the 3 % houses for the elderly poor.

However, during the course of the study, we did find some cases where the beneficiaries of the housing scheme were senior citizens. This selection was not done on the basis of their age, but other factors of selection. It is mere co-incidence.

ii) ***District Grievance Redressal Cell for Older Persons***

A notification was issues on 17th July 2003 to constitute the District Grievance Redressal Cell for the welfare of senior citizens in all the four districts of the state. The redressal Cells have ten members each, headed by the DM & Collector of the District as Chairman. The District Inspector of Social Welfare and Social Education of the district acts as Member Secretary.

The Grievance Redressal Cell has been constituted to act as the nodal agency at the district level for looking into the various grievances and problems the elderly will be possibly facing. The cell will also act as a forum for grievance redressal and take necessary action accordingly. Coordination of schemes and programmes being implemented for the senior citizens in the district is also to be coordinated by them.

The formation of the District Grievance Redressal Cell for Senior Citizens remains a piece of document in records only. Neither the members nor the senior citizens are aware of the existence of the Grievance Redressal Cell for Senior Citizens. Since the formation of the Grievance Cell in all the four districts, no complaints or grievances have been received by the cells in particular. Even if any complaints that may have been lodged by Senior Citizens have been registered and treated like any other general complaint. The Grievance Redressal Cell for the Older Persons is found to be non functional in all the four districts.

Awareness level of the existence of the District Grievance Redressal Cell for Older Persons among the public in the study was nil. Among the government officials too, it was found that, only 3 (2.56 %) knew that there was a grievance cell for senior citizens but, they too were not very sure of themselves. In fact, the members themselves were neither aware that there is a grievance cell for the older persons nor the fact that they are members of the cell. As for the members who are political representatives, elections were conducted in July 2004 and thereby the representatives have also been changed. They too are not aware of the existence of the cell and their membership.

iii) ***Senior Citizens Forum***

In the Agartala Municipal Council (AMC) and 12 Nagar Panchcyat areas, *Senior Citizens Forums* are yet to be formed. It was found that neither the AMC nor the thirteen Nagar Panchcyats were aware of the matter as they had not received any information regarding the formation of the senior citizens councils and therefore, the senior citizens forums have not been formed in any of the Municipal Councils and Nagar Panchayat areas.

At the village level, informal neighborhood groups of elderly were not found. Friends and acquaintances did exist but there were only two or three friends who met once in a while that too not all at the same time, so as to be able to discuss problems of old age and get solace from each other etc, thereby acting as an informal old age forum at the village level. No one, among the respondents both the public and officials were aware about the formation of such informal groups by older persons at the village level.

iv) ***Information, Education and Communication***

IEC is a very important tool for making any action to be taken or programme to be implemented a success. In the study, it was found that the concerned agencies like ICAT, local press, Doordarshan, cable TV, All India Radio, Panchayats etc. are not aware of their role in the process of sensitisation of welfare schemes / programmes facilities available, problems faced and needs of older persons. They were not aware of any instructions regarding their role in the sensitization and awareness issues and programmes relating to senior citizens.

In the action plan, it is mentioned that assistance of Doordarshan, AIR and Cable TV may be taken for generating awareness on programmes for Senior Citizens at frequent intervals. Press release is to be issued for awareness programmes by Social Welfare Department on Senior Citizens which has not been done so far. ICA T is supposed to take steps in inculcating the values of love and respect for the elders and take adequate care for them. They are also to take steps for supply of information about ageing process and changing role responsibility and relationship at different stages of human life cycle. But, due to not being informed and therefore unaware of their role in the IEC process for Senior Citizens, no action has so far been taken by any of the agencies of mass communication.

Social Welfare and Social Education Department along with GA (P& T) Department are responsible to take necessary steps for informing rights of parents without means, to be supported by their children. GA Department is to issue a G.O in this regard and Social Welfare and Social Education Department is to circulate the legal provisions among the PRI bodies for disseminating information through awareness programmes which is yet to be done.

Social Welfare and Social Education Department is to collect information from banks and other organizations about savings under their existing functionary scheme. They have to then request the PRI bodies to undertake awareness programmes to inculcate among the self-employed and salaried non government employees the need for savings for their old age under the existing functionary scheme run by Public Sector financial institutions. But no such exercise of collecting information from banks and informing the PRI bodies has been undertaken. The PRI bodies are therefore unaware about their role in awareness creation regarding encouraging savings amongst the public and thus no action has been undertaken so far. Among the public, no one has seen any programme aired by Doordarshan, Agartala regarding old age. However three people of whom one is from the public and two from the officials' category claimed to have seen documentary film on old age pension etc. aired on Doordarshan National Channel. No IEC committees/teams etc. were found at any level nor posters, hoardings, slogans etc. were found regarding the sensitization on issues of older persons.

v) *Old Age Homes and Day Care Centers*

There are presently five full time old age homes in the state of which one is a State Infirmary Home on the outskirts of Agartala under West District run by the Social Welfare and Social Education Department. The home has a capacity to accommodate 200 persons. Presently, the home houses 65 persons of whom 50 are women and 15 are men. In the infirmary there are also three physically handicapped women. One of them is a girl who is less than 18 years old. The infirmary can not house more inmates due to want of maintenance of the buildings and lack of infrastructure facilities including sanitation.

There are also four number of Oldage Home run by the NGOs. It is noticed that, all the old age homes that are presently running are located in and around Agartala. No other old age home is found in the other three districts. One NGO is planning to open two of its old age home branches in Dhalai and North Districts.

From the total sample 94.10 % of the respondents from the public were unaware about the existence of old age homes and amongst the officials, 83.76 % were aware. Those who knew about the existence of the old age homes among the Government officials were mostly aware of the Govt. run home but were not sure about its exact location. Those among the public, who were aware of the old age homes were mostly from the West District.

vi) ***Day Care Centers***

There are also five day care centers for the Older Persons run by the same NGO. The day care centers are located in three districts of the state except for Dhalai District having capacity for caring for 50 old persons in each of the centers. The NGO also provides geriatric care facilities.

There is also a NGO run home for destitute women called *Nirmalaya Hridalaya* run by the Sisters of Charity. Presently there is one old destitute lady. Though not declared an old age home, from time to time they do have destitute old women under their care.

The old age homes and day care centers run by the NGOs are well maintained and clean. The inmates were happy. The institutions run with the help of funds from Ministry of Social Justice and Empowerment, Government of India besides their own funds through donations from the public.

97 % of the respondents from both the categories were unaware about the existence of day care centers for older persons.

vii) ***Priority Queues for Senior Citizens***

A Government Order was passed in 2004 by the Social

Welfare and Social Education Department to six departments i.e. Transport, Health and Family Welfare, Food, Consumer Affairs and Civil Supplies, Telecommunication, Banks, and Postal Departments, regarding the formation of separate queues for senior citizens. Priority queues for the senior citizens have been asked to be provided by these different departments and agencies as payment for their services is needed. The priority queues therefore are to be provided by the mentioned departments and agencies at their payment/ service counters as shown below:

a. Transport Deptt. - Ticket counters (road (bus), train, air)

b. Food Deptt. - Gas distribution centers

c. Power Deptt. - Bill Payment and complaint counters

d. Telecom Deptt. - Bill payment and complaint centers

e. Banks - Service counter

f. Post Office - Service counter

g. Health Deptt. - Registration and Medicine distribution counters

h. State and District Treasury Offices - Queues for pension matters etc.

In the *transport sector,* it was found that only the *railway* ticket booking counter at Agartala had converted one of their existing counters exclusively for the older persons. The railway ticket counter in the Kumarghat railway station however, did not have a separate queue for the older persons. There is no separate counter for purchase of *bus* ticket as there is no rush for the tickets.

The *Indian Airlines* did not have separate counters for the senior citizens at the TRTC booking office nor at the airlines City Office. They don't feel the need for a separate counter as there are travel agents allover the state.

Food Department had on issued a memorandum to all the *Gas agencies* in the State to have separate counters for the senior citizens. However, no separate counters were found in any of the distribution agencies. When asked about the counter, they said that they gave priority to the senior citizens when ever they came and thus there was no need for a separate counter. Besides most of the distribution centers provide home delivery and therefore the need for separate counter is not felt.

Gas pipeline connections are now being provided to households in some areas of Agartala town by GAIL They do not come under the control of the Food, Civil Supplies and Consumer Affairs Department. Here too, the queues at the payment counters are long and there are no separate older persons counter provided. Besides, the authorities are not aware of the provision for a separate counter for older persons.

In 2004, Commissioner and Secretary, *Health* Department instructed the provision of separate registration counters for the senior citizens on two days of the week i.e. Wednesdays and Saturdays to function during scheduled OPD hours.

Though orders in this regard has been issued by the different authorities at different levels, in the department, and claims of providing the queues for senior citizen's have been made, in reality, the queues or no counter for senior citizens have not been found in any of the hospitals including the big hospitals in the state like Govind Ballab Pant (GB) Hospital (till 20.4.2005), Indira Gandhi Memorial (IGM), Cancer Hospital and Dr. Ambedkar Hospital at Hapania, Regarding Govind Ballab Pant (GB) Hospital. But a sign board specifying separate queue for senior citizens on Wednesdays and Saturdays. In the Udaipur District Hospital, a separate queue was made at the hospital.

In IGM hospital, which caters mainly to women and children, there are no queues for Senior Citizens. They said that they mainly received delivery cases and very few old women come to them for treatment.

Some of the other reasons cited for not maintaining separate queues are lack of staff, not being aware of the order (especially at the sub-divisional and PHC levels). Many doctors expressed that there was no need for a separate counter for the older persons at the hospitals especially PHC level as there were not many patients who visited the hospitals and PHCs on a regular basis.

Power Department is also unaware about the provision for a separate counter for the elderly. There are long queues in their payment counters. In fact, one senior citizen in Agartala, during our presence in the area, asked for preference to be given to him due to his age, and he was instead mocked at.

Telecommunication Department i.e. BSNL is also supposed to provide separate counters for the aged which is not found in any of their counters despite letter sent to GM, Telecommunication from the Deptt. of SW & SE, Govt. of Tripura .

Separate service counters for older persons were not found in any of the *Banks* visited including State Bank of India, Main Branch at Melarmat, Agartala and other banks i.e. Union Bank of India (UBI), UCO Bank, Bank of Baroda, Punjab National Bank, including LIC.

It is found that, only UCO Bank has, in 2004, informed their rural/semi urban branches and also urban branches to give special assistance to senior persons in terms of assisting in filing forms/vouchers/slips and not let them stand in a queue in case of the rural/semi urban branches. In the case of urban branches, separate counters are to be provided for older persons/customers for pension payment and bank service, which was not found in the different branches throughout the state.

UBI Bank also has issued a circular to all its branches in Tripura to ensure arrangement of queues in counters both for ledger counters as well as in cash counters (recipt/ payment). Here again, no counters were found for the senior citizens in any of the branches.

Situation in the *Post Offices* is no different. In the GPO, Agartala, it was seen that only one separate counter was found for senior citizens, that too only for SA/TO/NSS/PPF,SC Deposit, MIS withdrawal and not for other post office transactions such as buying stamps, sending registered post. In the smaller post offices this counter is not provided.

All the surveyed public and 97.43 % of the officials in the study were unaware of the existence of priority queues as there are none to be found in any of the service centers. Further, the people and the officials are not even aware that separate counters are to be provided for senior citizens as they are unaware about the existence of older person's policy.

viii) ***Barrier free environment***

Provision of barrier free environment in the Government buildings at present has not been implemented. The Public Works Department, have received intimation to provide barrier free environment in all Government buildings keeping in mind the disabled and not the elderly. The PWD has however expressed their inability in providing barrier free environment to all the Government buildings keeping in mind the structural plan and huge cost to be incurred in additional construction as not feasible. They however have adopted in their building laws through the Tripura Building Rules - 2004 which came into effect since 20th December 2004, the provision of barrier free environment for all future constructions.

As per the action plan, Revenue Department has been requested by Social Welfare and Social Education Department to issue suitable instruction in 2005 to the DM & Collector of the four districts to make the District Treasury building barrier free. But the Revenue Department did not receive the information and has asked the Social Welfare and Social Education Department to send the letter again in reply to the request of Commissioner Social Welfare and Social Education Department to send a copy of the instructions sent by Revenue Department to DM and Collectors of the four districts to make the treasury office barrier free. Therefore, no action is found to have been taken in making the treasury office barrier free until now.

ix) ***Financial Security***

Since 1978, old age pension is being given to the senior citizens. Till today, it is being given only to those who are living below the poverty line and are senior citizens i.e. above 65 years. But not all the elderly who are above 65 years and are living below the poverty line are getting the old age pension. Due to limited funds, the old age pension under the National Old Age Pension Scheme (NOAP) is being given according to *quota*. The eligibility criterion in terms of age for the senior citizen to avail old age pension has been reduced from 65 years to 60 yrs. On 27th January, 2005, 23,560 persons were added to the existing list of 60,412 persons receiving old age pension, totaling the list to 83,972 persons in the state of Tripura.

Besides the *National Old Age Pension (NOAP)* scheme, there is the Annapurna scheme from which 17,351 families are receiving help in the form of receiving 10 Kgs of rice freely every month. Those who are eligible to receive help under this scheme are the BPL families and also senior citizens who could not be covered under the NAOP scheme. Senior destitute persons above 65 years are also covered under this scheme.

Old age pension is to be disbursed by the 7th of every month as directed by the Supreme Court Order. The Finance Department was requested to release the amount for old age pension regularly so that there is no interruption for payment of old age pension within the first week of every month. Government of India was also requested to release the pension fund for three months in advance.

Funds are being received on time in quarterly installments from the Ministry of Social Justice and Empowerment. But despite earnest efforts by the Finance Department at times delay takes place in sanctioning funds from the state share. The fund is placed to the DM & Collector of the Districts who in turn place the money to the BDO thereby causing some delay at times. Many a times, disbursement is not possible within the first week of the month as funds are received in the middle of the month making it impossible for the BDOs to disburse the old age pension within the first week of the month as per Supreme Court directive.

Old age pension at the block level is distributed to the beneficiaries by the concerned Panchayat Secretaries at the Panchcyat Ghar. It is practically not possible for a Panchayat Secretary to go house to house distributing the old age pension as suggested by the Social Welfare Department, as the Panchcyat Secretary is the implementing officer of many works at the GP/VDC level.

A *Government Order* was issued by General Administration (Administrative Reforms) Department instructing the rights of parents unable to support themselves to be supported by their children especially government servants. Any violation by a government servant regarding the issue can be deemed as an act unbecoming of a government servant and misconduct within the meaning of Rule-3(1) (iii) of the Tripura Civil Service (Conduct) Rules, 1988 and action can be taken against the government servant accordingly.

More than 77 % of the public and 100% of the officials who responded in the study was aware of the existence of old age pension scheme. No one among the public nor the officials were aware of the existence of the G.O about right of poor parents to be looked after by their children and none among the two categories are aware about the need to save for old age as mentioned in Policy for Older Persons. (i.e. Self-employed and salaried non government employees are to be sensitized about the need for saving under the existing functionary scheme run by Public Sector financial institutions for their old age.)

x) ***Mobile Geriatric Units and Health Workshops***

As for mobile geriatric units to be attached to the District hospitals, it has been expressed that the provision cannot be made at the moment as basic facilities are not available. But in due course, it will be considered as the facilities available will improve. However, one NGO has geriatric service facilities and also imparts training on geriatric care with financial assistance from Ministry of Social Justice and Empowerment.

As for the provision of ramps in all the State level hospitals and District level hospitals, the engineering wing of the department has been asked to prepare plan and estimate which is still in progress.

Workshops at regular intervals on the health and nutrition of the older persons and their family members are to be conducted which is not being done so. On October 1st 2004, the International Day of Older Persons, a health camp was organized at Udaipur Nagar Panchayat Office for the elderly. No other health camps or workshops have been arranged so far only for the older persons in any of the

However, the Police Department during the Police Week celebrations in 2004, called a meeting with prominent senior citizens and a senior citizen cell was set up which started functioning since December 2004 at the Police Head Quarters headed by Additional IGP. But until 2005, only one complaint has been received by the cell. General vigil goes on as usual and any complaints that are being received from older persons in other parts of the state outside Agartala, are being treated like any other case.

xi) ***Identification of 60 and BPL persons in GPs/VDCs***

Rural Development (Panchayat Department) has been asked to undertake an exercise to identify the number of persons 60+ in the Panchayats living below poverty line by maintaining registers for Old Persons of more than sixty years in the State. Three correspondences were sent to the various Blocks in this regard, on 3rd April 2004, 5th June 2004 and 26th March 2005. As on 15.4.2005, 15 R.D.Blocks had submitted the number of 60+ living Below Poverty Line.

The Gram Panchayats and Village Development Councils in the ADC areas besides identifying the number of senior citizens(60+) and senior citizens who are also BPL by maintain senior citizens' register are supposed to sensitise and promote savings especially among non-government employees through Public Sector Institutions such as National banks, Post Office, LIC etc. which has not been done as the Gram Panchayats and *VDCs* have not received any information regarding their role in promoting the habit of saving for old age.

As for sensitisation on rights of old parents (without means of support) to be supported by their children, the GPs and *VDCs* are unaware of the issue as no intimation has been received from the Social Welfare and Social Education Department.

Suggestions and Recommendations

The issues concerning the aged needs to be looked into by initiating a number of activities in interrelated fields, which are as follows:

1 Health and Nutrition

i) The elderly should be encouraged to lead independent lives in their own family and communities through proper health care and counseling instead of being cut off from society.

ii) There should be proper coordination between health care and welfare measures for more cost effective and efficient programmes.

iii) The elderly should be educated in self care with proper diagnosis of nutritional requirements as an integral part of health care.

iv) Health services should include a broad range of ambulatory services such as day care centers, outpatient clinics medical and nursing care and domestic services.

v) In the case of institutional care, isolation of aged from the society should be avoided.

vi) Provision of ambulance service during emergency for the elderly, especially after identifying the dwellings of the elderly is an important exercise. The hospitals and local NGOs also should have phone numbers and addresses of the elderly where ever possible. The police should also be able to send ambulance during emergency at late nights when ever needed by citizens calling the police emergency number/control room by dialing 100. There should therefore be coordination between the police, hospitals, NGOs, Senior Citizens Forum, Old Age homes and day care centers etc. in dealing with the problems of the senior citizens especially during emergency.

vii) For ambulance service during late nights on emergency, the police control room also should have the ability to send ambulance and therefore Geriatric care facilities should be given priority and efforts should be made to provide the proper health services to Senior Citizens at the earliest.

viii) Simple to remember hospital emergency numbers and ambulance call numbers should be made popular through wide publicity.

ix) Workshops and health awareness camps should be conducted frequently by hospital authorities in collaboration with local NGOs and local clubs. The District Administration at the Sub-Divisional and Block levels also frequently conducts health camps. During these camps, it should be made mandatory to conduct awareness campaign about health problems during old age and nutritional needs of the aging.

x) NGOs and local clubs can be trained and encouraged in conducting awareness camps on nutrition in general and nutritional requirements of the elderly and old age related health problems.

2. Housing and Barrier Free Environment in Govt. Buildings

i) Providing barrier free environment in the existing government buildings is not possible in all cases as said by the PWD due to enormous cost factor and other issues. Therefore, simple low cost additions to make the environment senior citizen friendly like making low angled slopes at the entrance of the building along with the existing steps at the entrance of the building instead of high costing ramps being constructed can be thought of.

ii) All important sections of the office should be shifted near the entrance of the building on the ground floor as far as possible for the convenience of s~nior citizens where ever possible

iii) To the extent possible, the aged should be given opportunity to associate themselves with such policy and plan formulation.

iv) 3 per cent reservation in housing scheme under IAY/ PMGY should be provided and made effective at the earliest by earmarking in the beginning itself.

3 Social Welfare

i) Young people through schools and local clubs should be encouraged to involve themselves in providing social services for the aged to promote inter generational ties.

ii) Ensure higher quality of institutional care certain minimum norms for services to be provided by the institution should be specified.

iii) Fiscal and other incentives should be given and controls and regulations relaxed to encourage the involvement of voluntary agencies in social welfare activities for the aged.

iv) Social policies should pursue in the maintenance of and strengthening family ties among generations.

v) Suitable incentive schemes should be formulated to encourage low income families to cover and maintenance cost for the aged.

4. Education and Information, Education & Communication

i) Continuing adult education at all levels should be encouraged.

ii) Mass media should undertake a coordinated effort to

highlight the positive aspects of aging by educating the general public to problems of aging.

iii) Local clubs should be encouraged in taking part in activities of the elderly and participate in IEC activities and monitoring programmes for the elderly.

iv) Involvement of NGO's, especially those working with senior citizens, PRIs, SHGs, school children, local clubs etc. should be given great responsibility and active role in the IEC activities and monitoring programmes for the elderly including, inculcating love for elders, encouraging savings for old age etc.

v) Awareness building measures for both senior citizens and common people for developing their understandings about need for giving physical and mental solace to Senior Citizens Forum (SCF).

vi) Making the issue of senior citizens a part of the school curriculum.

vii) Observing senior citizens day/week regularly.

viii) Through television and radio give wide publicity on the plight of elderly and the need to provide physical and psychological comfort.

ix) The State Policy on Older Persons should be published in the local dailies from time to time. It should also be made available on the website of Social Welfare and Social Education Department, in the citizens' charter of the department. It should also be made available either free of cost or on payment of a minimal amount of Re.1.00 at the GP, Block, Sub Divisional and District levels.

5. Protection of Elderly

i. Measures to ensure house hold products, medicines,

hearing aids, dentures, glasses etc. supplied to the aged conform to the required safety standards and the aged are not exploited by unscrupulous traders.

ii) Help lines for the elderly should be set up by the police where simple and easy to remember phone numbers can be given (preferably, the numbers should be in serial).

iii) Measures for prevention of crime against the elderly should be taken so that the aged do not suffer from fear psychosis.

iv) Identifying the dwellings of the elderly and keeping a police beat book at every house where constables on night rounds would visit the identified houses and sign on the beat books, will increase a sense of protection among the elderly community. This will be applicable in the Nagar Panchayats and Municipal areas.

6. Income Security and Employment

i) The elderly should get an appropriate minimum income either in the form of social security benefits or retirement benefits or through some other devices.

ii) There should be an opportunity for participation of the elderly persons in the economic life of the society by providing them suitable employment avenues

iii) Amount of the Old Age Pension Scheme Should be increased in consonant with the rise of market prices of commodities.

iv) The quota of the old age pension should be enhanced

7. District Grievance Cell and Senior Citizens Forum and Monitoring

i) Officers of Social Welfare Department should take

more responsibility in the implementation of welfare measures for the elderly persons right from the Director to the ICDS worker in terms of constituting forums for senior citizens, conducting meetings of forum and Grievance cell, monitoring progress involving participation of other line/concerned departments, receiving redressal, IEC campaign, distribution of old age pension, keeping every department involved in welfare activities of elderly informed about progress made, actions taken etc.

ii) Director should take complete responsibility for implementation of welfare schemes for the old in the whole state and DISE will be in charge for activities in the District, CDPOs in the Blocks and ICDS workers in the GP/VDC levels. (Each officer will be fully responsible and accountable in coordinating all the activities of the welfare programmes for the elderly in their respective jurisdiction right from formation of committees, forums/ groups etc. IEC, formation of team/s at various levels with other concerned departments, PRIs, SHGs, NGOs etc. reporting progress made etc.)

iii) The issues of older persons can be included in the agenda of the existing Social Justice Standing Committee in each Block which can be a monitoring agency at the Block level. It should also be made a part of the agenda of the GP and *VDC* meetings in every sitting. They should also be given the responsibility to monitor the activities regarding the senior citizens at the village level.

iv) The District Inspector of Social Education (DISE), in the present District Grievance Cell for the welfare of senior citizens is the member secretary. He/she should be made responsible regarding the activities of the

Cell and supervise the formation and functioning of the forums at the Nagar Panchayat and Municipal Councils.

They should give quarterly report to the Commissioner Social Welfare with copies to Director, Social Welfare and Social Education, DM and Collector who will remain Chairman of the Committee, SP of the district and also Chairman/Chairperson ZPs.

v) All Nagar Panchayats, Municipal Councils and District Administrations should be informed about the formation of the forum in Nagar Panchayat and Municipal Council areas and Nagar Panchayats for Senior Citizens. They should be asked to give a quarterly report to the Social Welfare and Social Education Department with copies to Commissioner Social Welfare and Social Education Department and Chief Secretary of Tripura.

vi) Social Welfare and Social Education Department should also give a quarterly report to the District Administrations, Nagar Panchayats and Municipal Councils on actions taken up by the department regarding grievances received through the forums and district grievance cells. This correspondence from both sides (i.e. Social Welfare and Social Education Department and forums for Older Persons in Nagar Panchayats, Municipal Councils and District Grievance Cell for senior citizens in the Districts Administrations) will give a sense of purpose and motivation for undertaking the exercise of forming the forums and grievance cells for senior citizens.

vii) Senior Citizens Forum (SCF) has immense potential to establish and strengthen older people's rights. But this can hardly be organized by government machinery. The need is to involve genuine NGOs who have experience in working with elderly like running old age homes, day care centers etc.

viii) PRIs, SHGs, NGOs, school children, local clubs etc. should also be involved in the monitoring activities of the old age programme implementation.

ix) Legal cell may be opened for obtaining and lessening their problems.

x) The role of the GP members especially the Pradhans, becomes very important when we want to involve the people in the process of development for the elderly. The motivation level of the Panchayat Pradhans and members towards the issue of the elderly should always be kept high through conscious effort of the monitoring cells especially at the higher level especially the Social Welfare and Social Education Department.

Conclusion

The success of any programme depends mainly upon the implementation which revolves around a strong awareness campaign, strong monitoring structure and active participation of the people. The elderly citizens should take part actively in their own welfare activities. This can be done only by making them aware of their rights and facilities available for them and encouraging them to take up their issue actively.

The District Grievance Redressal Cell for Senior Citizens is non functional in all the four districts. It is also practically very difficult for the DM and Collector of the District who is presently Chairman of the District Grivance Redressal Cell for the older persons to conduct meetings of the cell on a regular basis. Therefore, it is suggested that, the District Inspector of Social Welfare and Social Education (DISE) who is presently the member Secretary in the present District

Grievance Redressal Cell for the older person, should play an active role in the review of the implementation of the welfare measures for the senior citizen District. Members of the NGOs, SHGs, and Local Clubs working with the elderly are to be encourdswd to. involve themselves in IEC activities. Senior Citizens Forum at the Municipal Council and Nagar Panchayat levels has so far not been formed. Here again, the issue of and implementation of welfare programmes for senior citizens should be made a part of the agenda in every meeting agenda of the Municipal Council and Nagar Panchayat meetings.

The Standing Committee for Social Justice at the Samity/ BAC level should have the issue of senior citizens as part of their agenda in every meeting and members of the NGOs, SHGs, Local Club working with the elderly can be included in the meeting.

Programmes of older persons should not be done with a sympathetic attitude but with empathy having constitutional backing as a right of the elderly.

REFERENCES

Aguilar, M., ed. (1998). *The Politics of Age and Gerontocracy in Africa: Ethnographies of the Past and Memories of the Present.* Lawrenceville, N.J.: Africa World Press.

Albert, S., and Cattell, M. (1994). *Old Age in Global Perspective: Cross-Cultural and Cross-National Views.* New York: G. K. Hall.

Amoss, P., and Harrell, S., (eds.) (1981). *Other Ways of Growing Old: Anthropological Perspectives.* Stanford: Stanford University Press.

Barker, J. "Between Humans and Ghosts: The Decrepit Elderly in a Polynesian Society." In *The Cultural Context of Aging: World-Wide Perspectives,* 2d ed. Edited by J. Sokolovsky. Westport, Conn.: Bergin and Garvey, 1997. pp. 407-425.

Bernardi, B. (1985). *Age Class Systems.* Cambridge: Cambridge University Press.

Bever, E. (2000). "Witchcraft Fears and Psychosocial Factors in Disease." *Journal of Interdisciplinary History* 30: 573-590.

Census of India, (2001): *Report and Tables on Age*, C-14, C-14 SC, C-14 ST.

Cattell, M. "African Widows, Culture and Social Change: Case Studies from Kenya." Edited by J. Sokolovsky. *In The Cultural Context of Aging: World-Wide Perspectives, 2d ed.* Westport, Conn.: Bergin and Garvey. pp.71-98.

Counts, D., and Counts, D., eds. *Aging and Its Transformations: Moving Toward Death in Pacific Societies.* New York: University Press of America, 1985.

Cowgill, D. *Aging Around the World.* Belmont: Wadsworth, 1986.

Cowgill, D., and Holmes, L. D., (eds.) (1972). *Aging and Modernization.* New York: Appleton-Century-Crofts.

Debbarma, S. (2008). *Elderly People in the Tribal Society of Tripura- a case study of the Kokborok Speaking People* " Aging in North East India"

Glascock, A. "When Killing is Acceptable: The Moral Dilemma Surrounding Assisted Suicide in America and Other Societies." In *The Cultural Context of Aging: World-Wide Perspectives,* 2d ed. Edited by J. Sokolovsky. Westport, Conn.: Bergin and Garvey, 1997. pp. 56-70.

Glascock, A., and Feinman, S. (1981). "Social Asset or Social Burden: Treatment of the Aged in Non-Industrial Societies." In *Dimensions: Aging, Culture and Health.* Edited by C. Fry. New York: Praeger.

Gutmann, D. (1987). *Reclaimed Powers: Toward a New Psychology of Men and Women in Later Life.* New York: Basic Books, 1987.

Halperin, R. (1987). "Age in Cross-Cultural Perspective: An Evolutionary Approach." In *The Elderly as Modern Pioneers.* Edited by P. Silverman. Bloomington, Ind.: Indiana University Press. pp. 283-311.

Haviland, W. (2000). *Anthropology,* 9th ed., New York: Harcourt.

Kaberry, P. (1939). *Aboriginal Women.* New York: Gordon Press,

Keith, J.; Fry, C.; et al. (1994). *The Aging Experience: Diversity and Commonality Across Cultures.* Thousand Oaks, Calif.: Sage.

Kerns, V., and Brown, J., (eds.) (1992). *In Her Prime: New Views of Middle-Aged Women,* 2d ed. Urbana: University of Illinois Press, 1992.

Kertzer, D., and Madison, O. B. B. (1981). "Women's Age-Set Systems in Africa: The Latuka of Southern Sudan." In *Dimensions: Aging, Culture and Health.* Edited by C. Fry. Brooklyn, N.Y.: J. F. Bergin. pp. 109-130.

Putnam-Dickerson, J., and Brown, J., (eds.) (1998). *Women Among Women: Anthropological Perspectives on Female Age Hierarchies.* Champaign, Ill.: University of Illinois Press.

Poddar, S. (2008). *Problem of Lonliness Among the Elderly Persons of Tripura,* Aging in North East India".

Rhoads, E., and HOLMES, L. D. *Other Cultures, Elder Years,* 2d ed. Thousand Oaks, Calif.: Sage, 1995.

Sangree, W. (2001). "The Childless Elderly in Tiriki, Keyna, and Iriqwe, Nigeria: A Comparative Analysis of the Relationship Between Beliefs about Childlessness and the Social Status of the Childless Elderly." *Journal of Cross-Cultural Gerontology* 2: 201-223.

Silverman, P., (ed.) (1987). "Comparative Studies." In *The Elderly as Modern Pioneers.* Bloomington: Indiana University Press, pp. 312-344.

Simic, A. (1978). "Introduction: Aging and the Aged in Cultural Perspective." In *Life's Career Aging: Cultural Variations on Growing Old.* Edited by B. Myerhoff and A. Simic. Beverley Hills, Calif.: Sage, pp. 9-22.

Sokolovsky, J., (ed.) (1997). *The Cultural Context of Aging: World-Wide Perspectives,* 2d ed. Westport, Conn.: Bergin and Garvey.

Spencer, P. (1965). *The Samburu: A Study of Gerontocracy in a Nomadic Tribe.* Berkeley: University of California Press.

Sreedhara Swamy,S. (2005). "Population and Development Education" Voll-2, Neelkamal Publications PVT. LTD. Educational Publishers, New Delhi.

Van Arsdale, P. (1981). "The Elderly Asmat of New Guinea." In *Other Ways of Growing Old: Anthropological Perspectives.* In P. Amoss and S. Harrell. Stanford: Stanford University Press, pp. 111-123.

Warner, L. *A Black Civilization: A Social Study of an Australian Tribe,* rev. ed. New York: Harper and Brothers, 1958.

Weiss, K. (1981). "Evolutionary Perspectives on Aging." In *Other Ways of Growing Old.* Edited by P. Amoss and S. Harrell. Stanford, Calif.: Stanford University Press, pp. 25-58.

Index

■■■